S0-ABC-692

Medical Informatics:
An Executive Primer

Edited by
Kenneth R. Ong, MD, MPH

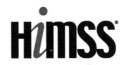

HIMSS Mission

To lead change in the healthcare information and management systems field through knowledge sharing, advocacy, collaboration, innovation, and community affiliations.

© 2007 by the Healthcare Information and Management Systems Society.

All rights reserved. No part of this publication may be reproduced, adapted, translated, stored in a retrieval system, or transmitted in any form or by any means, electronic, mechanical, photocopying, recording, or otherwise, without the prior written permission of the publisher.

Printed in the U.S.A. 5 4 3 2 1

Requests for permission to reproduce any part of this work should be sent to:

Permissions Editor
HIMSS
230 E. Ohio St., Suite 500
Chicago, IL 60611-3270
cmclean@himss.org

The inclusion of an organization name, product or service in this publication should not be construed as an endorsement of such organization, product or service, nor is the failure to include an organization name, product or service to be construed as disapproval.

ISBN: 0-9777903-3-9

Code: 501

For more information about HIMSS, please visit www.himss.org.

About the Editor

Kenneth R. Ong, MD, MPH, FACP, FIDSA, is the Director of Medical Informatics at Saint Vincent Catholic Medical Centers. In addition to strategic planning and managing clinical applications, Dr Ong's past projects at Saint Vincent's include developing and implementing the clinical decision support for the ambulatory EMR in the HIV clinic (Epicare) and the hospital pharmacy system (Pharmnet); implementing web-based results review, and physician charge capture (PatientKeeper).

Dr Ong is the President of the New York State chapter of the Health Information Management and Systems Society (HIMSS); Past President of Medical Informatics New York; a board member of the New York Clinical Information Exchange (NYCLIX); a member of the advisory board of the Doctors Office Quality IT (DOQ-IT) initiative of the Island Peer Review Organization (IPRO); a member of the client advisory board of PatientKeeper; and, a reviewer for the Informatics Review and the International Journal of Medical Informatics.

Dr Ong is a senior lecturer at Columbia University's Mailman School of Public Health. His medical informatics seminar was among the top rated in 2005. He is an assistant professor at New York Medical College. He is a previous recipient of the AMDIS Award In Applied Medical Informatics and the Centers for Disease Control Charles C. Shepard Science Award. Dr Ong is a former deputy commissioner in the New York City Department of Health and Mental Hygiene.

Dr Ong is residency-trained and board certified in family practice, internal medicine, and infectious disease. He is a fellow of the American College of Physicians, the Infectious Disease Society of America, and the New York Academy of Medicine. He received his MPH at Columbia University, MD at Wayne State University, and BS at University of Michigan.

Dr Ong can be reached at kong@svcmcny.org.

Contributors

Abha Agrawal, MD, FACP, is the director of medical informatics and associate medical director at Kings County Hospital, Brooklyn, New York. Dr Agrawal is an associate professor of clinical medicine at the State University of New York Downstate College of Medicine, Brooklyn, New York. She is a commissioner on the Certifying Commission for Healthcare Information Technology (CCHIT).

Rachel Block is the project director for the United Hospital Fund's Quality Strategies Initiative where she has been developing and implementing coordinated efforts to measure, report on and improve healthcare delivery and outcomes across New York's healthcare system since 2003.

Prior to joining the Fund, Ms. Block was vice president in the Health Services Group at MAXIMUS, where she directed strategic planning and development of products and services to improve the effectiveness and efficiency of state health programs. She also worked from 1994–2002 at the Centers for Medicare & Medicaid Services (previously Healthcare Financing Administration), where she held several senior management positions directing policy development and operations of Medicaid, State Children's Health Insurance and Federal Survey and Certification Programs, with particular emphasis on quality improvement, data and systems issues. During this time, she worked closely with CDC and HRSA to improve coordination across federal and state health programs.

From 1992–1994, Ms. Block worked for then-Governor Howard Dean in the development of a comprehensive health reform plan for the state of Vermont. She also worked for the New York State Legislature from 1978–1992 where she concentrated on Medicaid, coverage for the uninsured, public health and professional licensing issues. She is a member of the eHealth Initiative Foundation Board, and she currently serves as their secretary. She is also a member of the American Medical Informatics Association, the Academy for Health Services Research and Policy and the national advisory committee for the Robert Wood John Foundation's Depression in Primary Care Initiative.

Janet Bowen, MBA, PMP, Janet Bowen is currently employed with Siemens and serves as a Project Manager for clinical systems on the Saint Vincent Catholic Medical Center account. She is responsible for managing implementation of PatientKeeper and leads the selection committee for SVCMC's OR and ED systems. Ms. Bowen started in healthcare IT in 1985 at New York University Medical Center as a business analyst where she conducted business process reengineering studies in financial, procurement and clinical departments and as a project director developed business strategies and service contracts to deployed outpatient clinical systems for private physician practices and clinics. Her previous career in respiratory care services led to a supervisory position a cardiopulmonary department of EKG, EEG, cardiac stress testing and respiratory care services at Riverside General Hospital in Secaucus, New Jersey.

Ms. Bowen holds a B.S. from NYU Stern School of Business, an MBA from Montclair State University. Janet is a member of the Project Management Institute, New Jersey Chapter (PMINJ), and the PMI Healthcare Special Interest Group and is a certified Project Management Professional (PMP). She also received Information Technology Infrastructure Library (ITIL) certification.

Neil S. Calman, MD, is a board certified family physician who has been practicing in the Bronx and Manhattan for the past 30 years. He is president and a co-founder of the Institute for Urban Family Health. Since 1983, Dr Calman has led the Institute in developing family health centers in the Bronx and Manhattan and in establishing health professional training in medicine, nursing, administration and mental health. He is currently chair of the Health Reform and Finance Subcommittee of the New York State Council on Graduate Medical Education and serves on the Pediatric Advisory Committee of the State Department of Health. He is also currently chair of the Clinical Committee of the Community Healthcare Association of New York State. This year, he was appointed to the Health Policy Roundtable of the Aspen Institute—a group charged with delineating the values and principles on which the U.S. must base its future healthcare system.

Dr Calman is the recipient of many national awards for his work in public health including the Robert Wood Johnson Foundation's Community Health Leadership Award, the American Academy of Family Physicians' Public Health Award and the Pew Charitable Trusts' Primary Care Achievement Award. In September 1999, he became the project director of a multi-year grant from the Centers for Disease Control to work towards eliminating racial and ethnic differences in health outcomes in the Bronx. Dr Calman's published essay "Out of the Shadows" (*Health Affairs*, Jan/Feb 2000) details his experiences in dealing with racism in the care of his patients. "Making Health Equality a Reality: The Bronx Takes Action" (*Health Affairs*, Mar/Apr 2005) describes the community-based legislative action that has evolved from this grassroots effort to address institutional racism in medical care.

In 2002, the Institute became one of the first community health center networks in the country to implement a fully integrated electronic medical record and practice management system, improving both preventive and chronic care treatment outcomes throughout its centers. In recognition of this achievement, he received the prestigious 2005 Physician's Information Technology Leadership Award, presented annually by the Healthcare Information and Management Systems Society. Dr Calman serves on the executive committee of the newly established citywide Primary Care Health Information Consortium (PCHIC) and on the New York State Department of Health's Information Technology Stakeholder Group Planning Committee as well as on the Board of the New York Clinical Information Exchange (NYCLIX).

Janet L. Carr, MD, is senior medical director at Group Health Incorporated (GHI). She is responsible for clinical programs for utilization, quality and disease management, physician profiling, and medical claim administration. She leads GHI's patient safety activities and coordinates activities for physician electronic prescribing.

Prior to joining GHI, Dr Carr was medical director at United HealthCare and clinical director at Anchor Rush Prudential Health Plan in Chicago, Illinois. She is a board certified pediatrician.

Dr Carr serves on the Board of Women in Health Management.

Curtis L. Cole, MD, is the director of information services for Weill Cornell Physicians, the faculty practice of the Weill Medical College of Cornell University (WMC). He practices internal medicine at Cornell Internal Medicine Associates at the New York Presbyterian Hospital. He is an assistant professor of medicine and an assistant professor of public health at Weill Cornell. Dr Cole is also the WMC University Overseer of New York Presbyterian's outsourced information systems department. After medical school at Cornell and residency at the-then New York Hospital, he was a clinical investigator in Medical Informatics at NYH. He has led the implementation of several EMR systems. Dr Cole is also responsible for the other core information systems that service the practices. These include access management, revenue cycle, managed care, an interface engine, a home-grown data dictionary called TruData, a data warehouse, www.CornellPhysicians.com, as well as a variety of smaller commercial and home-grown applications and databases. Dr Cole can be reached at ccole@med.cornell.edu.

Leanne M. Currie, RN, DNSc, is an assistant professor of nursing, Columbia University School of Nursing; affiliated faculty, Department of Biomedical Informatics, Columbia University; and nurse researcher, New York Presbyterian Hospital. She received her Master's of Science in Nursing Informatics from University of California, San Francisco, and her Doctorate in Nursing Science from Columbia University School of Nursing (Hons). While at Columbia, Ms. Currie was a National Library of Medicine Trainee in Informatics via the Department of Biomedical Informatics. She is currently conducting research in the following areas: clinical decision support and patient safety; informatics in collaboration with leadership at New York Presbyterian Hospital; decision support via mobile devices for advanced practice nursing students; information retrieval at the point-of-care in collaboration with the Infobutton project; and fall and injury prevention in the acute care setting.

Maxine L. Golub, MPH, is Senior Vice President, Planning and Development at the Institute for Urban Family Health in New York City, a primary care organization dedicated to the development of innovative ways to provide primary health services to underserved urban populations. The Institute also provides education and training to health professionals, and participates in health services research and policy development.

Ms. Golub provides leadership for the Institute's fundraising, organizational development, and communications activities. She has served as a trainer in the Institute's diversity training program since 1997, and as a leader in the Bronx Health REACH Coalition, a group dedicated to eliminating racial disparities in health outcome since 1999. In 2003, she received the Rosemarie Forstner Award "for outstanding dedication to making health care more accessible to the medically underserved" from the Community Health Care Association of New York State.

Ms. Golub holds a master of public health degree from the Hunter College School of Health Science and a bachelor of science in human development and family studies from Cornell University.

George T. Hickman, FHIMSS, CPHIMS, is responsible for overseeing all information technology activities throughout Albany Medical Center. Prior to joining AMC, he was a vice president with Cap Gemini Ernst & Young and a partner for Ernst & Young LLP. He also has worked with PriceWaterhouseCoopers and started his career as a project engineer for a health provider. He has performed consulting engagements across the U.S., the Ministry of Health in Singapore and the U.K. Health Authority. Mr. Hickman frequently publishes on healthcare IT and operational change topics. This is his third academic health system CIO post.

Mr. Hickman is 2007 Chairman of the Board of Directors and is a Fellow for the Healthcare Information and Management Systems Society (HIMSS). He is a past member of the HIMSS Analytics Board and also sits on the University Healthsystems Consortium (UHC) CIO Forum and the Executive Council for the Editorial Advisory Board of *ADVANCE for Health Information Executives*. He holds a BS and an MS in engineering.

Joseph Kannry, MD, has dual appointments in IT and Medicine at Mount Sinai Medical Center. He is chief, Division of Clinical Informatics, Mount Sinai Medical Center. He is director of the Center for Medical Informatics and Director of IT for Department of Medicine. Dr Kannry is an assistant professor in medicine, and a practicing board certified internist at IMA. He is a graduate of the Yale Center for Medical Informatics, a National Library of Medicine training program in Informatics.

Dr Kannry is a frequent contributor to AMIA and HIMSS, and was/is a member of the AMIA Task Force on Guidelines for the Clinical Use of Electronic Mail with Patients; AMIA Task Force on Applied Informatics; AMIA's Education Committee; HIMSS' Ambulatory EMR Knowledge Resource Task Force; HL7 EHR Ambulatory Care Large Minimum Function Set: Ambulatory Care-Large; Greater New York Hospital Association IT Steering Committee; Chairman of Clinical Advisory Group for NYCLIX (New York Clinical Information Exchange); and member of NYCLIX Steering Committee/Board. He has presented at several conferences and has been cited by the *Journal of the American Medical Association, Medinfo, PC Week, Washington Post* and the *New York Daily News*.

Dr Kannry's paper "The Relationship of Usability to Medical Error: An Evaluation of Errors Associated with Usability Problems in the Use of a Handheld Application for Prescribing Medications" won the silver medal at the 11th World Congress of Informatics, Medinfo 2004. His research has focused on patient-provider identification, clinical notification and messaging, CPOE, Ambulatory EMR, and usability. In 2004, Dr Kannry successfully led the Ambulatory EMR Selection process for Mount Sinai Medical Center. He has been the Informaticist in charge of EMR implementation since 2005.

Kwame Kitson, MD, is a family physician at the Urban Horizons Family Health Center in the Bronx, NY. Dr. Kitson is medical director of the Center's COMPASS program for HIV+ patients in the Bronx. He has a special interest in sports and fitness as a way to promote good health for his patients. Dr. Kitson received his medical degree from Howard University in Washington, DC.

Mark Leavitt, MD, PhD, FHIMSS, is considered one of the pioneers of electronic health records in ambulatory care. Dr Leavitt is the chair of the Certification Commission for Healthcare Information Technology. Previously, he was the medical director at the Healthcare Information and Management Systems Society (HIMSS). He is actively engaged in a number of national initiatives to accelerate the adoption of robust, interoperable electronic health records to improve the quality, safety, and efficiency of healthcare.

Dr Leavitt received his BSEE from the University of Arizona, his PhD from Stanford University, his MD from the University of Miami, and Board Certification in Internal Medicine from the Oregon Health and Sciences University, with subsequent Added Qualifications in Geriatrics. He practiced internal medicine full-time for ten years in Portland, and led a project to launch the implementation of system-wide electronic records at Providence Health System in Oregon. In 1985 he founded MedicaLogic, a pioneering developer of ambulatory electronic health records, leading the company as its CEO and Chairman for 15 years. In 2002 GE Healthcare acquired MedicaLogic, and Dr Leavitt served as Vice President of Clinical Initiatives for GE.

In addition to being a Fellow in HIMSS, he holds a Clinical Assistant Professorship in the Department of Medical Informatics at the Oregon Health and Science University. Dr Leavitt is a past president of the Oregon chapters of HIMSS and the Society of Internal Medicine.

Jonathan Leviss, MD, is medical director, Healthcare Strategies, Sentillion Inc., where he is responsible for spearheading Sentillion's activities in community-based and national healthcare information initiatives in the U.S. and Canada. Additionally, he provides clinical and informatics expertise in Sentillion's ongoing focus to develop and deliver caregiver-centered identity, and to access management solutions to the industry.

Prior to joining Sentillion, Dr Leviss was a senior manager in the Deloitte Consulting Healthcare Practice. His medical informatics leadership experience includes serving as the director of medical informatics at Bellevue Hospital, New York, NY; and as chief medical informatics Officer for the New York City Health & Hospitals Corporation, the largest US municipal hospital system. He also was a physician executive with Cerner Corporation. He has used advanced information technologies in direct clinical care for over ten years, including computerized practitioner order entry and computerized clinical documentation. Dr Leviss has held faculty positions at the NYU School of Medicine and the Columbia University College of Physicians and Surgeons, co-authored papers in several peer-reviewed academic medical journals, and frequently presents at academic and industry conferences and forums. He continues to practice as a primary care internist at the Thundermist Health Center in Rhode Island.

Mark Lipton, MD, is the vice chairman of the Board of Directors and chair of the Business Committee of the New York Clinical Information Exchange. He is the director, clinical informatics, New York University Medical Center and a clinical associate professor of medicine at New York University School of Medicine. Dr Lipton earned his AB at Cornell University and MD at New York University. He completed an internal medicine residency at Bellevue Hospital and a cardiology fellowship at New York University Medical Center.

Dr Lipton is a member of the voluntary faculty of NYU, where he served as the Interim Chief Medical Officer in 2004 and Chair of the Executive Committee of the Medical Board in 2002 and 2003. He currently chairs the Quality Improvement Committee at NYU.

In addition to his clinical responsibilities, as director of clinical informatics at NYU Medical Center, Dr Lipton researches the integration of information technology with innovation in patient treatment and medical research. He is the principal investigator of a National Institutes of Health grant to plan for health information exchange in the NY metropolitan area. He has lectured about health information exchange and authored a book chapter on ambulatory medical records.

Glenn Martin, MD, is director of medical informatics for the Davies award-winning Queens Health Network. QHN is composed of the two public hospitals in the borough of Queens. While providing clinical direction to the implementation of the electronic medical record, he has also been actively involved in deploying smart card technology in the form of patient ID cards containing extracts of the medical record. He is president of Medical Informatics New York.

Dr Martin matriculated at the University of Rochester where he received a BA with high honors in biology. He received his medical degree from the Université de Liège, Belgium. He is a board certified psychiatrist and a distinguished fellow of the American Psychiatric Association. Before becoming CMIO, Dr Martin was the deputy director of psychiatry at Queens Hospital Center. He is also Vice Chair of the Institutional Review Board and Associate Dean for Research at the Mount Sinai School of Medicine and a practicing psychiatrist.

Dov Rothman, PhD, is currently an associate at the Analysis Group, Inc., an economic, financial and strategy consultancy. Prior to joining Analysis Group, he was an assistant professor in the Department of Health Policy and Management at the Mailman School of Public Health, Columbia University. Dr Rothman has a PhD from the Haas School of Business at the University of California, Berkeley.

Charmaine Ruddock, MS, is the Project Director at Bronx Health REACH. She has been involved in the design, development and operational oversight of Managed Care Organizations serving underserved communities in New York City, Long Island and Connecticut for the past 10 years. She joined the Institute for Urban Family Health in 2000 to direct the Bronx Health REACH Coalition. The Institute leads a coalition of community, faith-based and healthcare organizations in implementing a plan to eliminate racial disparities in health outcomes for diabetes and cardiovascular disease in the Southwest Bronx.

Ms. Ruddock received a BA degree from the University of the West Indies in Jamaica, and a master of science in management and policy analysis from the New School for Social Research, Graduate School of Management and Urban Policy.

Kimberly A. Spire, BA, BSN, MS, RN, is Director of Information Services - Program Development and Transformation at the Albany Medical Center in Upstate New York. Ms. Spire's previous role was Director of Operations for a private consulting firm with oversight for software development, network services and information technology staffing lines of business.

Ms. Spire served as the Chief Information Officer for a leading behavioral health firm with three corporate locations spanning Westchester and Saratoga Counties. Ms. Spire is a Registered Nurse in the state of New York. She received an undergraduate degree in Political Science from SUNY Albany; an undergraduate degree in Nursing from Florida Atlantic University; and a Masters degree in Nursing Administration from PACE University.

Dedication

To Donna, Kimberly, Ryan, Fawn, Jo, and, of course, Edwin

Acknowledgment

*Thanks to Pete Garrison who has always
encouraged me to excel.*

Contents

Foreword

Sherry Glied, PhD, MA
Professor and Chair, Department of Health Policy and Management
Mailman School of Public Health, Columbia University

Healthcare is an industry characterized by revolutionary technological advances. From the smallpox vaccine to coronary angioplasty, the nature and quality of medical care are regularly transformed through innovation. As healthcare advances, it also becomes increasingly information intensive. Providers must keep up with the rapid flow of new knowledge and incorporate a vast range of information about each specific patient into their treatment choices. New developments in information technology place new and transformative technical capabilities at the service of managing healthcare information.

Developments in information technology promise to transform our healthcare system in many dimensions. Information technology may be the key element in allowing consumers to be more engaged in their own healthcare, making appropriate choices among the options available to them. Champions of healthcare quality improvement see the electronic medical record and the possibility of electronic prescribing as a crucial component of efforts to reduce errors and improve the match between patient and treatment. Those concerned about rising healthcare costs see developments in information technology as a promising counterweight to the continual deployment of costly medical treatment technologies.

All of these objectives are worthy—and increasingly, they are technically possible. New technologies by themselves, however, do not translate into improvements in the health of the public. The degree to which information technologies realize their considerable promise depends critically on how these technologies are deployed and managed. The particular nature of information technology—which operates at the level of a practice, institution or system—makes the quality of management especially critical in this area.

Medical Informatics: An Executive Primer offers healthcare executives an opportunity to learn how to make these exciting new technological advances work toward improving system functioning and population health. Kenneth Ong, MD, MPH, the volume's editor, is one of the nation's leading experts in medical informatics, with considerable expertise in implementing effective information systems. He is a prized member of the Mailman School's Department of Health Policy and Management. The volume, which grew out of a top-rated seminar in our department, is designed and organized to provide healthcare leaders with the information they need. Dr Ong has drawn on the expertise of scholars and practitioners to collect, in a single volume, information on a wide range of medical informatics applications, technologies, and strategies.

We are far from realizing the enormous potential of medical information technologies. To get where we want to go will take resources, both financial and intellectual. The financial resources are in the hands of healthcare decision-makers— Federal, state, and local policymakers, senior executives in healthcare institutions levels, private payers, even office-based physicians. They need to make medical information a pocketbook priority. But money is not enough. The management of medical information will also require an infusion of intellectual resources. So far, our technical capacity to collect and analyze data far exceeds the managerial capacity to put that capacity to good use. This volume helps to bridge that gap and bring the promise of medical informatics closer to reality.

Preface

Kenneth R. Ong, MD, MPH

"Health informatics or medical informatics is the intersection of information science, medicine and healthcare. It deals with the resources, devices and methods required to optimize the acquisition, storage, retrieval and use of information in health and biomedicine. Health informatics tools include not only computers but also clinical guidelines, formal medical terminologies, and information and communication systems."[1]

Wikipedia

It is inescapable. The growth of medical informatics in our daily lives can be found everywhere. Information technology in healthcare is increasingly being applied at the hospital bedside at point-of-care, at the doctor's office and in our homes no more than a click a way.

Terms like electronic health record, health information exchange and electronic prescribing are no longer exclusively the purview of research papers or policy recommendations. An entirely new menagerie of acronyms and abbreviations has blossomed. CPOE with CDS, BCMA, ASP, PAC and RHIO have insinuated themselves into our daily conversations in the hallways between patient rooms, executive suites and board rooms. The new vocabulary resides not in the family's hide-bound dictionary but virtually in Google.

In this storm of new technology, many healthcare managers and clinicians have to learn when and how best to use it. They must decipher what works and what does not. The economic environment for healthcare delivery organizations continues to be challenging and resources for capital are dear, especially for information technology. There is scant room for investments that fail to return on investment.

Yet the newspaper and literature are replete with the value that IT can bring to quality of care and improved efficiency. The drivers for IT are ubiquitous. The FDA promotes bar coding medications and blood.[2] Pay-for-performance encourages electronic reporting and the greater adoption of the electronic health record.[3] Smart cards are making their way into our patients' wallets and purses.[4]

This book was written in a way much like Tom Sawyer's picket fence was white-washed. It started with a seminar on medical informatics at Columbia University's Mailman School of Public Health. The seminar served as an excellent opportunity to invite friends and colleagues to not only share their knowledge and expertise within the classroom but to create a book for that larger audience outside the classroom. The corps of volunteer writers was recruited in a variety of venues throughout New York in the course of talking about, doing or collaborating in the work of applying IT to healthcare.

Ultimately, the book was a natural outgrowth from the same source it seeks to serve—the ferment of medical informatics in our daily lives.

REFERENCES

1. Wikipedia. Definition of health informatics. Available at: http://en.wikipedia.org/wiki/Medical_informatics. Accessed on October 3, 2006.

2. Federal Drug Administration. Bar coding sample. Available at: http://www.fda.gov/cber/barcode/bldreg011706dm2.htm. Accessed on October 3, 2006.

3. Bridges to Excellence homepage. Available at: http://www.bridgestoexcellence.org/. Accessed on October 3, 2006.

4. Briggs B. Are cards finally a good bet? There's no consensus on whether smart cards have a role to play in an increasingly connected industry. *Health Data Management.* 2006; November 9. Available at: http://www.healthdatamanagement.com/html/current/CurrentIssueStory.cfm?articleId=12884. Accessed on October 3, 2006.

CHAPTER 1

Electronic Prescribing

Janet L. Carr, MD

The electronic transmission of a prescription to a pharmacy delivery system, whether by facsimile or wireless, has become a critical tool in the medical arena. As improvements to the process occur, the information conveyed electronically will serve a more functional component with the transmission of patient demographic and clinical information to help with prescription generation, as well as with the use of computer devices to enter, review, modify, output and communicate drug prescriptions. It is a functionality in medicine long overdue.

WHY ELECTRONIC PRESCRIBING IS IMPORTANT

The impetus for electronic prescribing was the November 1999 Institute of Medicine report, *To Err Is Human,* that described the industry problem of medical errors.[1] With more than 3 billion prescriptions written annually and more than 60% of the population receiving prescriptions, there is no room for mistakes in this arena. Yet, the report described medication errors as the cause of death for more than 7,000 Americans with a financial cost of nearly $77 billion dollars. A significant portion of the errors are due to handwritten prescriptions, most of which could have been prevented.[2] In addition to poor handwriting, the issue of drug-drug and drug-allergy interactions is also a contributing factor in medical errors. The Center for Information Technology Leadership reports more than 8.8 million adverse drug events each year.[3] Absence of all drug information except from the patients' memory has always been a factor in increased hospitalization and mortality. To ensure appropriate dosing—and for patients' convenience—information regarding the price of the prescription would improve the process for physician and patient. In 1998, Schiff and Rucker announced "there should not be another paper prescription."[4]

THE ART OF PRESCRIPTION WRITING

The process of prescription writing is complex. The physician, patient, pharmacist, and payor are the key players in the dynamic. This process includes diagnosis, prescribing, dispensing and administering medications. The information necessary to complete the process comes from multiple sources. The provider must diagnose a condition and determine the appropriate drugs necessary. Optimal frequency is a memory-dependent value. A 1970 recommendation from the American College of Family Practice recommended the use of three to seven references to appropriately prescribe the correct drug and the right dose. Patient allergies and other prescribed medications are additional points of information that impact the outcome of the prescription process. In many cases, the patient is not a reliable source of this information. With this many variables, the patient-physician encounter is ripe for errors.

HISTORY OF TECHNOLOGY:
HOW ELECTRONIC PRESCRIBING EVOLVED

These concerns regarding medication errors have been noted in the literature for decades. In 1967, Hyman and Land proposed the application of computerized technology to outpatient pharmacy services. A 1976 study using a prototype of a computerized pharmaceutical services support system providing drug history caused the MD to change therapy in 73% cases. In 1987, a study of family physicians using a computerized drug interactions screening systems (CDISS) found 79% of the drugs prescribed had potential drug interactions of varying clinical significance. In addition, the study concluded that exposure to a CDISS tool was both educational and of clinical value to the physician. In 1998, the use of computerized systems in the hospitals that utilizes drug alerts was shown to reduce medication errors and adverse events. In 1991, the Physician Desk Reference was available as the first electronic version small enough to put into a lab coat pocket.

In the late 1980s, early electronic prescribing software development was attempted by programs such as Rx Writer and Medication Manager. Rx Writer's primary function was to print prescriptions from a prepared list of up to 200 medications as defined by the physician. Medication Manager was a total medication management system without clinical information.[5] These preliminary attempts at electronic prescriptions were utilized for maintaining, viewing and printing prescriptions, and they were one of the first attempts to address handwriting errors. However, these software tools were cumbersome and did not allow multiple user access.

Other systems and industries have addressed the issue of error reduction. Both the airline and banking industries are touted as examples of successfully approaching a total reduction in errors. The healthcare industry will be playing catch up for a significant amount of time.

In the United States, healthcare is provided by either an employer or the government with approximately 40 million uninsured. This segmentation causes lack of continuity for physicians and their patients. Each major managed care organization aligns with different pharmaceutical benefit management (PBM) vendors to manage a select number of drugs available, known as formularies, for the assigned patients.

Commercial insurers use pharmacy benefit managers to contract with manufacturers to provider drugs for the insured. These companies have valuable data: all the drugs written by any practitioner and presented to the insurance for payment. The physician is faced with different formularies and different electronic tools/devices for each major insurance carrier. This has been a significant barrier to the advancement of electronic prescribing, as a physician needs access to individual programs for each insurer.

In 2001, three of the major PBMs: Advance PCS, Medco Health Solutions and Express Scripts, founded Rx Hub to develop a common data warehouse and a single point of contact for a major portion of patients covered by commercial insurance.[6] Therefore, how a patient's insurance is covered, be it commercial or governmental, affects the dynamics of the delivery of care. Other similar companies soon developed, including ProxyMed, Gold Standard and Tricare which provides military pharmacy benefits. Today, this accounts for nearly 150 million members in 50 states. Electronic prescribing made a significant leap with the formation of Rx Hub and similar companies.

The challenges in the existing prescription writing process are daunting. As Figure 1-1[1,2,3,4] shows, sheer volume alone plays a significant role in its success or failure.

- Estimates of 150–900 million calls annually from pharmacists to physicians for clarification[1] on formulary and drug-drug interactions

- Practices reporting almost 30% of prescriptions required pharmacy callbacks[2,3]

- Requesting and receiving approval for refills alone, estimated at nearly 500 million per year, adds to the telephone and fax burdens[4]

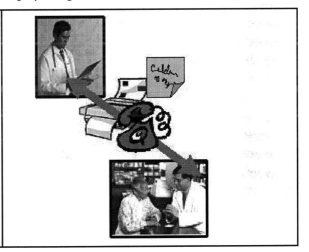

Figure 1-1: The Challenges.

The Center for Medicare and Medicaid Services' (CMS) Medicare Modernization Act of 2003 addressed objectives for patient safety, quality of care and cost savings in the delivery of care. The Act noted that Rx and certain other information for covered Medicare Part D drugs that are transmitted electronically should comply with formal standard uniform standards to be adopted by CMS. Because most major commercial insurers also covered Medicare Part D, these standards were significant and included:

- Provider eligibility and benefits, including formulary requirement for prior authorization
- Medication history
- Drug interaction
- Dosage adjustments
- Lower cost alternatives

Functionality

In response to these and other drivers for transforming the prescribing system (see Figure 1-2), electronic prescribing company start ups were formed and software developed. The initial products were basic, but the access to Rx HUB data allowed only for that level of prescribing functioning. In recent years, the number of e-prescribing software vendors and their capabilities have increased significantly. The top vendors offer the most valued services for electronic prescribing and can be categorized in ten capabilities—seven are related to patient medication safety medication and the others related to cost. The clinical capabilities are described as clinical decision support tools (CDS) that provide the clinical information that helps the physicians make the right choice and decreases the chance of medical errors.

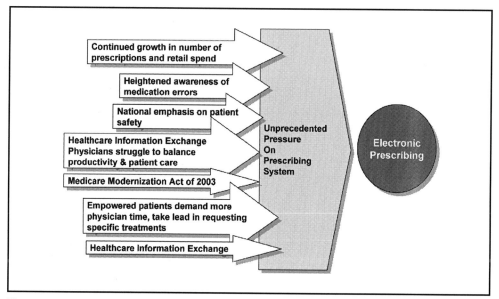

Figure 1-2: Drivers for Electronic Prescribing.

Electronic prescribing systems are described in numerous ways by level of functioning (Table 1-1). In most large markets, there are at least top 5 vendors that maintain the most valued services and Clinical Decision Support (CDS) tools for electronic prescribing. There is significant competition in the marketplace, but none of the software companies have developed capabilities too far beyond the demands or mandates of consumers, payors or government.[3] Recommendations for advances in CDS are anticipated in 2008. These recommendations were commissioned by the Agency for Healthcare Research and Quality (AHRQ) and submitted to the National Committee on Vital Health Statistics Subcommittee on Standard and Security for approval.

As described by the eHealth Initiative, clinical decision support is: *Proactive,* occurring at the beginning of the process to assist decision-making based on clinical criteria; *Reactive,* giving information presented after the decision is executed and gives the practitioner additional information about the choice of medication such as drug alerts; and *Informational,* providing references for making a decision or educating the patient to assist in the plan of care.[3]

Table 1-1: Descriptions of Functionality for Software E-prescribing Programs.

Patient identification	Patient demographics, formulary, allergies, and age that can generate alert. Information includes patient's name, address, gender, age, and insurance eligibility, all downloaded from an electronic billing format existing with practice. Key demographics should be visible throughout the Rx process.
Access historical data	Current medication should include all drugs prescribed, including those by other providers from both the inpatient and outpatient settings. This should allow for manual additions of medication.
Medication selection	Most programs list medication by alpha or from a "favorite list" formatted by the practitioner. Higher level of functioning may list by diagnosis. Medication should be identified by cost and formulary compliance.
Medication alerts	Safety alerts including drug interactions and allergies, as well as drug-diagnosis contraindications. Certain alerts are usually categorized by severity level with black box warnings the most severe level. Physician can continue with the selected drug (override) or choose another medication.
Patient education	Ability to send via e-mail or print education regarding medication diagnosis and/or compliance.
Data transmission and storage	Transmission of prescription should comply with HL7 standards minimally and bidirectional transmission failures can be immediately addressed.
Monitoring and renewals	Patient adherence and alert for non-renewal.
Transparency and accountability	Full disclosure for any third party support or messaging.
Provider feedback	Providers could access their own aggregate data, i.e., self profiling and registry documentation.
Security and confidentiality	Adherence to HIPAA, as well as sign on and access security. Use of structured signature.
Library of medications	Provides standard unit doses that can be accessed and sorted in numerous categories. Basic Rx entry with medication dose check. Allows dose search by name and creates a prescription without medication history.
Reference	Access to Rx reference information without actual prescribing capabilities.

Clinical decision support is developing and its maturity varies by application and setting of care. For example, weight-based dosing and prescribing is poorly developed at present and may be the reason for low utilization by pediatric practices. This has been successfully deployed in certain major academic centers.[7]

STANDARDS AND MANDATES

HIPAA

The Health Insurance Portability and Accountability Act of 1996 (HIPAA), and revisions in 2000, is considered the landmark legislation for patient privacy. The establishment of protections for personal health information is a significant advancement as medicine evolves to patient centric models and technology-assisted activities continue to develop. HIPAA mandates and provides standards for policies and processes to protect the patient. This protection, however, potentially prevents communication between healthcare providers, and therefore can hamper improved quality of care. Exemptions were established to allow disclosure of protected health information as necessary for treatment, payment and healthcare operations (TPO). The conversion of medical information to a digital format creates new possibilities for breach of patient privacy and confidentiality. Most experts agree that the present functionality of electronic prescribing falls into the regulatory exemption to TPO. HIPAA regulations do not impose much incremental burden to the current form of electronic prescribing over that of conventional practice. There is interest and concern regarding future developments to electronic prescribing with the growing understanding of the need for confidentiality safeguards inherent in most electronic transmission. The practitioner may incorporate the "e-consent" both electronically and by hard copy into the practice workflow for all new patients and encounters. There certainly will be a need to define HIPAA more clearly as the future of e-prescribing moves toward wider scope in distribution of Personal Health Information and network information exchange.[8]

National Standards

The industry recognizes the need for standards in order to advance electronic prescribing. Without these, the process will continue to be fragmented which will prevent real large scale adoption of electronic prescribing. The standard setting agencies for the last five years have worked in developing standards for all components necessary for the transfer of electronic data for prescribing.

The American National Standards Institute (ASNI) is a private, non-profit organization dedicated to the development of accrediting the procedures of standards of membership organizations. ANSI is the only accrediting body that coordinates the development of voluntary consensus standards in the United States.[9]

The National Committee on Vital and Health Statistics (NCVHS) is the Department of Health and Human Service's advisory body on healthcare data statistics and national health information policy. The NCVHS, a member of ANSI, developed recommendations after consulting with practicing physicians, hospitals, pharmacies, pharmacists, PBMs, state boards of pharmacy and medicine and industry experts. The NCVHS standards must be ANSI accredited and implemented successfully by more than one healthcare partner, interoperable and recognized as a standard by key stakeholders in the industry.

Mandates and State Legislations

In April 2005, CMS promulgated rules for electronic prescribing and proposed standards under the Medicare Modernization Act of 2003 (MMA). These are known as foundation standards which are those that are widely accepted in the industry. Therefore, anyone utilizing e-prescribing for a patient eligible under Medicare Part D will have to comply with these standards which supersede state laws. The proposed standards are the first step toward a more complete set of standards required for e-prescribing. The criteria must include at a minimum: the ability to transmit a prescription and information on eligibility, benefits, medication history, drug–drug interaction, dosage adjustment and low-cost alternatives, as well as medical history concerning the patient and related to a covered drug prescribed upon request to the pharmacist

ELECTRONIC PRESCRIBING: THE PROCESS

The patient–physician visit is the point-of-care for most initial prescriptions. Following the exam and discussion with the patient, the physician determines the diagnosis and decides which medication(s) should be ordered. The physician may enter a diagnosis into the handheld device or PC and a list of drugs is presented. A drug selection, dose and frequency are displayed. The provider may make a change if necessary. Once drugs are selected, alerts may be displayed regarding a conflict due to conditions, current or past medications, or allergies. The practitioner may select another drug or override the conflict alert. In addition, the selected drug is noted as included or not in the patient's insurance company's preferred drug or formulary list. This allows the patient and physician to make prescription choices based on the patient's relative cost burden for the prescription. The provider will pick the patient's choice of pharmacy and location, which has been loaded into the system by the software vendor. The prescription is sent electronically through a server or faxed to the pharmacy. If the provider or patient prefers, the prescription can be printed in the office as well as sent electronically to the pharmacy. The provider potentially may also print additional educational information for the patient and/or instructions for compliance. Figure 1-3 and Figure 1-4 outlines the electronic prescribing process from both the physician and Rx points of view.

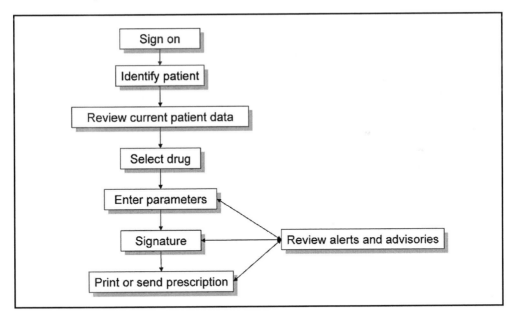

Figure 1-3: The Physician Process.

In order to complete this process, there is a connection to the data warehouse to determine eligibility, provide the clinical decision support feedback and send back the data to the device or PC. These data repositories were mentioned earlier (Rx Hub) and each state may have a similar repository available for their government program enrollees. The prescription is sent electronically through a service that connects pharmacies wirelessly. The retail pharmacy must apply for membership to a network that allows them to receive these electronic prescriptions. Companies such as Quality Systems Incorporated and Surescripts developed networks allowing two-way electronic exchange of prescription information between physician and pharmacies. The prescription, once final selection is made, is sent electronically though a secure system connection to the pharmacies.[3,9]

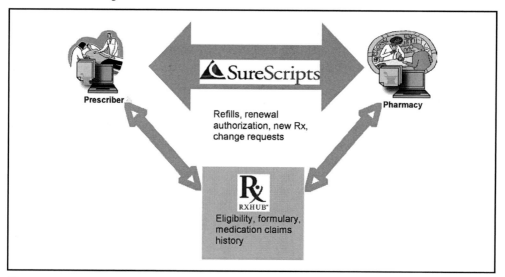

Figure 1-4: Electronic Prescription Process Flow.

IMPLEMENTATION

Getting Started

The Boston Consulting Group found that 16% of US physicians are using e-prescribing and another 21% said that they plan to start within eighteen months. The lead person for implementing an electronic prescribing process in a medical practice should be the physician-practitioner. In group practices, a lead physician champion should be identified to oversee the implementation and maintenance of the process and to act as a liaison between vendors and partners. An assessment of the practice type and office workflow should be completed prior to choosing an electronic prescribing package. All of the office staff should be involved when a physician or group practice decides to adopt electronic prescribing. The least intrusive plan for starting electronic prescribing is refill management using a PC Web-based program. In that situation, the office staff can place all refill requests in the PC system in a queue and the provider(s) can respond at their convenience. The savings for refill management are a significant portion of the overall savings from electronic prescribing.

Formulary Management

The inclusion of a dataset of drugs is key to the prescribing process, whether paper or electronic.

In most cases, patients are associated with a health plan or government-funded program for coverage for medications. These health plans have their own list of drugs or formulary that is most economical for the health plan and patient. The health plan manages its own formulary or partners with a PBM. The electronic Rx software vendor acquires data directly from either source and is available to the practitioner at the point-of-care. For drug, allergy and condition conflict alerts, the software vendor purchases additional databases with drug information from third party commercial entities such as Multum, MicroMedex, or First Data Bank. The formation of PBM collaborations such as RxHub had provided a more consolidated source of information, but single source formulary vendors are also prevalent in the market. A practice should review its patient mix and determine which formulary source best suits the practice. Because Medicaid programs are administered by each state, there is not a consolidated source for Medicaid and commercial formularies at this time. This may be a significant barrier to a practice evenly split between commercial and Medicaid patients.

The predominant electronic prescribing software vendors are listed in Table 1-2. All of the major software products are certified and comply with latest interoperability and Medicare standards.

Table 1-2: Software Vendors.

Vendors	Software
Allscripts	TouchScript
DrFirst	Rcopia
InstantDx	On Call Data
RxNT	RxNT
ZixCorp	PocketScript
Gold Standard	eMPOWERx
ePocrates	ePocratesRx

Hardware

The hardware necessary for these functions is basic and easily accessible. The physicians have access to these functions via web-based Internet products utilizing a Personal Computer (PC), Tablet PC, or a handheld device such as a PDA or Blackberry. Most software can be downloaded easily to a PC and many are at no cost. PDAs are hand-held devices that were originally designed for personal organizing, but have evolved as the most significant hardware tool supporting electronic prescribing. They can be either wireless or local server based. The server-based system frequently requires local system/server updates. Tablet PC is a mobile computer with digitalization allowing the user to utilize a stylus or digital pen instead of a keyboard or mouse. This allows for the ease of a mobile unit in the exam room, but it must be attached to a local server. An individual or small group practice may choose wireless handheld devices. Either PDA or Tablet will support the various software programs. However, these devices require back-up batteries for longer availability.

Blackberrys are wireless devices that allow the transmission of data utilizing the wireless data networks of cellular telephone carriers. While mostly known for e-mail capabilities, the Blackberry has its usefulness for physicians as it has the capability to electronically prescribe from multiple offices and the hospital setting. All locations should be assessed for wireless reception. Physical requirements in the practice and practice facility may cause interference with reception (ie, MRI equipment and concrete walls). In those cases, the practitioner may have to use a PDA single server system with daily synchronization.

Bluetooth functionality allows communication via radio frequency with a Bluetooth card or handheld. A Bluetooth-enabled printer can increase printing range to up to 30 feet, making it convenient for in-office printing.

Device Compatibility

Below are the hardware specifications necessary for electronic prescribing that are compatible with most software products.

Palm OS 5.0 or higher
8.0 MB minimum available memory
Microsoft Pocket PC 2002/2003
Microsoft Internet Explorer 5.0 or Netscape Communicator 6.0
Mac OS 9.2/X (10.x)
Palm Desktop 4.01 or higher

COSTS

Hardware

Hardware needed includes handheld devices such as a PDA, tablet or Blackberry. Software costs vary depending on other features desired such as a scheduler or access to additional references. The average cost for a PDA, tablet, or Blackberry is approximately $300–500.

Software Rental

The monthly software expenses range from $50 to $70 per month depending on whether or not additional programs are included.

Ancillary Charges

For high speed Internet service, the costs are approximately $50 to $60 per month. For an individual practice, the estimated cost may total $1,200 to $1,500 per year.

Training

The entire office staff should be familiar with the basic elements of electronic prescribing, while dedicated key staff should be trained regarding their roles in the electronic process. Practitioner training is variable. For physicians with considerable computer and technical experience, the initial training may be minimal. They would need on-site training or Web. For providers with little previous experience, on-site training would be given over a one-to-two month timeframe. In addition, repeated refresher sessions may be necessary for the majority of practitioners.

The most significant issue with training is managing expectations for the physician and staff. There is reduced productivity during the ramp up and training periods. There are two key benchmarks for adoption status: (1) at least 50% of all prescriptions are provided electronically and (2) at least fifty prescriptions per week per provider. The practice workflow should be adjusted to these expectations, including scheduling fewer patients per day, with more down time between patients.

Workflow

The workflow for the practice will be modified to delete steps in the prescribing processes while adding more efficient steps. For instance, calls for refills may be typed into the computer rather than handwritten. The display of the patients' medication history may eliminate the need for full chart retrieval for all refills. This allows the physician to designate chart retrieval for certain medications. All of the steps in the new workflow should be documented for staff to refer to as needed. For fax and printed prescriptions, the staff will decide if the printer will be close to examination rooms or with the clerical staff in case copies are required for charting. This again may be dependent on size of the practice. There must be a resolution of some of the workflow issues and concerns such as strategic location of work stations and integration of prescription reminders.

Incentives

One of the key factors toward adoption is the existence of incentives. As mentioned, there are savings in the reduction of duplicate prescriptions. These savings are appreciated by all of the stakeholders in the prescribing process. Physician office efficiency is improved by reduction in office calls. Health plans realize a savings from increases in generic prescribing and formulary compliance. These savings are passed to the health plan and employer. Physicians think this savings model is the most profitable, so they are looking to health plans to fund and support electronic prescribing. Various health plans are realizing incentives are the key towards widespread adoption and are funding provider incentive programs based solely on electronic prescribing or as a part of one that is more comprehensive. In early electronic prescribing pilot projects, all components of the e-prescribing process were given free of charge to providers by the health plan. This proved to yield less than expected results, so incentive programs are now maturing toward a tiered structure requiring: (1) implementation, (2) utilization targets, and (3) outcomes.[10]

Health plans are using electronic prescribing alone, or in conjunction with utilization and quality measures such as the Health Plan Employer Data and Information Set (HEDIS), for a comprehensive pay for performance program. One of the most known is the P4P collaboration, a program of the Integrated Healthcare Association, a California non-profit leadership organization comprised of more than 30 employers, health plans, pharmaceutical and consumer groups. Now in its fourth year of measurement, electronic prescribing is one of the measures for technology implementation.[11]

Another program, Bridges to Excellence, was created by a multi-state, multi-employer coalition to encourage significant leaps in the quality of care by recognizing and rewarding healthcare providers who demonstrate that they deliver safe, effective, efficient, and patient-centered care. This program rewards physicians using information technology. Via its Physician Office Link, it enables physician office sites to qualify for bonuses based on their implementation of specific processes to reduce errors and increase quality, including the adoption and use of electronic medical records. They can earn up to $50 per year for each patient covered by a participating employer or plan. In addition, a report card for each physician office describes its performance on the program measures and is made available to the public.[12]

OUTCOMES

Effectiveness, Efficiency and Savings

Recently, pilots and programs have been studying the actual effectiveness and efficiency of electronic prescribing, as well as identifying the direct recipients of the savings. In a study to determine the efficiency of electronic prescribing, 48% of inbound calls to a physician office were pharmacy-related prior to implementation. Electronic prescribing resulted in a 42% reduction in pharmacy-related calls overall. Specifically, formulary-related calls decreased, while maintaining compliance with the benefit's formulary and constant generic prescribing rates. In addition, physician and pharmacy rework was reduced. Formulary-related calls per 1000 prescriptions fell 84% and clarification calls (because of illegibility) per 1000 prescriptions written declined 30%. Because of the use of an automated prescription renewal system, renewal calls decreased 42%. The prescribing rates for generic drugs remained unchanged. Providing information regarding availability of a home delivery pharmacy benefit during the patient encounter also increased the use of home delivery—an obvious financial benefit for the patient, health plan and/or employer. The ability to transmit a prescription directly to the home delivery pharmacy from the physician's office via this technology led to a 10% increase in home delivery use that was twice the increase seen for the control group for the same period.[13]

A study conducted by BCBS, Allscripts (TouchWorks) and Express Scripts, Inc. looked at 687 physicians to evaluate cost savings and adoption. The physicians included 343 electronic prescribing users to serve as the test group and 344 paper prescribers to act as the control group. The results were normalized for specialty, geography, total retail prescription volume and percent of prescription by third party payors. Results showed a potential savings of $.75 to $3.20 per electronic (TouchWorks) prescription from increases in generic prescribing rates and greater formulary compliance, with no change in the number of prescriptions written. The electronic technology prompted the behavior change because the physician that stopped prescribing electronically reverted back to the level of control group. Figures 1-5 and 1-6 show the results of this study.

Government Programs

Since implementing eMPOWERx—the Florida state-sponsored electronic prescribing software with access to a Medicaid drug data warehouse to more that 1,000 physicians—Florida Medicaid has benefited from a significant cost savings, fraud reduction and a decline in dangerous drug events. To extend these benefits, Florida approved expansion of the system from 1,000 to 3,000 physicians that represents physicians writing 80% of all Medicaid prescriptions in Florida, approximately twenty-five million transactions.

The Medicare Prescription Drug and Improvement Modernization Act of 2003 created a new voluntary prescription drug benefit under Medicare that is administrated by CMS. Although electronic prescribing will be optional for physicians and pharmacies, Medicare will require drug plans participating in the new prescription benefit to support electronic prescriptions. By January 2006, drug plans had to comply with standards defined by the National Council for Prescription Drug Programs and

Accredited Standards Committee (ASC). These standards apply to prescription refills, change requests, cancellation requests, eligibility, and benefit queries and responses.

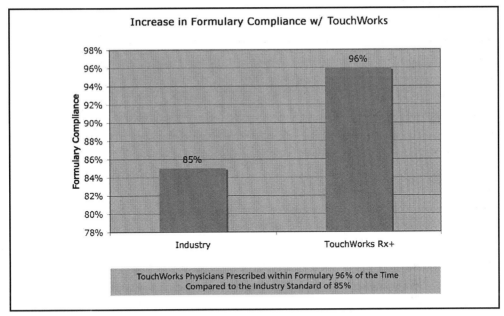

Figure 1-5: Increased Formulary Compliance.

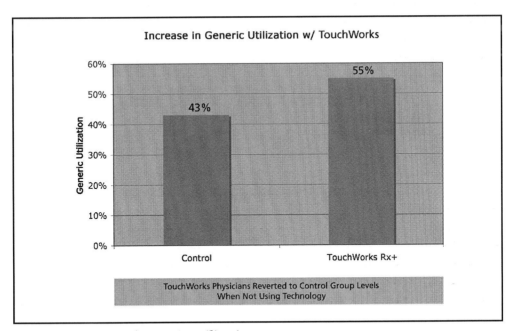

Figure 1-6: Increased Generic Utilization.

THE FUTURE

In the coming years, the landscape for electronic prescribing will significantly improve. A 2005 study reported that 52% of traditional prescribers are either considering or ready to implement electronic prescribing technology in their practices, but competing priorities have gotten in the way.[14] As more clinical research validates savings, incentives will become more accepted by more health plans and employers. In many practices, electronic prescribing is the initial step to be followed by electronic medical record implementation. Collaborations of health plans, such as the Massachusetts' Health Data Consortium's MA-SHARE initiative, have demonstrated the value of such alignments. As the saving models are being validated, software companies, health plans and PBMs are entering into risk arrangements based on generic and formulary adherence.

Patient Compliance

A significant advancement in electronic prescribing is the concept of feedback to the physician regarding patient compliance. Did the patient fill the prescription? Is the patient compliant with the treatment plan and continuing the medication as prescribed? At present, the physician does not have this information until the patient returns for a follow visit, potentially too late to prevent an adverse event caused by non-compliance. Just as the practitioner calls the patient to remind him/her of a missed appointment, the physician should know if the patient failed to fill or is not compliant with medication. This will be a significant improvement in the management of chronic diseases such as diabetes and asthma. Pilot studies are ongoing to measure physician acceptance and effectiveness of this added capability.

Barriers

Despite the recent results of effectiveness and efficiency studies, there remain significant barriers to rapid electronic prescribing adoption. In a survey by Quest Diagnostic Labs, no IT initiative received more that 50% of responding health plans willing to provide incentives to ensure the physicians are using the technology available to them— including electronic prescribing.[15]

Similar to implementation of most new technology, electronic prescribing causes a decrease in productivity as the office staff and physician adjust the workflow and the psychological mindset to accept the new processes and interfaces. There can be as much as 10–20% decreases in office productivity, depending on size of the practice and its previous utilization of computer technology. This element is one of the physicians' arguments for health plan support for implementation of electronic prescribing.

Medicare requires drug plans participating in the new prescription benefit, Part D, to support electronic prescribing. CMS has awarded funding for pilots to test standards for electronic prescribing. The pilots will test initial e-prescribing standards for information on formulary and benefits, patient instructions on how to take their medications, prior authorization messages, drug product information, patient medication histories and clinical drug terminology. The grants, worth nearly $2 million each, were awarded to the following: (1) Rand Corporation in New Jersey, (2) SureScripts, a multi-state collaboration, (3) Boston's Brigham and Women's Hospital in Massachusetts, and (4) Achieve Healthcare Information Technology in Minnesota. Results of the standards testing due in 2007 are expected to assist in determining the final specifications for electronic prescribing in 2008.[16]

Functionality

In the recent years, technology has allowed the development of online communications between physician and patients. Founded in 1999 and based in Emeryville, California, RelayHealth is a provider of secure online healthcare communication services linking patients, healthcare professionals, payors and pharmacies. A physician survey sponsored by Blue Cross of California and conducted by the University of California and Stanford University evaluated the satisfaction of online visits. Results showed the majority of the physicians responded were satisfied (63%) and thought it was easy to use (72%). Over half of the respondents (56%) preferred the Web visit for handling non-urgent patient health needs. A survey of over 380 thought leaders predicted that more that 20% of all office visits could be replaced by an online equivalent by 2010. To be successful, however, the system must have a clinical structure, optimize office work flow and increase physicians' reimbursement.[17]

Other Electronic Prescribing Activities

Additional healthcare companies are entering into the electronic prescribing space. Laboratory companies are developing integrated portals for physicians to allow access via the Web. Physicians can review laboratory results and prescribe online the needed medication based on the results.[18] In addition, messages for disease management activities and results of interventions will assist in determining the appropriate prescribing steps to take for that specific patient. This captures the spirit of the patient-centric model that is more effective in producing positive clinical outcomes

SUMMARY

The writing of prescriptions is a function of healthcare delivery that reaches back to ancient medicine. In the last 30 years, the significant improvements brought about by technology are well known. Despite this, there have been relatively small rates of adoption of electronic prescribing as compared to the number of prescriptions written daily. Early individual and community adopters have shown the value of electronic prescribing. However, cost and the ownership of those costs are significant barriers that have made stakeholders very cautious. The next step toward revolutionizing the process may be mandates at the state and federal levels. The Federal government has taken a role in implementation of standards in order to move towards greater adoption. Health plans generally have taken a "wait and see" approach in the recent past, but more incentive programs are supported by the health plans and PBMs as the cost saving data emerges. Within the next five to seven years, the landscape should be immensely different.

REFERENCES

1. Institute of Medicine. *To Err is Human: Building a Safer Health System*. Washington DC: National Academies Press; November 1999.

2. eHealth Initiative. Toward maximum value and rapid adoption: a report of the electronic prescribing initiative. April 14, 2004. Available at:
   http://www.ehealthinitiative.org/assets/documents/eHIFullReport-ElectronicPrescribing2004.pdf. Accessed November 9, 2006.

3. Center for Information Technology Leadership. The value of computerized provider order entry in ambulatory setting, 2003. Available at: http://www.citl.org/research/ACPOE_Executive_Preview.pdf. Accessed November 9, 2006.

4. Schiff GD, Rucker TD. Computerized prescribing: building the electronic infrastructure for better medication usage. *JAMA*. 1998;Apr 1;279(13):1024–9.

5. Epinette WW. RXWriter and Medication Manager. 1: *MD Comput*. 1987 Mar–Apr;4(2):29–32.

6. RxHub homepage. Available at: www.RxHub.net. Accessed on November 9, 2006.

7. Potts AL, Barr FE, Gregory DF, Wright L, Patel NR. Computerized physician order entry and medication errors in a pediatric critical care unit. *Pediatrics*. 2004 Jan;113(1 Pt 1):59–63.

8. Greenberg MD, Ridgely S, Bell DS. Electronic prescribing and HIPAA privacy regulations. Inquiry. 41:461–468.

9. American National Standards Institute homepage. Available at: www.ANSI.org. Accessed on November 9, 2006.

10. Gartner Industry Research, August 4, 2006.

11. Integrated Healthcare Association homepage. Available at: www.iha.org. Accessed on November 9, 2006.

12. Bridges to Excellence homepage. Available at: www.bridgestoexcellence.org. Accessed on November 9, 2006.

13. McMullin ST, Lonegan TP, Rynearson CS. Twelve month drug cost savings related to use of an electronic prescribing system with integrated decision support in primary care. *J of Man Care Pharm*. 2005;May;11(4):322–32.

14. Pizzi LT, Suh DC, Barone J, Nash DB. Factors related to physicians' adoption of electronic prescribing: results from a national survey. *Am J Med Qual*. 2005 Jan–Feb;20(1):22–32.

15. Special Report : The HealthCare Information Technology Gap. February 2006. http://www.questdiagnostics.com/brand/business/health_plan/white_papers/healthcare_tech_gap.pdf [Accessed 11/22/06]

16. http://www.cms.hhs.gov/EPrescribing/ [Accessed 11/22/06]

17. The RelayHealth Web visit study report. Available at: https://www.relayhealth.com/rh/general/studyResults/webVisitStudyResults.pdf. Accessed on November 9, 2006.

18. Federal Register rule: Medicare and state health care programs: fraud and abuse; safe harbor for certain electronic prescribing arrangements under the anti-kickback arrangement. Available at: http://www.ashp.org/emplibrary/Proposed%20Rule%20re%20Safe%20Harbor%20for%20the%20Anti-Kickback%20Statue.pdf. Accessed on November 9, 2006.

ADDITIONAL READING

1. Bell DS, Cretin S, Marken RS, Landman AB. Conceptual framework for evaluating outpatient electronic prescribing systems based on their functional capabilities. *J Am Med Inform Assoc*. 2004;January–February;11(1):60–70.

2. Stephen E. Wogen, MHA, George Fulop, MD, MS, Judith Heller, RN. Improving the Efficiency of the Prescription Process and Promoting Plan Adherence. *Drug Benefit Trends* 15(9):35–40, 2003.

3. Proposed E-prescribing Rules. Federal Register/Vol. 70, No. 23/Friday, February 4, 2005. http://a257.g.akamaitech.net/7/257/2422/01jan20051800/edocket.access.gpo.gov/2005/pdf/05-1773.pdf [Accessed 11/21/06]

4. Bates DW, Kuperman GJ, Wang S, Gandhi T, Kittler A, Volk L, Spurr C, Khorasani R, Tanasijevic M, Middleton B. Ten commandments for effective clinical support: making the practice of evidence-based medicine a reality. *J AM Med Inform Assoc*. 2003;November–December;10(6):523–30.

5. Scheck McAlearney A, Schweikhart SB, Medow M. Doctors' experience with handheld computers in clinical practice: qualitative study. *BMJ*. 2004:328:1162–5.

6. Wogen S, Fulop G, Heller J. Improving the efficiency of the prescription process and promoting plan adherence. *Drug Benefit Trends*. 2003;15(9):35–40.

7. Johnston D, Pan E, Middleton B. Finding the value in healthcare information technologies. ©2002. Center for IT Leadership. http://www.citl.org/research/articles.htm# [Accessed 11/21/06]

8. Teich JM, Osheroff J. Clinical Decision Support and Electronic Prescribing: Recommendation and an Action Plan Report of the Joint; Clinical Decision Support Work Group. 2005; March.

9. Miller RA, Gardner RM, Johnson KB, Hripcsak G. Clinical decision support and electronic prescribing system: a time for responsible thought and action. *J Am Medical Inform Assoc*. 2005;12:403–409.

10. Proposed E-prescribing Rules. Federal Register/Vol. 70, No. 23/Friday, February 4, 2005. http://a257.g.akamaitech.net/7/257/2422/01jan20051800/edocket.access.gpo.gov/2005/pdf/05-1773.pdf [Accessed 11/21/06]

11. The Federal Register. 2005;October 11. http://a257.g.akamaitech.net/7/257/2422/01jan20051800/edocket.access.gpo.gov/2005/pdf/05-20322.pdf [Accessed 11/21/06]

12. Hammond WE. The role of standards in electronic prescribing. *Health Aff* (Millwood). 2004:January–June(suppl);Web Exclusives:W4-325–7.

13. Formulary compliance, patient safety to improve as physicians take up e-prescribing. Drug Cost Management Report, Oct, 2002. ©2002 Atlantic Information Services, Inc. http://findarticles.com/p/articles/mi_m0NKV/is_10_3/ai_92712189 [Accessed 11/21/06]

14 Marken RS, Meili RC, Wang CJ, Rosen M, Brook RH. Recommendations for comparing electronic prescribing systems. HEALTH AFFAIRS Web Exclusive:W4.305–W4-317 ©2004 Project HOPE.

CHAPTER 2

Computerized Practitioner Order Entry and Patient Safety: Panacea or Pandora's Box

Joseph Kannry, MD

Scenario: The Chief Executive Officer of Mega Hospital offers you the job of Chief Quality Improvement Officer (CQIO). Your mission, should you decide to accept it, is to improve patient care and safety any way you can. Should you fail, the CEO will disavow all knowledge of this task. You agree anyway to take the job. As you reach for the doorknob, the CEO proudly tells you they have a Computerized Practitioner Order Entry. Does this help or hurt you?

In order to answer this question, it is important to understand how information technology in general can improve patient safety. More specifically, how does the use of a Computerized Practitioner Order Entry (CPOE) factor in this issue? Does it automatically lead to improved safety, or does it come with its own potential for medical errors? How would one best mitigate these concerns? And what factors lead to successful CPOE implementation?

QUESTION #1

You've just been appointed Chief Quality Improvement Officer (CQIO). What do you need to know about computerized practitioner order entry (CPOE) and health information technology (HIT)?

Patient Safety: Why now?

It is obvious that the CEO feels that patient safety is a major issue for Mega Hospital in that he created a new post CQIO, but why is this a priority now? We all have seen multiple headlines and studies proclaiming that healthcare is rife with errors and well-intentioned healthcare professionals are killing patients. The headlines began to mushroom after the results of the Harvard Medical Practice became public.[1] This study of over one million patients found a medical error rate of 27.1%, an adverse event rate of 3.7% and a mortality rate of 13.6% . A key take-home point of this study is that not all medical errors lead to adverse events and not all adverse events lead to death. Later studies on adverse events would also demonstrate that not all events were preventable or caused harm.[2] The Harvard study was not without controversy. One question was how long would patients have lived had care been optimal? What mortality could be attributed to the errors themselves? Many of the patients examined had serious underlying disease. Other studies have since asked if the error rate was over reported.[3,4]

An Approach for Assessing the Role and Use of HIT (Health Information Technology)

Healthcare is an industry that at its very core is built around science: the Science of Medicine. Scientific research is translated into breakthroughs in patient care at the bedside.[5,6,7] One would expect the assessment of HIT interventions to be scientific as well.

Medical Informatics is the interdisciplinary science of information management in medicine.[8,9] Medical informatics has a rich and long history of scientifically evaluating the role of the information technology in healthcare. The science of informatics provides the evidence needed to make informed decisions about the efficacy and effectiveness of HIT Interventions.[10,11,12] This chapter uses an Informatics framework to focus on how inpatient clinical information systems—and in particular, a computerized practitioner order entry (CPOE) system—can improve patient safety.

The Case for HIT and Patient Safety

Evidence suggests several HIT interventions may improve patient safety. Specifically these interventions include: access to reference information at the point-of-care,[13,14] remote monitoring in critical care units to address the shortage of intensivists,[15,16,17,18] smart monitoring,[19] smart intravenous pumps that control flow rates,[20] and bar code medication administration (or bar code at point of service).[21,22] There is a great deal of reasoned thought and suggestive evidence on how HIT interventions can prevent or intercept medical errors and thereby reduce adverse events. For example, physicians do not have access to reference material needed to make informed clinical decisions at the point-of-care.[23,24] Personal digital assistants (PDAs) can bring reference knowledge to the point-of-care.[25,26] For example, the Leapfrog Group has identified the need for more intensivists.[27] Remote monitoring is thought of as a means of addressing the intensivist shortage by enabling fewer intensivists needed to monitor more patients. Smart telemonitoring can alert physicians to changes in patient condition and better display information used to make decisions. However, there is a paucity of published and scientifically-conducted studies. Fischer et al reviewed the literature and found no convincing evidence that handhelds improved patient care or patient safety.[13] There is not only a shortage of studies on the bar coding of medications but among the few conducted, there have been conflicting results. This has lead all to agree that bar code technology requires a carefully thought-out workflow.[28,29,30]

To date, the vast majority of published and peer-reviewed informatics research on the use of HIT to improve patient safety has concentrated on medication errors and, in particular, adverse drug events (ADEs).[31] Perhaps the most compelling reason for this emphasis is that ADEs are the most common type of adverse events.[32]

Before proceeding any further, we need to review the definitions of medication error and adverse drug event and examine the relationship between the two. A medication error is any error that occurs during the process of ordering, dispensing or administering a medication regardless of whether harm occurred to the patient or if there was the potential for harm.[33] Adverse drug events are medical errors that cause harm to the patient or have the potential to cause harm. Medication errors do not automatically result in corresponding adverse drug events. A study by Bates determined that seven in every hundred medical errors have the potential to cause an ADE,[34] while a study by Brennan found one in every hundred medical errors actually causes an ADE.[1] Not all adverse drug events are preventable and not all adverse drug events result in harm.[2]

Adverse drug events have a significant impact on healthcare as a whole. Bates et al estimate that ADEs cost $2,595 per admission, increase length of stay (LOS) by 2.2 days per patient and result in a national cost of $2 billion per year.[35] A study by Classen at Intermountain Health found similar numbers. Each ADE added a cost of $2,262 to each admission and increased LOS 1.91 days per patient.[36] An earlier study done in 1992 by Evans at LDS Hospital established that the severity of the ADE affected average LOS as well as cost. Patients suffering a severe ADE had an average LOS of twenty days, less severe ADEs thirteen days and patients without an ADE had an average LOS of five days. Total hospitalization costs per patient were $38,007, $22,474 and $6,320 respectively.[37] All three studies, Bates, Classen and Evans, looked at ADEs in the inpatient setting. More importantly, the specific HIT intervention for reducing medication errors and ADEs was CPOE with CDSS (Clinical Decision Support System).

QUESTION #2

There's so much information about CPOE. What's fact and what's fiction?

Fiction 1: CPOE is the hospital's clinical information system.

CPOE is mistakenly thought of as the hospital information system (HIS). In reality, it is but a module or portion of the bigger HIS. The HIS is an information system used to collect, store, process, retrieve and communicate patient care and administrative data. CPOE is the part of HIS that handles the physician and nursing orders sent to the laboratory, radiology, pharmacy and other ancillary departments.[38] CPOE uses and adds to the information already stored in HIS. This relationship can be seen in Figures 2-1 and 2-2. Because of this architecture, results review and other modules that support CPOE can be activated before physicians go live on CPOE, as part of a CPOE rollout.

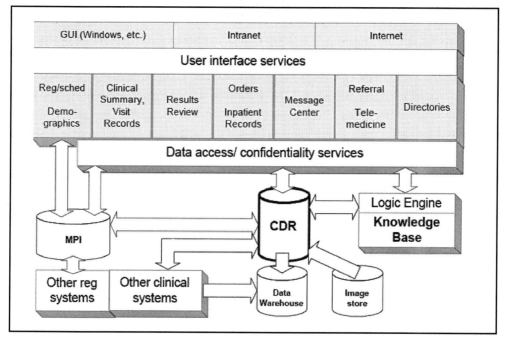

Figure 2-1:   BICS: Example of a Non-commercial CPOE and HIS.

(From Teich JM. Clinical information systems for integrated healthcare networks. Proc AMIA Symp *1998: 19–28.)*

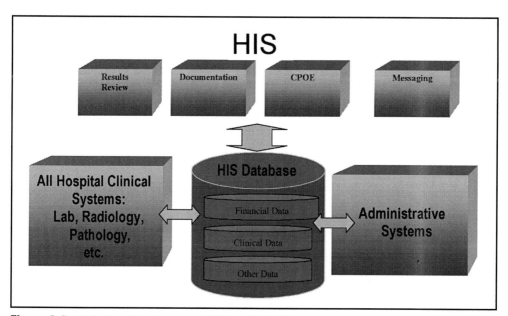

Figure 2-2:   Relationship between HIS and CPOE.

Fiction 2: Only physicians place electronic orders.

When physician assistants, nurses, dieticians, respiratory therapists and other care givers are placing and retrieving orders, they are doing so in COE (Computerized Order Entry). As shown in Figure 2-3, CPOE is actually a subset of computerized order entry (or electronic order entry) that supports the electronic entry by physicians of patient orders for diagnostic and treatment services, such as medications, laboratory and other diagnostic tests.[39] While the terms CPOE and COE are frequently used interchangeably, the significance of the difference in meaning is in functionality and usability. Successfully developing orders for physicians in CPOE does not mean the ordering needs of nurses, nurse practitioners, physicians assistants, nutritionists, physical therapists, and social workers have been either adequately assessed or met.

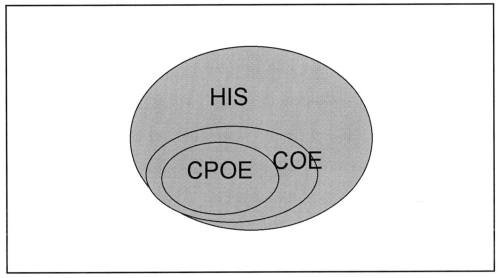

Figure 2-3: Relationship between HIS, CPOE, and COE.

However, the majority of orders are written by physicians. At Vanderbilt, physicians place 70% of the total orders while other clinicians write the remainder.[40] At Brigham and Women's Hospital, physicians place 80% of the total order, while other clinicians place the rest.[41] The balance of this chapter will accordingly concentrate on the physician portion of computerized order entry. Unfortunately, physicians are also one of the biggest barriers to CPOE diffusion.[42,43,44,45,46,47]

Fiction 3: CPOE improves patient safety.

Like Microsoft's Office products, commercial CPOE has gone through an evolution. The first version of CPOE, version 1.0, by itself could do little to improve patient safety except standardizing orders through the use of order entry screens and order sets, improving legibility, reducing order transmittal time, rapid retrieval and centralization of orders and, in some cases, useable checking for drug allergies.[48] The next iteration, version 1.5, introduced some elements of clinical decision support, such as drug-drug, drug-allergy, drug-food interaction checking and medication dose calculators.

Six short years ago at the turn of the century, CPOE version 1.x was the state of the art. Both versions of CPOE are still in operation in many sites. Screenshots of first generation CPOE can be seen in Figure 2-4.

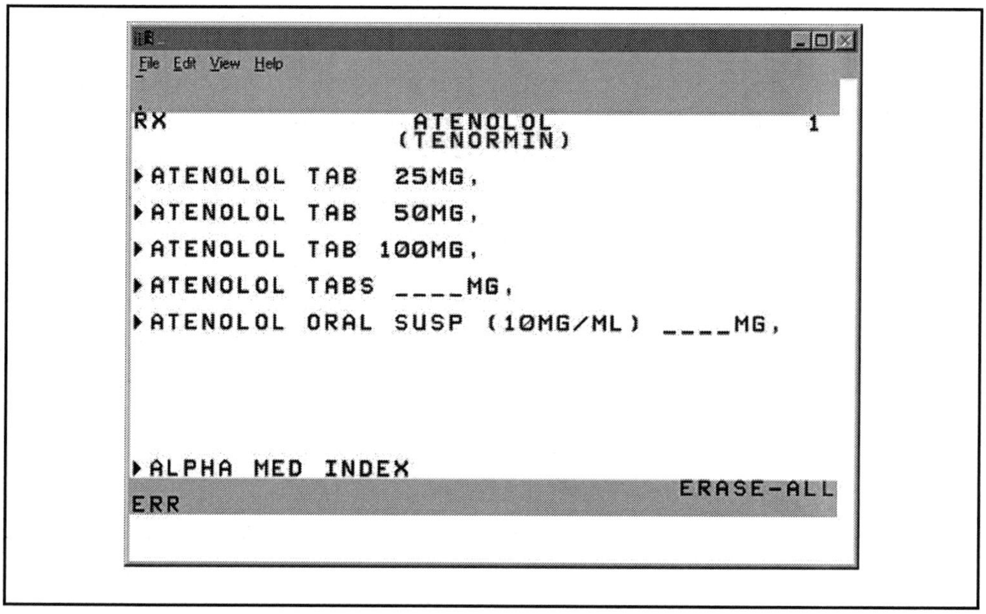

Figure 2-4: First Generation CPOE.

The second version of CPOE, version 2.0, introduced CPOE with CDSS. The components of CDSS consisted of a clinical event monitor, a rules (logic) engine and a medical knowledge base.[49,50,51,52,53] To function correctly, CDSS requires both an EMPI (enterprise master patient index) and a data dictionary. An EMPI identifies each patient uniquely so all healthcare information about a single patient will be correctly associated with him/her. A data dictionary is required to create a shared medical vocabulary for decision report rules. See Figure 2-1 for an example of CDSS architecture, e.g., logic engine and knowledge base. It is CDSS that accounts for the vast majority of improvements in patient care and patient safety.[54,55,56,57]

The architecture and extensibility of the CDSS determines the extent that a CPOE system can improve patient safety. A key caveat worth repeating is that the studies that reported successful use of CPOE with CDSS for patient safety were done with non-commercial systems built in-house. These non-commercial CPOE systems had CDSS five to ten years earlier than their commercial counterparts.[58,59,60] In contrast, two of the highly publicized studies demonstrating medical errors attributable to CPOE were conducted using CPOE systems with minimal capacity for[61] or implementation of CDSS.[62] In 2006, almost every commercial CPOE system has a CDSS.

Implementation of CDSS is both time and labor intensive as it includes such non-technical tasks as the selection and writing of rules, and maintenance of the knowledge base.[63,64,65,66,67,68,69] Physicians, nurses and quality assurance experts are required to supply the necessary domain expertise and knowledge.

QUESTION #3

Your CEO proudly proclaims we have a CPOE system. Your job is going to be easy, isn't it?
(Making the case for CPOE with and without CDSS)
Your first instinct is to be very happy because you have a CPOE system. Nationally, the diffusion of CPOE is quite low.[70,71,72] You quickly look at the CPOE system and

determine you are dealing with a first generation commercial system, version 1.x. Beyond drug-allergy, drug-drug, drug-food checking, any and all improvements are going to require significant IT resources. An example of this kind of work was done at Mount Sinai. We implemented intravenous to oral (PO) substitution of the antibiotics Ciprofloxacin, Levaquin and Fluconazole by sending data back and forth to a pre-existing data warehouse.[73] These three drugs were chosen because in almost all cases the efficacy of administering the antibiotic orally is equal to administering the drugs intravenously. The oral route is also associated with fewer complications and costs. We wrestled with issues such as who should receive the alert (i.e., anyone viewing that patient in CPOE or only physicians attempting to write pharmaceutical orders). CPOE version 1.x provides limited options for delivering clinical decision support.

How do you make the case for upgrading your CPOE to version 2.0, CPOE with CDSS? Your CEO instructs you to first review the benefits to date of the CPOE system you have. Let's first look at the general case for all CPOE, and then the particular case for CPOE alone without CDSS. Table 2-1 shows the benefits of CPOE without CDSS for decision makers to appreciate the concrete efficiencies CPOE can bring.

• **Elimination of "lost orders"**
• **Elimination of illegible handwriting**
• **Reduction of duplicate orders**
• **Improved/consistent documentation**
• **Reductions in variances in care**
• **Reduced order processing time**
• **Reduced order verification time**
• **Improved charge capture**
• **Length of stay reduction**
• **Reduced malpractice exposure**
• **Reduced data entry needs**

Table 2-1: Benefits of CPOE without CDSS for Decision Makers.

(Adapted from Sittig DF, Stead WW. Computer-based physician order entry: the state of the art. J Am Med Inform Assoc *1994;1(2):108–23; Remmlinger E. Functionality of computerized physician order-entry systems. In: Paper presented at VHA New England, editor. Practitioner Computer Order Entry Symposium; 2001 Mar 9, 2001; Boston, MA; 2001.; Gray MD, Felkey BG. Computerized prescriber order-entry systems: evaluation, selection, and implementation.* Am J Health Syst Pharm *2004;61(2):190–7.)*

There are some important caveats about the list of CPOE benefits. For example, improved charge capture is frequently listed but there are no published studies showing significant improvements in revenue from it. Charge capture is dependent on process and nursing documentation. A problematic area of charge capture for CPOE is test ordering in emergencies. For example, an EKG is commonly performed for a patient in cardiac arrest without an order. Without an order for the EKG, there will be no charge for the procedure or reimbursement.

Reducing order verification and processing time require interfaces to other systems, particularly the pharmacy system. Full integration with the pharmacy system is far from an easy task and may be the source of medication errors in CPOE systems.[2,61,74,75,76]

A length of stay reduction of .89 days, not related to reduction of medical errors, has been shown in only one study. This study, however, was with a version 2.0 system that the author noted may not be statistically significant and that the system had to be fully replicated.[77] Finally, reduced exposure to malpractice has yet to be realized. Please note that patient safety is not listed above as a benefit of a CPOE system without CDSS, as major improvements in safety come with the CDSS feature.

Making the argument for CPOE with CDSS, there are two significant additional benefits of relevance to decision makers: major improvements in patient care and patient safety. Studies of CPOE with CDSS do not consistently show changes in patient outcomes. Some studies were designed to demonstrate feasibility and use, as opposed to measurable improvements in patient safety, prevention of adverse events and medical errors. Other studies were underpowered. One of the challenges facing these earlier CPOE-CDSS studies was the number of patients involved. A rather larger number of patients need to be treated to show changes in outcomes due to CPOE with CDSS.[78] Improvements in patient care, while noble and desirable, do not readily convert into reduction of medical errors.

A frequent source of confusion, often exploited commercially, is that the terms "clinical decision support" and "clinical decision support system" are used interchangeably. Clinical decision support is defined as anything that directly aides in clinical decision making about individual patients. Decision support can include collegial advice, text references, Web sites and computer systems.[79] A CDSS (Clinical Decision Support System) is a computerized system that directly aides in clinical decision making about individual patients. Specifically, CDSS incorporates individual patient data, a rules engine and a medical knowledge base to produce a patient-specific assessment or recommendation for clinicians.[54,55] It is CDSS that makes it possible to deliver the clinical decision support to the user in the CPOE system. For example, when the physician sees a clinical decision support message in CPOE instructing him/her to change medication dose due to renal failure, it is the CDSS generating the message that appears to the physician in CPOE.

There are two types of clinical decision support. The first type is passive, in which the user has to input data and then request help from an online source like the National Library of Medicine's Medline (http://www.pubmed.org). CDSS may or may not be present. In contrast, the second type—active decision support—automatically produces suggestions and presents them to the user for action and almost always implies the presence and use of a CDSS. Active decision support is triggered by an event and delivers information to the physician that was not requested by the provider, but is relevant and of interest.[80,81] The physician may or may not have taken an action to initiate the trigger. For example, a physician may order a nephrotoxic medication and trigger a CDSS-generated alert that recommends a dose appropriate to the patient's kidney function and enables ordering a corollary order for blood levels of the medication. We will only discuss the active type of clinical decision support, which is the type that has been studied the most and shown to be responsible for most of the improvements in patient safety.

The active form of clinical decision support can be delivered as push or pull. Pull means the physician logs on to the system, CPOE in this case. Push, however, means the physician receives messages sent to him regarding orders on CPOE via wireless device.

To be successful, active decision support must be delivered at point-of-care, relevant to patient, in clinical context, timely, delivered to the right provider(s), automated as much as possible, allow explanation for override and is both tested and validated.[82] However, it should be noted that overrides can become a source of error. In a study on the effect of overrides on ADEs, one out of thirty overrides resulted in an ADE.[83,84]

CDSS can generate active decision support in several ways: alerts, reminders, corollary orders and guidelines (see Figures 2-5, 2-6, 2-7, 2-8 and 2-9).[54,55] An alert is a suggestion requiring immediate response or action. For example, an inappropriately high dose of a medication or dangerous interaction between a medication and the value from lab test would trigger an alert (e.g., Digoxin and low potassium). A reminder is a suggestion not requiring immediate response or action. For example, a reminder may caution that the increased risk of heart disease associated with Celebrex must be balanced with its pain relieving benefit. Reminders are frequently used more in ambulatory care but have been successfully used in the inpatient setting.[85] The success of a reminder is often proportional to the difficulty of the task that the user is being reminded to do. For example, reminders for vaccination and monitoring lipids have a higher success rate of patient and physician compliance than those reminding the user to arrange screening colonoscopy.

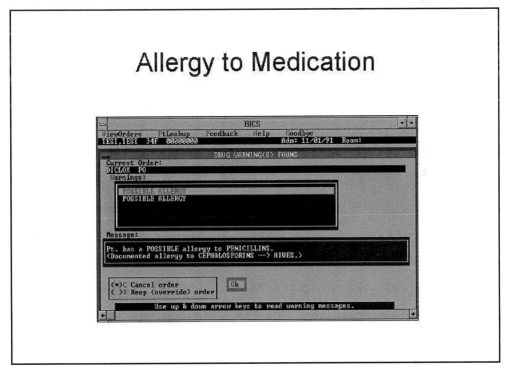

Figure 2-5: **Drug-Allergy Interaction Alert (BICS-Brigham Integrated Computer System).**

Corollary orders refer to "orders required to detect or ameliorate adverse reactions that may result from the trigger order."[86] For example, if a physician ordered a nephrotoxic drug such as Amphotericin, he/she would be prompted with an order to check the serum creatinine a minimum of two times per week This second order is not mandatory, but is ready to be added with the physician's approval.

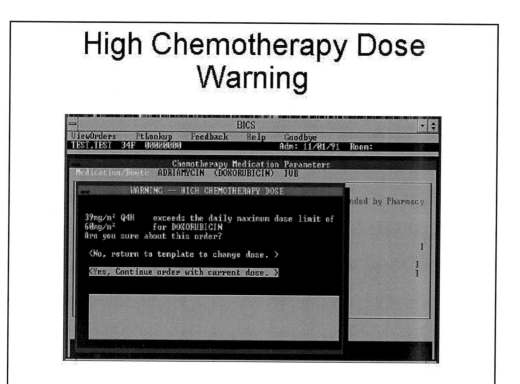

Figure 2-6: Excessive Dosing Alert-BICS.

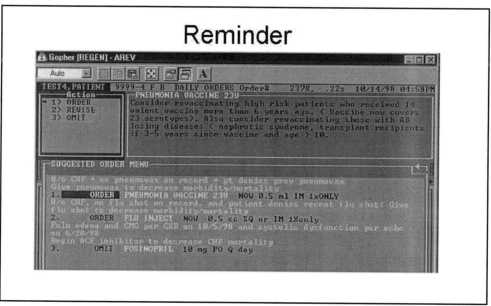

Figure 2-7: Reminder-Regenstrief Medical Record System.

(From McDonald CJ, Overhage JM, Tierney WM, Dexter PR, Martin DK, Suico JG, et al. The Regenstrief Medical Record System: a quarter century experience. Int J Med Inform 1999;54(3):225–53.)

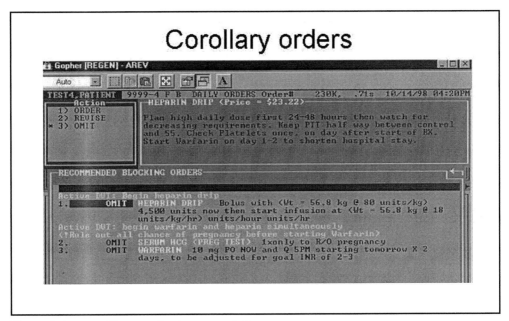

Figure 2-8: Corollary Order-Regenstrief.

(From McDonald CJ, Overhage JM, Tierney WM, Dexter PR, Martin DK, Suico JG, et al. The Regenstrief Medical Record System: a quarter century experience. Int J Med Inform 1999;54(3):225–53).

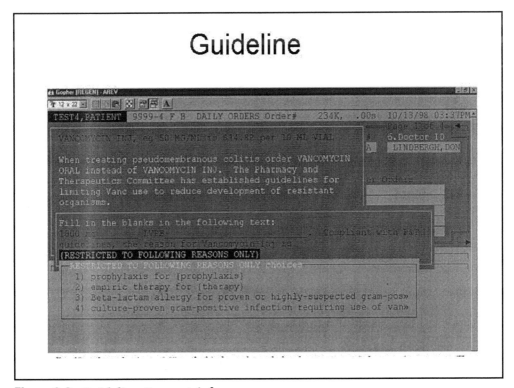

Figure 2-9: Guideline-Regenstrief.

Guidelines are a series of instructions on how to care for the patient based on information about the patient's clinical status. In contrast to alerts and reminders, there are several pieces of information required for a guideline to fire. If a physician orders

Metformin, a medication used to control blood sugar in diabetes, a guideline might fire that prompts the optional ordering of hemoglobin A1C and calculates the estimated creatinine clearance.

The benefits of CDSS "patient care" section of this table is a partial survey of improvements in patient care (see Table 2-2).[31,57,56] Cited references provide a more extensive list. The benefits of CDSS "patient safety" section of this table is a partial survey as well; consult references for additional information.

Table 2-2: Benefits of CPOE with CDSS for Decision Maker.

Category	Intervention	Findings/Outcome
Patient Safety	Reduction of Medical Errors and Adverse Drug Events at Brigham and Women's[2]	• Serious medication errors decreased 55%, 10.7 events per 1000 patient-days to 4.86 events per 1000 patient days • Decrease in ADEs was larger for potential ADEs than for errors that actually resulted in an ADE
	Reduction of Adverse Drug Events at Brigham and Women's[33]	• Serious medication errors fell 86% from baseline to study conclusion • Large differences were seen for all types of medication errors including dose errors, frequency errors, route errors, substitution errors and allergies (adapted from original abstract)
	Reduction of Adverse Drug Events: LDS Hospital[89]	• The control group had forty-one and CPOE had twelve severe ADEs • The control group had fifty-six and CPOE had eight drug-allergy interactions
	Reduction of Adverse Drug Events and Medication Errors at Vanderbilt Children's Hospital (a non-commercial system)[87]	• ADEs reduced from a rate of 2.2 per 100 orders to 1.3 per 100 orders • Medication errors reduced from rate of 30.1 per 100 orders to 0.2 per 100 orders • ADEs were reduced by 40.9%, and medication errors were reduced by 99.4%
Patient Care	Doubled compliance with corollary orders (orders that should occur at the time of another order) at Wishard Memorial Hospital[88]	• 46.3% compliance with CPOE versus 21.9% without CPOE • One-third fewer interventions by pharmacists with CPOE
	Improved Response Time To Critical Labs at Brigham and Women's Hospital[78]	• CPOE was associated with a shorter response time to critical laboratory values (38% shorter median time interval)
	Improved compliance with antibiotic guidelines at LDS[89]	• CPOE improved use of antibiotics: surgical patients receiving appropriately timed preoperative antibiotics (40% to 99.1%) • Reduced costs: per patient costs decreased from $122.66 to $51.90 • Stabilization of resistant strains of organisms

It is worth noting the differences in the Bates' medical error studies of 1998 and 1999 as the studies looked at no CPOE, CPOE without CDSS and CPOE with CDSS. Specifically, the Bates study in 1998 compared no CPOE to CPOE without CDSS. In contrast, the Bates study in 1999 compared no CPOE to CPOE with CDSS. Interestingly, one the earliest mentions of CPOE-related medical errors is when an early version of CPOE with CDSS introduced a new error involving potassium chloride. This error was later fixed in a subsequent version of the software.

QUESTION #4

Does CPOE with CDSS eliminate all medication errors?

The medication process is a process that starts with a physician ordering a medication and ends with the patient receiving the medication. This process has three distinct pieces: ordering, dispensing and administration. The ordering component for the most part can be either done directly by physicians or can involve transcription by clerical staff. Dispensing involves the pharmacy receiving the order, verifying the medication and then sending the medication to the nursing unit. Once on the nursing unit, the medication is administered, the nurse documents administration in a MAC or medical administration record (e.g., medication Cardex), and, last but not least, the hospital generates a charge for the medication.

The bulk of the medication errors occur in ordering, 56% by physicians and 6% by clerical staff.[34,90] Another 34% occur in medication administration. Only 4% of the errors occur in the pharmacy while dispensing the medication (see Figure 2-10).

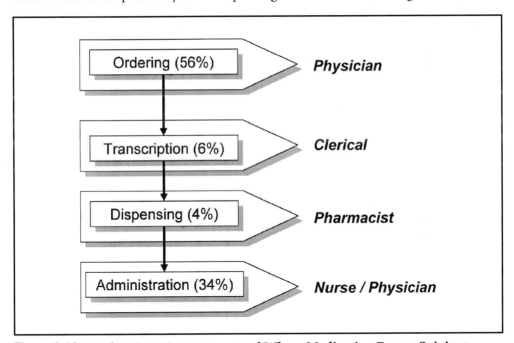

Figure 2-10: **Medication Management and Where Medication Errors Originate.**

(Adapted from Bates DW, Cullen DJ, Laird N, Petersen LA, Small SD, Servi D, et al. Incidence of adverse drug events and potential adverse drug events. Implications for prevention. ADE Prevention Study Group. JAMA. 1995;274(1):29–34.[34])

Assuming 100% efficacy, CPOE with CDSS can prevent more than half of the medication errors, with the bar coding of medication administration preventing another third. However, studies by Bates have demonstrated less than 100% efficacy for CPOE with CDSS, with error reduction rates of 55–86%.[2,91]

QUESTION #5

Does the reduction in ADEs provide a significant ROI (Return on Investment)?

The bottom line for a decision maker comes down to dollars. In this case, they are looking at the dollars saved from the reduction of medication errors and ADEs versus the dollars spent for the HIT intervention, CPOE with CDSS.

The estimated savings that might accrue from reducing medication errors varies. David Bates estimates that the annual costs of ADEs are $5.6 million per each 700-bed hospital for all ADEs and $2.8 million per each 700-bed hospital for preventable ADEs. The aggregate savings nationally could be $2 billion.[35]

While the estimated costs for CPOE with CDSS vary, the cost is quite high due to the cost of hardware, people, software licenses and interfaces.[70,60] In a report prepared by First Consulting Group for Advancing Health in America and the Federation of American Hospitals, the estimated cost of CPOE with CDSS for a 500-bed hospital is $8 million to implement and $1.3 million per year to maintain.[92] In this author's own experience, the cost to implement may be as high as $20 million or more for a 700-bed hospital with a maintenance cost of $2 million per year. Any of these commercial cost estimates for CPOE with CDSS pose a significant barrier to adoption.

In contrast, Kaushal reported a significantly lower cost for Brigham's non-commercial system, BICS than a commercial counterpart. Over a ten-year period, 1993–2002, the total cost of the BICS system was $11.8 million to develop, implement and maintain. Of the $11.8 million, $3.7 million was capital while maintenance was $600,000 to $1.1 million per year. The reported costs for BICS did not include the costs of the internally developed pharmacy system,[93] medication administration system, and clinical data repository, or the costs of IT personnel and knowledge engineering by Informaticists. Both a medication administration system and clinical data repository are standard part of commercial CPOE. The cost was also further reduced by building only what was needed when it was needed.[94]

This is the dilemma decision makers face whenever any attempt is made to portray a cost savings from reduction of medication errors and ADEs. The cost of the CPOE system significantly outweighs any money saved.

While the impact of CPOE with CDSS on overall patient safety may not be sufficiently convincing from a return on investment perspective, it is compelling from the viewpoint of patient safety and quality of care. ADEs occur in 6.5% of all admitted patients.[34] From a physician and patient point of view, CPOE with CDSS is a worthy intervention as morbidity and mortality from errors and corresponding adverse events is reduced. The math suggests it may cost millions of dollars in healthcare information technology to reduce ADEs.

At the time of this chapter, national, regional and local report cards are coming out on quality. This may better align the financial with the quality driver.

QUESTION #6

As CQIO you breathe a sigh of relief. The CEO and board approved the CPOE with CDSS. Quality does matter. Now comes the easy part……..convincing the doctors and nurses?

As Table 2-3[47,95,96,97] shows, the potential benefits and barriers to CPOE with CDSS for physicians and nurses should be appreciated to enlist their support.

Table 2-3: Benefits and Barriers.[47,95,96,97]

	Benefits	Barriers
Physician	• Remote Order Entry • Summary Reports • Patient Lookup/Lists • Personal Order Sets • Clinical Decision Support	• Learning Curve • Time Consuming – Payback never equals time saved • Fragmented Information • Rigidity of Orders • Time on Phone Clarifying Orders
Nurse	• Less Calls to MD • Decreased Variability • Decreased Time Transcribing and Creating Medical Administration Record (e.g., medication cardex) – Depends on system implementation	• Increased Time Charting • Decrease Time Communicating with MD

However, benefits can bring new sets of problems. For example, personal orders sets that provide speed and efficiency in ordering, can grow to a volume that makes them hard to administer, maintain and monitor—and may not even represent best practice.[98]

It may seem contradictory that nurses cite fewer calls to the physician as a benefit and decreased time communicating with physicians as a barrier. In practice, phone calls clarifying orders are frequent opportunities to discuss other issues requiring clarification or input, not only by the nurse calling but by other personnel on the floor. After CPOE implementation and the decreased need for order clarification, the nurse no longer finds it comfortable or efficient to page the physician about these other issues.[97]

One of the arguments put forth regarding physician benefits of CPOE is that order entry saves time. In any side by side or time motion study, it is always faster to write orders with pen on paper than it is to enter them electronically.[77,99,100] Studies do show time saving in some tasks but the time saved by these tasks are frequently balanced by the increased time it takes to enter orders.[101,77]

For example, Tierney showed an almost even trade off of time, but noted that it was a reflection of the system design, might be hard to reproduce and was not readily acknowledged by physicians.[77] The lack of acknowledgement is not hard to understand. Physicians do not spend the day tallying up where time was saved and time lost. What physicians will remember is that orders take longer to do with CPOE with CDSS. While time may be saved with remote order entry, information retrieval from one central system and patient lists, the perception is more time is spent. Of course, the physician view of time spent may be affected by who has to do the time-consuming portion of the work. At an academic medical center, housestaff frequently write the majority of orders. In one study, housestaff at an academic medical center wrote 76% (4,800/6,300) of physician orders in the CPOE system.[102]

What physicians want out of an order entry system—or for that matter any clinical information system—comes down to 3 things: ease of use, improvement in efficiency in daily work and perceived improvement in patient care.[97] Physicians view improvements in patient care as improvements that affect their patients and not the aggregate patient population.

QUESTION #7

One of the senior physician leaders approaches you and expresses significant concern over the CPOE project. With a very stern face, he asks, "Does CPOE with CDSS cause a whole new set of medical errors and ADEs?"

CPOE systems with and without CDSS can introduce their own set of medical errors and ADEs. The earliest published mention of medication errors caused by CPOE appears in Bates' second study regarding ordering of intravenous potassium.[33] The system allowed large doses to be ordered without making it explicit that these doses were to be given as divided doses. For example, an order of potassium chloride 120 meq should be divided into at least three separate runs of potassium chloride, such as 40 meq every one to two hours times three for a total of 120 meq. However, errors caused by CPOE really came to public attention due a succession of studies published during 2004–2005, as seen in Table 2-4.

Table 2-4: Errors Caused by CPOE.

Year	CPOE System Studied	Findings and Highlights
1999	BICS (non-commercial system) at Brigham and Women's Hospital[33,103]	• Study was looking at reductions in medication error and ADEs • Intercepted ADEs rose from baseline 15.8% per 1,000 patient days, to 31.3% and then 59.4% • Source of errors was ordering of Potassium Chloride and dose dividing • Error later fixed and essentially eliminated
2004	BICS (non-commercial system) at Brigham and Women's Hospital[83]	• A total of 6,182 (80%) of 7,761 alerts were overridden for 1,150 patients • In a random sample of 320 patients, nineteen (6%) experienced an ADE; with 9/19 (47%) were serious ADEs • One out of twenty drug allergies were overridden • Poor specificity of alerts blamed
2005	Commercial Order Entry System at the University of Pennsylvania[61]	CPOE facilitated 22 types of medication errors including: • Fragmented displays of patient medications • Pharmacy inventory displays mistaken for dosage guidelines • Ignored antibiotic renewal notices placed on paper charts and not in the CPOE system • Separation of functions that lead to double dosing and incompatible orders • Inflexible ordering formats generating wrong orders. • Weekly occurrence of errors • Adapted from original abstract
2005	VISTA at the VA Medical Center Salt Lake City[59]	• High rate of ADEs still occurring after CPOE implementation • Fifty-two ADEs per hundred admissions • Analysis suggests that problem was lack of clinical decision support for drug selection, dosing and monitoring
2005	Commercial System at the Children's Hospital of Pittsburgh[104]	• Increase in mortality associated from implementation of CPOE from 2.8% to 6.57% • Multivariate analysis confirmed CPOE independently associated with increased odds of mortality

It is beyond the scope of this chapter to review the numerous published rebuttals and discussions that occurred as a result of the Koppel article.[105,106,107,108,109,110] As noted earlier, Koppel's study was conducted on a first generation system with limited elements of decision support and this could have contributed to the errors.

However, Koppel's study suggests serious issues that could have been addressed post implementation through a software quality review process.

A continuing commitment to analyze and improve any healthcare information technology is critical to its ongoing success.[111,112,113,114,115] One of the considerations for a successful CPOE implementation is ongoing analysis and improvement post implementation.[65] The key components can be described as Learn, Evaluate, Feedback and Test, or L.E.F.T. In a sense, no CPOE system should be L.E.F.T. behind.

After implementation, Mount Sinai implemented a software quality improvement process called Optimization. Feedback was actively obtained, progress was reported back to the users and changes were made to the system.

Optimization came about as a result of an Informatics study demonstrating significant user dissatisfaction.[102] Upon reviewing the study results, the CIO charged one of the study authors to lead the post-implementation process that became known as "Optimization". The Optimization process made over 200 changes eliminating nuisances, modifying screens and pathways, adding functionality and improving overall utility. One innovation of Optimization was the optimization team actively and regularly sought out users to identify new concerns and issues. One of the problems identified early on in the previous study was that although users had issues, they stopped voicing them. The optimization team would take advantage of regularly scheduled meetings of users such as the Department of Medicine's housestaff noon conference. Additionally, all users were encouraged to inform designated team members of additional problems.

The group dynamics of user meetings highlights an interesting phenomenon where one user might be very vocal about a complaint, while other users in the room would indicate that this was not the case. One problem prior to optimization was the loudest issues sometimes received the greatest attention. Issues were reviewed and prioritized by a committee of physicians, nurses, Informaticists and Information Technology personnel. A key aspect of this committee is that IT personnel who could make changes to the system were present at the meeting. While not all identified issues resulted in changes, all issues were addressed and status with explanation was reported to the users. When appropriate, small sub-groups of users and team members would meet to design and implement changes. Progress reports from the subgroups were presented back to the optimization committee.

Optimization added additional functionality by revisiting issues such as drug allergy checking that had not been initially implemented. At the time of implementation in the late 1990s, there were significant functionality issues making drug allergy checking unusable. When Mount Sinai subsequently implemented drug allergy checking, the vendor was also revisiting functionality. As a result, Mount Sinai became one of the first sites to receive new functionality.

System functionality was also turned off. Nuisances that reduced efficiency and reinforced stereotypes of the system as being clumsy were eliminated. One such nuisance was the day of discharge screen. The screen was designed to have physicians enter an estimated day of discharge and then have this reported elsewhere for bed planning. Optimization found that while this might have worked for procedure-based specialties, the information obtained from the screen was not being used and was frequently useless or inaccurate for decision makers. The screen would prompt for a discharge date even when a discharge order had been written.

In conclusion, we would strongly recommend creating a software quality review process such as Optimization to reduce errors that are a direct result of CPOE, with or without CDSS.

QUESTION #8

You finally scream in desperation, "So just tell me already what I need to do to ensure a successful implementation of CPOE with CDSS?"

In an article summarizing considerations for a successful CPOE implementation, the nine factors listed in Table 2-5 were identified as being critical.

Table 2-5: Considerations for a Successful CPOE Implementation.

Component
1. Leadership, Organizational Culture and Personnel
2. Cost Analysis
3. Integration with Workflow and Healthcare Processes
4. Value to Users
5. Development and Maintenance of CDSS
6. Project Management and Staging of Implementation
7. Training and Support
8. Technology
9. Learning Evaluation Improvement

(Adapted from Ash JS, Stavri PZ, Kuperman GJ. A consensus statement on considerations for a successful CPOE implementation. J Am Med Inform Assoc *2003;10(3):229–34.)*

Leadership, Culture and Personnel

The role of leadership in a successful implementation cannot be underestimated. There is some evidence to suggest that leadership is an independent risk factor that correlates with success or failure.[116] Characteristics of such leadership include a clear and concise strategic vision for the enterprise, unwavering support, an understanding of the strategic value of information technology, an organizational culture that values constructive feedback and the ability to distinguish between issues and necessities. Perhaps most importantly leadership needs to identify the *raison d'etre* for selecting and implementing a CPOE. Unfortunately, leadership neither can be purchased with the system nor does it come as a standard feature.

The broad umbrella of leadership includes not only senior management but clinical, administrative and IT leadership.[117] Clinical leadership can be blamed for some of the difficulties Massaro cited in his installation of CPOE without CDSS.[42,43] Treister notes that poor IT leadership can result in clinical staff losing faith in an implementation.[118]

Organizational culture is a matter of both history and happenstance. How a CPOE project is perceived and prioritized is determined by: (1) past success or failure with clinical information systems, (2) the presence or absence of a learning culture and, (3) the success of major projects (IT or otherwise) in the recent past.[57] Culture affects the way an organization governs itself and makes decisions. Leadership and culture are intertwined, and good leadership can change culture or be fighting upstream against it.

An example of leadership and culture leading to a successful project can be seen in Evanston Northwest Healthcare. At Evanston, the EHR (Electronic Health Record) project included CPOE-HIS, ICU systems, ADT, registration, the ED system and the ambulatory Electronic Medical Record.[119] The project was done in a 'big bang' approach over three hospitals in the span of eighteen months. The 'big bang' is a project management term borrowed from cosmology that describes an installation timeframe that is relatively short. Leadership gave the EHR project the highest priority of any project. Leadership was both active and visible. Evanston's successful implementation won a Davies Award, an award given out every year for excellence in EHR implementation and improving the delivery of healthcare.[120]

Organizational culture also plays a role in the need to hire qualified personnel. If there is a culture of success, there is probably an abundance of qualified project managers and personnel that can be repurposed. However, if qualified personnel need to be hired, this can be a very difficult task as such personnel in healthcare are in short supply.[121]

Differences in culture and leadership may in part explain different outcomes with the same clinical information system. This author has seen the same system installed at similar institutions with different outcomes. There is even a study by O'Connell describing differing outcomes within the same institution attributable in part to leadership and culture. Specifically O'Connell describes two rollouts of the same EMR from a commercial vendor at the same institution. The two roll-out sites had significantly differing perceptions regarding the success of implementation, as well as which functionality did and did not work.[116]

Cost

Implementation begins when selection begins. The selection process determines the project's goals, institutional objectives, metrics, user expectations and total cost.[122] Portions of the rest of this discussion on cost have been taken from an article by Kannry.[10]

The Mount Sinai selection process for ambulatory EMR employed a meticulous total cost of ownership (TCO) analysis that assessed and compared real costs of implementing a vendor solution. Inaccurate TCO analysis affects the longevity and success of a project. It can lead to projects being accepted and then stalled or even cancelled if there are budget overruns.

One of the keys to successfully calculating the TCO is to realize the majority of costs are internal costs. While many vendors are willing to decrease software license fees or reduce the professional services rates, the vendor costs are a small portion of the overall project implementation costs. According to Informatics and healthcare IT professionals, 70% of the total cost of ownership are internal costs to the institution.[123] Other keys to successful calculation of TCO are: (1) clear understanding of implementation scope; (2) defining which costs are the vendor's and which are the client's; (3) reserving a contingency of budget of 10%; and, (4) working closely in tandem with the CEO or CFO.

Equally important is the decision to include or exclude a return on investment (ROI) analysis with the TCO analysis. The decision to include an ROI analysis with the TCO analysis should be made in consultation with senior management, particularly the CFO.

The practical shortcomings of ROI are well-illustrated by healthcare's chronic under investments in IT. Hospital financial officers have helped keep their organizations on an expensive paper trail because automated alternatives presumably did not have a positive ROI.[124] The direct financial ROI may sometimes be minimal or neutral.

Studies consistently show that CPOE with CDSS can improve quality, increase patient safety and facilitate regulatory compliance as baseline benefits.[48,49,50,51,53,58,59,60,70,57]

However, when measuring a return on investment, "one of the most serious problems is the absence of consistency." There is a paucity of published literature and studies on ROI, let alone consistent methodology for calculating the ROI of CPOE.[94] One of the most detailed published studies on ROI was done on BICS at Brigham and Women's (BWH). The study found that over a ten-year period, the BWH spent $11.8 million to develop, implement and operate the BICS CPOE system, saving $28.5 million for a cumulative net savings of $16.7 million and net operating budget savings of $9.5 million. The study notes that this was given the institution's 80% prospective reimbursement rate. The greatest cumulative savings were derived from "renal dosing guidance, nursing time utilization, specific drug guidance and adverse drug event prevention."[51]

The study has some limitations worth noting when the results are extrapolated to a commercial CPOE system. BICS is not a commercial system. BICS functionality was built when needed and paid for incrementally, as opposed to being purchased in advance in commercial systems. The cost of developing and maintaining a clinical repository, medication admitting record and internally developed pharmacy system[93] were not accounted for in the total cost nor were personnel costs such as Informaticists. A clinical data repository (CDR) would be a key component of any CPOE-HIS, as well as CDSS (see Figures 2-1 and 2-2). Medication administration is a standard feature of commercial CPOE. Costs incurred for BICS integration with an internally developed pharmacy system should be significantly less than that of commercial CPOE and pharmacy systems.

In contrast, the cost of a commercial system is fixed and spread out over years. The biggest limitation of this study is that the savings are related to cost avoidance, meaning money that would have been spent if the system was not in place.[94,125] For example, cost reduction from ADEs comes from avoiding the ADEs in the first place.

Most CFOs or CEOs are looking for increased revenue that can be subtracted from the cost of the system.[10,125] Mark Frisse notes that the problem in demonstrating increased revenue may be related to the Sokolow Productivity Paradox. This paradox postulates that it is hard to tease out productivity due to IT from the broader transformations that may be going on. For example, an ROI of the Internet would have to wrestle with productivity transformations that occurred because of the Internet, as well as subsequent and indirectly related transformations in business.

Integration with Workflow and Healthcare Processes

A successful CPOE implementation needs to account for and become part of existing workflow and processes. This need cannot be underestimated. Failure to integrate with existing processes has lead to significant difficulty and user dissatisfaction.[47,70,57,10,126,127,41,128]

CPOE doesn't just integrate with, but also significantly transforms, workflow and processes.[76] An example of transformation involves medical students. With paper ordering, there are shades of grey where medical students write orders for things like Tylenol, even though they are not officially licensed. On paper, medical students are undefined physician helpers. With CPOE, medical students may have to go through a cumbersome process of placing orders into suspension and awaiting co-signature. This new process becomes a significant barrier to education.[129] In CPOE, medical students are considered unlicensed physicians.

The key to ensuring integration with existing workflow and processes, as well as anticipating transformation, starts with fully mapping out existing workflow and then designing the future state.[126,127,130,131,132] This mapping needs to occur before implementation. Once implementation has occurred, these future workflows need to be compared to the new present state. This comparison can be used to identify new opportunities for integration and transformation.

Value to Users

User satisfaction is an important predictor of a system's success.[133] One of the biggest barriers to implementation of CPOE systems has been user dissatisfaction with CPOE, primarily physicians.[128,134,135,42,43,44,45,46,47]

Two rather infamous examples either stopped or nearly stopped a CPOE implementation.[42,43,44,45,46] It is beyond the scope of this chapter to analyze all the possible user-centered factors like age, computer proficiency, gender, etc., that may contribute to perceived value and satisfaction.[116] The bottom line is physicians are looking for systems that are easy to use, improve daily efficiency and provide perceived improvements in patient care.[116] Consistent with this bottom line is that user satisfaction seems to correlate with the ability to perform tasks efficiently.[102]

There is no commonly and consistently used scoring system for user satisfaction in regards to CPOE, though most users express more negative than positive emotions.[136] Physician satisfaction varies by CPOE system, and even with the same version of the same CPOE system. In a study by Murff et al, user satisfaction with the same user population was significantly higher (7.21 out of 10) with the Veteran Administration's CPOE system (CPRS at the time) versus (3.67 out of 10) with a commercial CPOE system.

Users need to be involved in the CPOE project as early as possible. Careful involvement of users during selection and implementation is critical and can be the difference between failure and success.[137,48,138,75,122,137] The inevitable and sometimes neglected question arises: Which population of physician users should be engaged?

As noted earlier, 76% of orders are written by housestaff at an academic medical center.[102] Capturing the attention and interest of housestaff is tricky from this author's experience and takes careful planning.[10]

Housestaff are very busy taking care of patients, as well as fulfilling education requirements. There is a need to identify housestaff both with system (i.e., healthcare system) and clinical experience, but who will still be around for the implementation. The ideal housestaff participant should know patient care and his/her needs better than the technology. One must avoid self selection in which housestaff are more interested in the technology and computers than patient care. They are frequently seen by their colleagues as the "technical gurus."

Engaging the housestaff in selection and implementation is fraught with one more difficulty—institutional interest and support. While they are performing the bulk of the work and the orders, housestaff are viewed as a captive and transient audience.[42]

In comparison, vocal attending physicians who account for a significant number of admissions are easier to identify.

In contrast, a community hospital has a smaller housestaff population. The focus may need to be more on the attending physicians, and the nurse practitioners and physician assistants who work for them.

Finally, it must be emphasized that physicians are not the only users of order entry as mentioned above. Nursing attitudes towards order entry are significantly different and their needs must be addressed as well.[95,97]

Development and Maintenance of CDSS

The requirements for developing and maintaining CDSS were discussed in a previous section. However, it worth emphasizing that CDSS development, implementation and maintenance takes a great deal of effort and thought. It is also worth repeating that this effort is not solely the province of IT and requires active involvement of physicians, nurses and quality improvement experts, to name a few.[63,64,65,66,67,68,69,94] If development and maintenance are done improperly, CDSS functionality could be undermined. CDSS provides some of the perceived quality and efficiency physicians look for by helping physicians with "their" patient.[97]

Project Management and Staging of Implementation

It is beyond the scope of this chapter to review project management as project management is a discipline in its own right.[139] Project management is critical to the success of the project, or for that matter any project involving significant sums of money and thousands of users. It is also beyond the scope of this chapter to contrast the different implementation approaches such as big bang, phased or unit by unit except to say there are examples of successful implementations using each of the approaches. Which approach works where depends on leadership, culture, and IT and non-IT personnel as well as whether or not there is a pre-existing CPOE system that will be replaced.

Training and Support

There is universal agreement on training as prerequisite for a successful implementation of CPOE.[48,70,75,57]

There is little difference of opinion on the need for 24/7 training, especially during the "go live" of CPOE and for ongoing support. The problem is in making the budget case for training as a sufficiently funded and resourced activity. Some oft heard urban legends to address insufficient funding and resources include: (1) "Everyone uses a computer today so there is a little need for training;" (2) "Train the trainers. Users should train each other;" (3) "The users will never sit still with training;" and, (4) "We can't lose valuable space to set up a training room." Every study suggests training is a crucial piece of the implementation process that can make or break the project. Poor training can result in inappropriate or under utilization of functionality.[119,140]

During Mount Sinai's selection process, we made sure that training was a clearly funded, properly resourced part of our budget and part of our total cost of ownership.[10] Evanston's Davies Award-winning implementation spent millions on training and adequate space to conduct it.[119]

Another frequently neglected area is post-implementation training. Previously, we discussed the value of reassessing the system post-implementation in processes such as Optimization. Post-implementation training processes are also necessary for success. Users forget lessons learned in training, are confused while using the system, want to learn more or receive advanced training and need to learn about new features added to the system. The concepts of yearly training assessments—along with need for further training, just in time training, refresher training and shadow trainers—have been used by some sites to great success.[141,142,119] However, these post-implementation approaches are not routinely part of most training plans because of funding, space and resource requirements.

Technology

Ash defines technology as access by role, functionality at user and system levels, remote access, integration with other systems, response time and assessment of user interface.[143] Access by role is complicated by the different roles one physician may have with different patients. A physician may be a patient's primary care provider, consultant, second opinion or covering physician. Remote access is always a desired and important feature of CPOE as physicians receive calls off site in an office or at home, and need to be able to write orders for hospital patients in both of these locations. Integration with other systems is critical because the absence of integration creates a fragmented record,[142] and medical errors, as in the case of pharmacy systems.[2,61,74,75,76] Response time and assessment of user interface and functionality would benefit from formal usability assessments in addition to the user feedback traditionally received by IT.[144,145] At least two studies suggest that usability and user interface can contribute to medical errors in CPOE systems and their CDSS components.[61,84,146]

Finally, the newest technology should not be seen immediately as the cure for under-utilization or implementation difficulties. For example, the World Wide Web was seen as the solution to the poor diffusion of EMRs. Less than a decade ago, a frequent refrain would be "the EMR is Web-based. It will require no training at all." If one looks at two exhaustive reports on the computerized patient record as snapshots, each report predicted that new technologies such as networks, personal computers, the Internet and laptops would have allowed for significantly increased use and penetration of EMRs, but this did not occur either in or after 1991 or 1997, the publication dates of each report.[147,148] Each of the technologies mentioned in the report eventually played a specific role in solving a problem. For example, the World Wide Web provided a consistent user interface and means of remote and secure access. But at the same time, it did not solve the underlying problems of usability and integration with complex workflow.

The method of inputting the data (e.g., keyboard, voice or mouse driven) has nothing to do with the requirements for data entry. The decision to have data entered as structured discrete data is driven by regulatory, research and performance improvement requirements. Voice recognition of late is being seen as the solution to every problem with data entry, including facilitation of the entry of structured data. Voice recognition will not necessarily make it any easier to enter and complete sections requiring structured data.[149,150]

Leaning Evaluation Improvement

As discussed previously, without post-implementation processes in place to assess software quality, users may be dissatisfied but otherwise silent. In such a setting, it is very possible that errors due to CPOE will either not be detected or fixed before a catastrophic event occurs.

QUESTION #9
What's a CQIO to do?

CPOE with Clinical Decision Support can improve patient safety by reducing medication errors and correspondingly adverse drug events. However, these improvements cannot make a compelling financial case and/or ROI. The argument must center on ROV (Return on Value) or what's best for the patient. Even if a CPOE with CDSS is purchased, implementing a CPOE system with CDSS is not a panacea for improving all patient safety issues related to the integrated medication process (see Figure 2-11). CPOE with CDSS addresses medication errors due to physician ordering that accounts for slightly more than half of the integrated medication process. There are parts of the integrated medication process such as medication administration that would benefit from other solutions such as bar coding. These solutions may complement CPOE, but can offer value independent of CPOE. Some patient safety issues either cannot be addressed through CPOE or would be better served by reengineering workflow and process while planning for CPOE strategically.

Implementation of CPOE is not an easy undertaking and requires unwavering support from senior and clinical leadership, careful study and understanding of workflow, the ability to develop and maintain a knowledge base of rules for CDSS and post-implementation quality improvement process. Without these requirements for successful implementation, CPOE can be both a Pandora's Box of patient safety errors and a panacea for the ills of errors.

REFERENCES

1.   Brennan TA, Leape LL, Laird NM, Hebert L, Localio AR, Lawthers AG, et al. Incidence of adverse events and negligence in hospitalized patients. Results of the Harvard Medical Practice Study I. *N Engl J Med* 1991;324(6):370–6.

2. Bates DW, Leape LL, Cullen DJ, Laird N, Petersen LA, Teich JM, et al. Effect of computerized physician order entry and a team intervention on prevention of serious medication errors [see comments]. *JAMA* 1998;280(15):1311–6.

3. McDonald CJ, Weiner M, Hui SL. Deaths due to medical errors are exaggerated in Institute of Medicine report. *JAMA* 2000;284(1):93–5.

4. McDonald CJ, Weiner M, Hui SL. How many deaths are due to medical errors? *JAMA* 2000;284(17):2187.

5. Weaver CA, Warren JJ, Delaney C. Bedside, classroom and bench: Collaborative strategies to generate evidence-based knowledge for nursing practice. *Int J Med Inform* 2005.

6. Horton B. From bench to bedside... research makes the translational transition. *Nature* 1999;402(6758):213–5.

7. Marincola FM. Translational Medicine: A two-way road. *J Transl Med* 2003;1(1):1.

8. Greenes RA, Shortliffe EH. Medical Informatics: An Emerging Academic Discipline and Institutional Policy. *JAMA* 1990;263.

9. Shortliffe EH. *Medical informatics : Computer Applications in Health Care and Biomedicine.* 2nd ed. New York: Springer; 2001.

10. Kannry J, Mukani S, Myers K. Using an Evidence Based Approach for System Selection at Large Academic Medical Center: Lessons Learned in Selecting an Ambulatory EMR at Mount Sinai Hospital. *Journal Of Health Information Management* 2006;20(2):84–99.

11. Glaser JP. Facilitating applied information technology research. *J Healthc Inf Manag* 2005;19(1): 45–53.

12. Murray MD, Smith FE, Fox J, Teal EY, Kesterson JG, Stiffler TA, et al. Structure, functions, and activities of a research support informatics section. *J Am Med Inform Assoc* 2003;10(4):389–98.

13. Fischer S, Stewart TE, Mehta S, Wax R, Lapinsky SE. Handheld computing in medicine. *J Am Med Inform Assoc* 2003;10(2):139–49.

14. Rothschild JM, Lee TH, Bae T, Bates DW. Clinician use of a palmtop drug reference guide. *J Am Med Inform Assoc* 2002;9(3):223–9.

15. Breslow MJ. ICU telemedicine. Organization and communication. *Crit Care Clin* 2000;16(4):707–22, x–xi.

16. Breslow MJ, Rosenfeld BA, Doerfler M, Burke G, Yates G, Stone DJ, et al. Effect of a multiple-site intensive care unit telemedicine program on clinical and economic outcomes: an alternative paradigm for intensivist staffing. *Crit Care Med* 2004;32(1):31–8.

17. Bria WF, 2nd, Shabot MM. The electronic medical record, safety, and critical care. *Crit Care Clin* 2005;21(1):55–79, viii.

18. Gingrich N, Pavey D, Woodbury A. Saving lives & saving money : transforming health and healthcare. Washington, DC: The Alexis de Tocqueville Institution; 2003.

19. McKeown K, Jordan D, Feiner S, Shaw J, Chen E, Ahmad S, et al. A study of communication in the Cardiac Surgery Intensive Care Unit and its implications for automated briefing. *Proc AMIA Symp* 2000:570–4.

20. Wilson K, Sullivan M. Preventing medication errors with smart infusion technology. *Am J Health Syst Pharm* 2004;61(2):177–83.

21. Wright AA, Katz I.T.. Bar coding for patient safety. *N Engl J Med* 2005;353(4):329–31.

22. Bates DW, Gawande AA. Improving safety with information technology. *N Engl J Med* 2003;348(25):2526–34.

23. Osheroff JA, Forsythe DE, Buchanan BG, Bankowitz RA, Blumenfeld BH, Miller RA. Physicians' information needs: analysis of questions posed during clinical teaching. *Ann Intern Med* 1991;114(7):576–81.

24. Covell DG, Uman GC, Manning PR. Information needs in office practice: are they being met? *Ann Intern Med* 1985;103(4):596–9.

25. Rothschild JM, Fang E, Gottschall J, Liu V, Bates DW. Use and perceived benefits of handheld PDA clinical reference applications. *AMIA Annu Symp Proc* 2005:1099.

26. Rothschild JM, Fang E, Liu V, Litvak I, Yoon C, Bates DW. Use and Perceived Benefits of Handheld Computer-Based Clinical References. *J Am Med Inform Assoc* 2006.

27. Milstein A, Galvin RS, Delbanco SF, Salber P, Buck CR, Jr. Improving the safety of health care: the leapfrog initiative. *Eff Clin Pract* 2000;3(6):313–6.

28. Puckett F. Medication-management component of a point-of-care information system. *Am J Health Syst Pharm* 1995;52(12):1305–9.

29. McDonald CJ. Computerization can create safety hazards: a bar-coding near miss. *Ann Intern Med* 2006;144(7):510–6.

30. Patterson ES, Cook RI, Render ML. Improving patient safety by identifying side effects from introducing bar coding in medication administration. *J Am Med Inform Assoc* 2002;9(5):540–53.

31. Oren E, Shaffer ER, Guglielmo BJ. Impact of emerging technologies on medication errors and adverse drug events. *Am J Health Syst Pharm* 2003;60(14):1447–58.

32. Leape LL, Brennan TA, Laird N, Lawthers AG, Localio AR, Barnes BA, et al. The nature of adverse events in hospitalized patients. Results of the Harvard Medical Practice Study II. *N Engl J Med* 1991;324(6):377–84.

33. Bates DW, Teich JM, Lee J, Seger D, Kuperman GJ, Ma'Luf N, et al. The impact of computerized physician order entry on medication error prevention. *J Am Med Inform Assoc* 1999;6(4):313–21.

34. Bates DW, Cullen DJ, Laird N, Petersen LA, Small SD, Servi D, et al. Incidence of adverse drug events and potential adverse drug events. Implications for prevention. ADE Prevention Study Group. *JAMA* 1995;274(1):29–34.

35. Bates DW, Spell N, Cullen DJ, Burdick E, Laird N, Petersen LA, et al. The costs of adverse drug events in hospitalized patients. Adverse Drug Events Prevention Study Group. *JAMA* 1997;277(4):307–11.

36. Classen DC, Pestotnik SL, Evans RS, Lloyd JF, Burke JP. Adverse drug events in hospitalized patients. Excess length of stay, extra costs, and attributable mortality. *JAMA* 1997;277(4):301–6.

37. Evans RS, Pestotnik SL, Classen DC, Bass SB, Burke JP. Prevention of adverse drug events through computerized surveillance. *Proc Annu Symp Comput Appl Med Care* 1992:437–41.

38. Bemmel JHv, Musen MA, Helder JC. *Handbook of Medical Informatics.* AW Houten, Netherlands. Heidelberg, Germany: Bohn Stafleu Van Loghum ; Springer Verlag; 1997.

39. Handler T FCG Clinical Strategy Discussion at Stonybrook University Medical Center, March 27, 2001.

40. Neilson EG, Johnson KB, Rosenbloom ST, Dupont WD, Talbert D, Giuse DA, et al. The impact of peer management on test-ordering behavior. *Ann Intern Med* 2004;141(3):196–204.

41. Kuperman GJ, Teich JM, Gandhi TK, Bates DW. Patient safety and computerized medication ordering at Brigham and Women's Hospital. *Jt Comm J Qual Improv* 2001;27(10):509–21.

42. Massaro TA. Introducing physician order entry at a major academic medical center: II. Impact on medical education. *Acad Med* 1993;68(1):25–30.

43. Massaro TA. Introducing physician order entry at a major academic medical center: I. Impact on organizational culture and behavior. *Acad Med* 1993;68(1):20–5.

44. Langberg M. Challenges to implementing CPOE: a case study of a work in progress at Cedars-Sinai. *Modern Physician* 2003;7(2):21–22.

45. Cedars-Sinai suspends CPOE use. *ihealthbeat* 2003. Available at http://www.ihealthbeat.org/index.cfm?Action=dspItem&itemID=98901. Accessed on March 10, 2003.

46. Cedars-Sinai Has No Plans to Restart CPOE Program. *ihealthbeat* 2004. Available at http://www.ihealthbeat.org/index.cfm?Action=dspItem&itemID=100658. Accessed on March 10, 2004.

47. Ash JS, Gorman PN, Hersh WR, Lavelle M, Poulsen SB. Perceptions of house officers who use physician order entry. *Proc AMIA Symp* 1999:471–5.

48. Sittig DF, Stead WW. Computer-based physician order entry: the state of the art. *J Am Med Inform Assoc* 1994;1(2):108–23.

49. Slack WV, Bleich HL. The CCC system in two teaching hospitals: a progress report. *Int J Med Inf* 1999;54(3):183–96.

50. Gardner RM, Pryor TA, Warner HR. The HELP hospital information system: update 1998. *Int J Med Inf* 1999;54(3):169–82.

51. Teich JM, Glaser JP, Beckley RF, Aranow M, Bates DW, Kuperman GJ, et al. The Brigham integrated computing system (BICS): advanced clinical systems in an academic hospital environment. *Int J Med Inf* 1999;54(3):197–208.

52. Kuperman GJ, Hiltz FL, Teich JM. Advanced alerting features: displaying new relevant data and retracting alerts. *Proc AMIA Annu Fall Symp* 1997:243–7.

53. Miller RA, Waitman LR, Chen S, Rosenbloom ST. The anatomy of decision support during inpatient care provider order entry (CPOE): empirical observations from a decade of CPOE experience at Vanderbilt. *J Biomed Inform* 2005;38(6):469–85.

54. Randolph AG, Haynes RB, Wyatt JC, Cook DJ, Guyatt GH. Users' Guides to the Medical Literature: XVIII. How to use an article evaluating the clinical impact of a computer-based clinical decision support system. *JAMA* 1999;282(1):67–74.

55. Hunt DL, Haynes RB, Hanna SE, Smith K. Effects of computer-based clinical decision support systems on physician performance and patient outcomes: a systematic review [see comments]. *JAMA* 1998;280(15):1339–46.

56. Chaudhry B, Wang J, Wu S, Maglione M, Mojica W, Roth E, et al. Systematic Review: Impact of Health Information Technology on Quality, Efficiency, and Costs of Medical Care. *Ann Intern Med* 2006:0000605-200605160-00125.

57. Kuperman GJ, Gibson RF. Computer physician order entry: benefits, costs, and issues. *Ann Intern Med* 2003;139(1):31–9.

58. Morgan MW. The VA advantage: the gold standard in clinical informatics. *Healthc Pap* 2005;5(4):26–9.

59. Brown SH, Lincoln MJ, Groen PJ, Kolodner RM. VistA—U.S. Department of Veterans Affairs national-scale HIS. *Int J Med Inform* 2003;69(2-3):135–56.

60. Lloyd SS. Automated information systems provide health information management support to veterans' healthcare. *JAHIMA* 1992;63(6):63–7.

61. Koppel R, Metlay JP, Cohen A, Abaluck B, Localio AR, Kimmel SE, et al. Role of computerized physician order entry systems in facilitating medication errors. *JAMA* 2005;293(10):1197–203.

62. Nebeker JR, Hoffman JM, Weir CR, Bennett CL, Hurdle JF. High rates of adverse drug events in a highly computerized hospital. *Arch Intern Med* 2005;165(10):1111–6.

63. Geissbuhler A, Miller RA. Distributing knowledge maintenance for clinical decision-support systems: the "knowledge library" model. *Proc AMIA Symp* 1999:770–4.

64. Hripcsak G, Johnson SB, Clayton PD. Desperately seeking data: knowledge base-database links. *Proc Annu Symp Comput Appl Med Care* 1993:639–43.

65. Ash JS, Stavri PZ, Kuperman GJ. A consensus statement on considerations for a successful CPOE implementation. *J Am Med Inform Assoc* 2003;10(3):229–34.

66. Goldstein MK, Coleman RW, Tu SW, Shankar RD, O'Connor MJ, Musen MA, et al. Translating research into practice: organizational issues in implementing automated decision support for hypertension in three medical centers. *J Am Med Inform Assoc* 2004;11(5):368–76.

67. Denekamp Y, Boxwala AA, Kuperman G, Middelton B, Greenes RA. A meta-data model for knowledge in decision support systems. *AMIA Annu Symp Proc* 2003:826.

68. Jenders RA, Dasgupta B. Challenges in implementing a knowledge editor for the Arden Syntax: knowledge base maintenance and standardization of database linkages. *Proc AMIA Symp* 2002: 355–9.

69. Jenders RA, Hripcsak G, Sideli RV, DuMouchel W, Zhang H, Cimino JJ, et al. Medical decision support: experience with implementing the Arden Syntax at the Columbia-Presbyterian Medical Center. *Proc Annu Symp Comput Appl Med Care* 1995:169–73.

70. Overhage JM, Middleton B, Miller RA, Zielstorff RD, Hersh WR. Does national regulatory mandate of provider order entry portend greater benefit than risk for health care delivery? The 2001 ACMI debate. The American College of Medical Informatics. *J Am Med Inform Assoc* 2002;9(3):199–208.

71. Ash JS, Gorman PN, Seshadri V, Hersh WR. Computerized physician order entry in U.S. hospitals: results of a 2002 survey. *J Am Med Inform Assoc* 2004;11(2):95–9.

72. Ash JS, Gorman PN, Hersh WR. Physician order entry in U.S. hospitals. *Proc AMIA Symp* 1998: 235–9.

73. Lowy I, Kesicier A, Conte U, Mehl B, Karson T, Kannry J. IV-to-Oral Antibiotic Conversion Using a Computerized Order Entry System: Rationale, Progress and Lessons Learned. In: Bakken S, editor. *Proc AMIA Symp* 2001;Washington, DC; 2001.

74. Lehman ML, Brill JH, Skarulis PC, Keller D, Lee C. Physician Order Entry impact on drug turn-around times. *Proc AMIA Symp* 2001:359–63.

75. Wu RC, Abrams H, Baker M, Rossos PG. Implementation of a computerized physician order entry system of medications at the University Health Network—physicians' perspectives on the critical issues. *Healthc Q* 2006;9(1):106–9.

76. Sittig DF, Ash JS, Zhang J, Osheroff JA, Shabot MM. Lessons From "Unexpected Increased Mortality After Implementation of a Commercially Sold Computerized Physician Order Entry System". *Pediatrics* 2006;118(2):797–801.

77. Tierney WM, Miller ME, Overhage JM, McDonald CJ. Physician inpatient order writing on microcomputer workstations. Effects on resource utilization. *JAMA* 1993;269(3):379–83.

78. Kuperman GJ, Teich JM, Tanasijevic MJ, Ma'Luf N, Rittenberg E, Jha A, et al. Improving response to critical laboratory results with automation: results of a randomized controlled trial. *J Am Med Inform Assoc* 1999;6(6):512–22.

79. Connelly DP, Rich EC, Curley SP, Kelly JT. Knowledge resource preferences of family physicians. *J Fam Pract* 1990;30(3):353–9.

80. Gilad J. Kuperman, Sittig DF, Shabot MM. Clinical Decision Support for Hospital and Critical Care. *Journal of Healthcare Information Management* 1999;13(2):81–96.

81. Broverman CA. Standards for Clinical Decision Support Systems. *Journal of Healthcare Information Management* 1999; 13(2):23–31.

82. Bates DW, Kuperman GJ, Wang S, Gandhi T, Kittler A, Volk L, et al. Ten commandments for effective clinical decision support: making the practice of evidence-based medicine a reality. *J Am Med Inform Assoc* 2003;10(6):523–30.

83. Hsieh TC, Kuperman GJ, Jaggi T, Hojnowski-Diaz P, Fiskio J, Williams DH, et al. Characteristics and consequences of drug allergy alert overrides in a computerized physician order entry system. *J Am Med Inform Assoc* 2004;11(6):482–91.

84. van der Sijs H, Aarts J, Vulto A, Berg M. Overriding of Drug Safety Alerts in Computerized Physician Order Entry.

85. Dexter PR, Perkins S, Overhage JM, Maharry K, Kohler RB, McDonald CJ. A computerized reminder system to increase the use of preventive care for hospitalized patients. *N Engl J Med* 2001;345(13):965–70.

86. Overhage JM, Tierney WM, McDonald CJ. Computer reminders to implement preventive care guidelines for hospitalized patients. *Arch Intern Med* 1996;156(14):1551–6.

87. Potts AL, Barr FE, Gregory DF, Wright L, Patel NR. Computerized physician order entry and medication errors in a pediatric critical care unit. *Pediatrics* 2004;113(1 Pt 1):59–63.

88. Overhage JM, Tierney WM, Zhou XH, McDonald CJ. A randomized trial of "corollary orders" to prevent errors of omission. *J Am Med Inform Assoc* 1997;4(5):364–75.

89. Pestotnik SL, Classen DC, Evans RS, Burke JP. Implementing antibiotic practice guidelines through computer-assisted decision support: clinical and financial outcomes. *Ann Intern Med* 1996;124(10):884–90.

90. Advisory Board Company. *Reducing Adverse Drug Events: Best Practices in Reporting and Prescribing.* Washington, DC: Advisory Board Company: Clinical Initiatives Center; 2000.

91. Bates DW. Frequency, consequences and prevention of adverse drug events. *J Qual Clin Pract* 1999;19(1):13–7.

92. First Consulting Group. *Computerized Physician Order Entry: Costs, Benefits, and Challenges—A Case Study Approach.* Long Beach, CA; 2003 January 2003.

93. Kuperman GJ, Cooley T, Tremblay J, Teich JM, Churchill W. Decision support for medication use in an inpatient physician order entry application and a pharmacy application. *Medinfo* 1998;9 (Pt 1):467–71.

94. Kaushal R, Jha AK, Franz C, Glaser J, Shetty KD, Jaggi T, et al. Return on Investment for a Computerized Physician Order Entry System 10.1197. *J Am Med Inform Assoc* 2006:M1984.

95. Lee F, Teich JM, Spurr CD, Bates DW. Implementation of physician order entry: user satisfaction and self-reported usage patterns. *J Am Med Inform Assoc* 1996;3(1):42–55.

96. Weir C, Johnsen V, Roscoe D, Cribbs A. The impact of physician order entry on nursing roles. *Proc AMIA Annu Fall Symp* 1996:714–7.

97. Weiner M, Gress T, Thiemann DR, Jenckes M, Reel SL, Mandell SF, et al. Contrasting views of physicians and nurses about an inpatient computer-based provider order-entry system. *J Am Med Inform Assoc* 1999;6(3):234–44.

98. Thomas SM, Davis DC. The characteristics of personal order sets in a computerized physician order entry system at a community hospital. *AMIA Annu Symp Proc* 2003:1031.

99. Shu K, Boyle D, Spurr C, Horsky J, Heiman H, O'Connor P, et al. Comparison of time spent writing orders on paper with computerized physician order entry. *Medinfo* 2001;10(Pt 2):1207–11.

100. Bates DW, Boyle DL, Teich JM. Impact of computerized physician order entry on physician time. *Proc Annu Symp Comput Appl Med Care* 1994:996.

101. Bates DW, Kuperman G, Teich JM. Computerized physician order entry and quality of care. *Qual Manag Health Care* 1994;2(4):18–27.

102. Murff HJ, Kannry J. Physician satisfaction with two order entry systems. *J Am Med Inform Assoc* 2001;8(5):499–509.

103. Horsky J, Kuperman GJ, Patel VL. Comprehensive analysis of a medication dosing error related to CPOE. *J Am Med Inform Assoc* 2005;12(4):377–82.

104. Han YY, Carcillo JA, Venkataraman ST, Clark RS, Watson RS, Nguyen TC, et al. Unexpected increased mortality after implementation of a commercially sold computerized physician order entry system. *Pediatrics* 2005;116(6):1506–12.

105. Safran C, Detmer DE. Computerized physician order entry systems and medication errors. *JAMA* 2005;294(2):179; author reply 180–1.

106. Hegedus SM. Computerized physician order entry systems and medication errors. *JAMA* 2005;294(2):179; author reply 180–1.

107. Levick D, Lukens H. Computerized physician order entry systems and medication errors. *JAMA* 2005;294(2):179–80; author reply 180–1.

108. Bierstock S, Kanig SP, Marcus E. Computerized physician order entry systems and medication errors. *JAMA* 2005;294(2):178–9; author reply 180–1.

109. Wears RL, Berg M. Computer technology and clinical work: still waiting for Godot. *JAMA* 2005;293(10):1261–3.

110. Duke University Hospital uses rapid deployment to implement CPOE, clinical decision support. *Perform Improv Advis* 2005;9(4):44–6, 37.

111. Abookire SA, Teich JM, Bates DW. An institution-based process to ensure clinical software quality. *Proc AMIA Symp* 1999:461–5.

112. Abookire S, Martin M, Teich J, Kuperman G, Bates D. *Analysis of User-Feedback as a Tool for Improving Software Quality.* In: Overhage JM, editor. 2000 American Medical Informatics Association Annual Fall Symposium; 2000; Los Angeles, Ca: Hanley & Belfus, Inc; 2000.

113. Cosgriff PS. Quality assurance of medical software. *J Med Eng Technol* 1994;18(1):1–10.

114. Miller RA, Gardner RM. Recommendations for responsible monitoring and regulation of clinical software systems. American Medical Informatics Association, Computer-based Patient Record Institute, Medical Library Association, Association of Academic Health Science Libraries, American Health Information Management Association, American Nurses Association. J Am Med Inform Assoc 1997;4(6):442–57.

115. McDaniel JG. Improving system quality through software evaluation. *Comput Biol Med* 2002;32(3):127–40.

116. O'Connell RT, Cho C, Shah N, Brown K, Shiffman RN. Take note(s): differential EHR satisfaction with two implementations under one roof. *J Am Med Inform Assoc* 2004;11(1):43–9.

117. Ash JS, Stavri PZ, Dykstra R, Fournier L. Implementing computerized physician order entry: the importance of special people. *Int J Med Inform* 2003;69(2-3):235–50.

118. Treister NW. Physician acceptance of new medical information systems: the field of dreams. *Physician Exec* 1998;24(3):20–4.

119. HIMSS. Transforming Healthcare with a Patient-Centric Electronic Health Record. Available at http://www.himss.org/content/files/davies2004_evanston.pdf. Accessed on April 16, 2006.

120. HIMSS. Nicholas E. Davies Awards of Excellence. HIMSS 2006. Available at http://www.himss.org/asp/daviesAward.asp. Accessed on April 16, 2006.

121. AHIMA and AMIA. Building the Work Force for Health Information Transformation; 2006.

122. McDowell SW, Wahl R, Michelson J. Herding cats: the challenges of EMR vendor selection. *J Healthc Inf Manag* 2003;17(3):63–71.

123. Quinn J Vendor Perspectives: Critical Do's and Dont's in: Spring AMIA 2004 2004. McClean, Va. April 28–29, 2004.

124. Bauer JC. Return on investment: going beyond traditional analysis. *J Healthc Inf Manag* 2003;17(4): 4–5.

125. Frisse ME. Comments on Return on Investment (ROI) as it applies to clinical systems 121.10.1197/jamia.M2072. *J Am Med Inform Assoc* 2006:M2072.

126. Teich JM, Spurr CD, Schmiz JL, O'Connell EM, Thomas D. Enhancement of clinician workflow with computer order entry. *Proc Annu Symp Comput Appl Med Care* 1995:459–63.

127. Ali NA, Mekhjian HS, Kuehn PL, Bentley TD, Kumar R, Ferketich AK, et al. Specificity of computerized physician order entry has a significant effect on the efficiency of workflow for critically ill patients. *Crit Care Med* 2005;33(1):110–4.

128. Mekhjian HS, Kumar RR, Kuehn L, Bentley TD, Teater P, Thomas A, et al. Immediate benefits realized following implementation of physician order entry at an academic medical center. *J Am Med Inform Assoc* 2002;9(5):529–39.

129. Knight AM, Kravet SJ, Harper GM, Leff B. The effect of computerized provider order entry on medical student clerkship experiences. *J Am Med Inform Assoc* 2005;12(5):554–60.

130. Payne TH. The transition to automated practitioner order entry in a teaching hospital: the VA Puget Sound experience. *Proc AMIA Symp* 1999:589–93.

131. Stablein D, Welebob E, Johnson E, Metzger J, Burgess R, Classen DC. Understanding hospital readiness for computerized physician order entry. *Jt Comm J Qual Saf* 2003;29(7):336–44.

132. Caudill-Slosberg M, Weeks WB. Case study: identifying potential problems at the human/technical interface in complex clinical systems. *Am J Med Qual* 2005;20(6):353–7.

133. Bailey JE. Development of an instrument for the management of computer user attitudes in hospitals. *Methods Inf Med* 1990;29(1):51–6.

134. Poon EG, Blumenthal D, Jaggi T, Honour MM, Bates DW, Kaushal R. Overcoming barriers to adopting and implementing computerized physician order entry systems in U.S. hospitals. *Health Aff (Millwood)* 2004;23(4):184–90.

135. Lawler F, Cacy JR, Viviani N, Hamm RM, Cobb SW. Implementation and termination of a computerized medical information system. *J Fam Pract* 1996;42(3):233–6.

136. Sittig DF, Krall M, Kaalaas-Sittig J, Ash JS. Emotional Aspects of Computer-based Provider Order Entry: A Qualitative Study. *J Am Med Inform Assoc* 2005.

137. Ahmad A, Teater P, Bentley TD, Kuehn L, Kumar RR, Thomas A, et al. Key attributes of a successful physician order entry system implementation in a multi-hospital environment. *J Am Med Inform Assoc* 2002;9(1):16–24.

138. Gray MD, Felkey BG. Computerized prescriber order-entry systems: evaluation, selection, and implementation. *Am J Health Syst Pharm* 2004;61(2):190–7.

139. PMI Standards Committee., Project Management Institute. *A Guide to the Project Management Body of Knowledge.* Upper Darby, PA: Project Management Institute; 1996.

140. Schectman JM, Schorling JB, Nadkarni MM, Voss JD. Determinants of physician use of an ambulatory prescription expert system. *Int J Med Inform* 2005;74(9):711–7.

141. Chin H. The Reality of EMR Implementation: Lessons from the Field. *The Permanente Journal 2004;8(4):43–48.*

142. Walker JM, Bieber EJ, Richards F. *Implementing an Electronic Health Record System.* London: Springer; 2005.

143. Ash JS, Bates DW. Factors and forces affecting EHR system adoption: report of a 2004 ACMI discussion. *J Am Med Inform Assoc* 2005;12(1):8–12.

144. Kushniruk AW, Kaufman DR, Patel VL, Levesque Y, Lottin P. Assessment of a computerized patient record system: a cognitive approach to evaluating medical technology. *MD Comput* 1996;13(5):406–15.

145. Patel VL, Bates DW. Cognition and measurement in patient safety research. *Journal of Biomedical Informatics* 2003;36(1-2):1–3.

146. Horsky J, Kuperman GJ, Patel VL. Comprehensive analysis of a medication dosing error related to CPOE. *J Am Med Inform Assoc* 2005;12(4):377–82.

147. Institute of Medicine (U.S.). Committee on Improving the Patient Record., Dick RS, Steen EB. *The Computer-Based Patient Record: An Essential Technology for Health Care.* Washington, D.C.: National Academy Press; 1991.

148. Institute of Medicine (U.S.). Committee on Improving the Patient Record., Dick RS, Steen EB, Detmer DE. *The Computer-Based Patient Record: An Essential Technology for Health Care.* Rev. ed. Washington, D.C.: National Academy Press; 1997.

149. Wormek AK, Ingenerf J, Orthner HF. SAM: speech-aware applications in medicine to support structured data entry. *Proc AMIA Annu Fall Symp* 1997:774–8.

150. Zafar A, Overhage JM, McDonald CJ. Continuous speech recognition for clinicians. *J Am Med Inform Assoc* 1999;6(3):195–204.

CHAPTER 3

Identity Management in Healthcare

Jonathan Leviss, MD

IDENTITY MANAGEMENT STORIES[1]

Case #1

A new physician at a hospital rounds on patients covered by her practice. While she has admitting privileges at the hospital, she has not yet received her access to the clinical information system. In order to review patients' lab results and order medications in the hospital information systems, she uses the username and password of one of the other physicians in her group.

Case #2

An information systems analyst saves to a memory stick several files of patient information from the hospital financial reporting system to work from home that evening. Her car is broken into and the memory stick is stolen, along with other personal items. The local newspaper reports the story, stating that up to 50,000 patients are now at risk for identity theft.

Case #3

A clothing store sales clerk who takes medications for Post-Traumatic Stress Disorder falls from a ladder and is taken by ambulance to the local emergency room for treatment of a compound fracture. On day #2 of hospitalization, the patient becomes irritable, then inappropriate, then uncontrollable, requiring medical sedation and transfer to the ICU. While the patient's medical record is accessible through the health system's electronic medical record, his psychiatric record is restricted and the clinical care team is unaware that he is withdrawing from a prescribed medication.

Case #4

A clinical case is presented to a group of medical students, housestaff, and faculty at a teaching hospital. After the conference, the patient's family is alarmed at the amount of personal information that was included in the academic case discussion and files a formal complaint with the hospital.

Case #5

Two hospitals that serve the same community have implemented a data interchange capability to share information about patients. At one hospital the caregivers are required to use fingerprint biometric scanners in order to sign on to the clinical information system and at the other using passwords. A particular patient's data can be accessed by caregivers at both institutions in spite of the different authentication processes.

Case #6

A leading health system initiates a project to evaluate emergency medicine physicians according to quality indicators for management of community acquired pneumonia. Because all medication orders are entered by physicians using a computerized practitioner order entry system (CPOE), the CPOE records are used to compare antibiotic selection and timing of orders with recommended guidelines.

Questions to Consider

- Which of these identity management cases are important to clinical care?
- Which of these cases are governed by regulations about patient confidentiality and the security of patient data?
- Which are important to your patients' desire for privacy of health data?
- Which of these identity management cases would provoke public concern and loss of confidence in your health system's ability to serve a community?
- What is *identity management*?

While the legal and ethical principles may not change, the risks to confidentiality and security of patient records appear to differ between paper- and computer-based records. Breaches of system security, the potential for faulty performance that may result in inaccessibility or loss of records, the increased technical ability to collect, store, and retrieve large quantities of data, and the ability to access records from multiple and (sometimes) remote locations are among the risk factors unique to computer-based record systems. Managing these risks will require a combination of reliable technological measures, appropriate institutional policies and governmental regulations, and adequate penalties to serve as a dependable deterrent against the infringement of these precepts.[2]

INTRODUCTION TO IDENTITY MANAGEMENT IN HEALTHCARE

As noted above in a statement issued in 1993 by the AMA's Council on Scientific Affairs, developing and maintaining policies, procedures and expertise to provide necessary Identity Management solutions is a complicated task; identity management has become increasingly important in healthcare over the past two decades. The public awareness of healthcare privacy issues, spurred in part by the HIV/AIDS epidemic and the passage of HIPAA, combined with the rapid growth of the electronic exchange of personal information by health systems, irreversibly elevated the importance of identity management in healthcare to regulators, privacy advocates and the lay public. Continued international, national and local news reports about identity theft have further enhanced the focus on this issue. The following chapter will serve to introduce and explain the core concepts of identity management in healthcare in 2006, and review best practices and solutions to address them.

Identity Management requires three specific qualities: (1) security—to help prevent unauthorized individuals from accessing patient data;[3] (2) privacy—to help prevent individuals authorized to access patient data from using or releasing that patient data inappropriately;[3] and, (3) efficiency to enable authorized individuals to appropriately access and share patient data quickly and easily, both individually and in groups.

There are many regulatory, cultural and quality of care drivers of identity management in healthcare, a detailed review of which is beyond the scope of this chapter. In general, HIPAA and other privacy and confidentiality regulations have required vigorous supervision of *who* is authorized to do *what* with *which* patient information, as well as raised public awareness of the ability for patient information to be exposed. Simultaneously, many quality improvement efforts in healthcare require that clinicians and patients have faster, less expensive and more complete access to the patient information that is currently captured in paper and electronic information. Much of this information is not integrated or able to be accessed from one computerized information system or paper record, requiring clinicians to access many different information systems and different paper records in order to gain a comprehensive view of a patient's record. These same quality efforts require that a health system be able to identify which treatments a patient has received, at what point in the care process, and by whom, so that care processes can be measured, analyzed and improved.

As Figure 3-1[3] shows, for identity management solutions to be effective in healthcare, security and privacy must be addressed while the main goal for healthcare—caring for patients—is recognized, respected and supported. The balance of providing effective identity management solutions within the healthcare world creates a tension between these different factors.

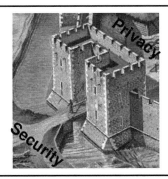

Figure 3-1: Security and Privacy.

Identity Management means:
- Knowing how to identify people, places and things
- Knowing someone is who they claim to be
- Knowing what they are allowed to do
- Knowing who they are related to
- Knowing what others are allowed to do in a manner related to the roles of others
- Knowing how to create identities
- Knowing how to maintain identities when circumstances change

Recognizing that the critical issue in delivering healthcare is treating the patient, addressing privacy and security effectively and efficiently can be daunting tasks.

IDENTITY MANAGEMENT LIFECYCLE

The components of identity management exist together in a continually revolving lifecycle as shown in Figure 3-2.

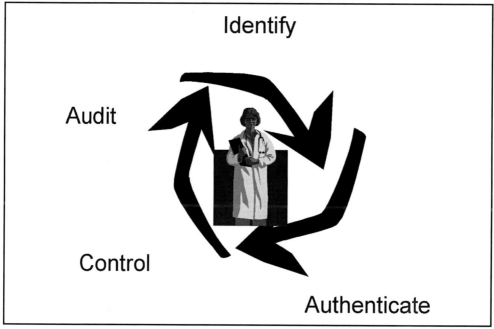

Figure 3-2: **Components of Identity Management.**

Let's examine each of these components in greater detail. First, a healthcare organization must *identify* those individuals who are entering their system. Consider the following examples:

Dr Gomez arrives at the Medical Staff Office with two photo IDs. The staff person retrieves her completed credentialing file, photocopies the ID cards, and hands Dr Gomez a letter to bring to the Security Office for a hospital ID to be issued. Mr. Marks presents to the Ambulatory Surgery Admitting Office on the day of an elective procedure. He shows the registration clerk a letter from his surgeon, his health insurance card, and a driver's license, after which he is registered as a patient. And Nurse Stephens administers an intravenous antibiotic to an inpatient and then returns to her mobile laptop. Her

RFID (radio frequency identification) active proximity badge presents her identity to the laptop and she logs the medication dose in the clinical information system.

➥ Identification is the first step for any person or thing to enter an identity management system. Health systems use many methods today to identify new individuals, whether the individuals are newly hired employees, newly credentialed physicians, patients to be admitted for care or visitors of patients. Most often, paper documentation is presented to a 'trusted' individual at an appropriate access point. The trusted individual reviews the relevant identification information or documents and then records that the individual is who he or she claims to be. An identification card with a photo, such as a state-issued driver's license, is commonly used to identify an individual. Other documentation might include a birth certificate, a passport or other government-issued document. A newborn infant upon delivery from the mother will often receive a hospital-issued bracelet or anklet even before leaving the delivery room; direct observation is used to determine that the infant is the same as the person named in the hospital's medical record. For a known individual within a health system, technology such as an RFID card or badge might facilitate how an individual is identified to an information system in order to provide an efficient workflow.

Once a health system identifies an individual, the health system must assign to that individual a role and access privileges. *Provisioning* is the act of assigning a role and granting user privileges, such as a case manager with access to patient information and care plans. One way that hospitals often provision staff is by creating and managing individual accounts in the hospital information systems. Roles and accounts may be provided for:

- **Access to paper or electronic medical records**—e.g., all physicians receive access to medical and general psychiatric records but only substance abuse treatment providers might have access to records from an alcoholism treatment program
- **Distribution of equipment**—e.g., all respiratory therapists receive mobile phones but only managers receive phones in the pharmacy department
- **Applications**—e.g., physician accounts in a CPOE system allow ordering and recording of administration of medications while nurse accounts only allow the recording of administration of medications
- **Relationships between individuals**—e.g., a physician admits a prominent member of the local clergy to the hospital and his entire physician coverage group receives access to the patient's medical record, while other physicians who are not part of the coverage group do not receive such access
- **Preferences**—e.g., a patient prefers for a primary care physician to order prescription medications from a pharmacy near the train station used to commute to work while another prefers to use the health system pharmacy

Through effective provisioning policies, procedures and technologies, a health system manages the roles and/or privileges of an individual, even as the roles and privileges evolve through the course of the individual's interaction with the health system. Patients are transferred from one provider to another or one inpatient unit to another; nurses and other employees change departments, responsibilities and roles, or might come from a staffing agency for a limited amount of time; and, physicians gain privileges to perform new procedures, or even retire or leave the health system.

Each step requires re-provisioning of an individual's role and account(s) within a health system; additionally, a process must occur to de-provision user accounts when an individual leaves a health system, either temporarily or permanently. Many departments are involved in the decisions and processes to provision and de-provision roles and privileges for individuals at a health system, such as Human Resources, a Credentialing or Medical Staff Office, a Clinical Department, a Security Office and Information Technology. A person's assigned department might have the responsibility of notifying another department of a change in role or a termination of employment; that department might process the change and then relay the new status to Information Technology or a Security Office. This final office might perform the actual modification of the individual's accounts and roles in the health system information systems.

Let's follow the imaginary Dr Gomez through the provisioning process. The Department of Medicine sends a request to the Information Technology Office for Dr Gomez to have accounts in the hospital e-mail, the clinical information system, and the quality reporting system, with privileges appropriate for an attending physician. The Clinical Information Systems Office creates a physician account for Dr Gomez in the requested information systems; a hospital-issued PDA is configured for Dr Gomez to securely download patient information from the hospital's electronic patient record. Dr Gomez is not alone. A recent HIPAA security audit by an outside firm reports that over 27,000 user accounts exist in a hospital's clinical information systems. The same audit reports that clinical, non-clinical, employed and affiliated staff only amount to 15,000 individuals. The Information Systems Office is not able to account for the difference.

The next step in the process is to *authenticate* or prove "you are who you say you are" to the healthcare system. An identified and provisioned user must still be authenticated to be able to exercise the privileges associated with a role. Depending on the role and the privileges associated, the authentication process might be simple or complex. The presentation of an ID bracelet attached to a patient's wrist, a typed username and password, RFID readers, biometric fingerprint scanners and smart cards that must be swiped through a card reader are all examples of different technologies and procedures for authentication. These examples illustrate how an individual can be required to authenticate using something *you have*, something *you know* or even something *that is part of you and unique to you*. The important principal is that only one identified individual is able to be authenticated as that individual. Depending on the need for security and privacy for a particular level of access, combined with a specialized workflow's need for efficiency, different technologies offer advantages and disadvantages. Just as a back room office staff is restricted so that only ICU staff are allowed to enter, a list of patients and bed numbers may be considered secure even if posted continuously on an open monitor screen; such a monitor might be important to providing care for the critically ill patients. Alternatively, a note in a child's medical record that documents suspected sexual abuse might only be accessible to a specific set of providers on a domestic violence team who have specific authentication credentials.

Examples of authentication include the following: (1) Nurse Kelly types his username and password to sign on to the computer so that he may record the medications he administers to patients on the Cardiology Unit; (2) In the ICU, Respiratory Therapist Staples approaches a bedside computer. The RFID card on his coat enables the computer to show his name on the sign on screen; he places his thumb on a biometric fingerprint reader and is signed on to the ICU information system; (3) A finance clerk has forgotten his password to the hospital billing system. On an intranet site, he answers questions about his dog's name, the color of his car and his favorite ice cream to reset his password and regain access to his accounts; and, (4) A nurse looks on the bottom of a keyboard to find a username and password that colleagues share to access the hospital's PACS in order to review a patient's chest x-ray.

Once a user has been identified, provisioned and authenticated, the user's actions within an information system must still be *controlled*. Different individuals within a health system need to enter, access and use patient information differently. Technologies offer many controls. Applications define individual roles with different privileges and capabilities, such as access to restricted antibiotic medications or the ability to sign off on test results. Devices allow for configuration settings that expand or restrict functions, such as a laptop that can be used to view patient information remotely via a hosted application but cannot be used to download patient information or a mobile phone that does not display a physician's number when calling a patient. Examples of control technologies can be found all over the hospital setting:

- A pediatric hospitalist has access to a standard list of antibiotics, listed by a menu in the hospital's CPOE system. In order to prescribe a new, restricted antibiotic, the hospitalist consults an infectious disease specialist about a patient. The infectious disease specialist concurs with the appropriateness of the antibiotic and orders the medication from a restricted antibiotics order menu in the CPOE system that is not available to the pediatric hospitalist.
- A Surgery Department Billing Staff person reviews a patient's visit history while substantiating a claim to Medicare for a recent procedure. The Finance Information System restricts her from seeing that the patient receives substance abuse counseling at the health center as the staff person does not need this information to process the Medicare claim.
- An Infection Control Officer frequently reviews reports and patient information from home, via his hospital laptop and a secure Internet connection. He is able to save aggregate reports with de-identified patient data to the laptop but not files that include identifiable patient information; such files only exist on the hospital's servers.

Auditing is the final component in the Identity Management Process. Audits in healthcare frequently require answers to six basic questions:

- *Who* had access to patient information?
- *What* information did the person access?
- *Where* was the person when accessing the information?
- *When* did the person access the information?
- *How* did the person access the information?
- *Why* did the person access the information?

A health system might perform an audit of information systems for a variety of reasons: to affirm or refute a violation of an identity management policy or process; to create reports for staff training, reinforcing that audits are possible and that violations of identity management policies and processes will be detected; to perform routine surveillance of access to records of VIPs treated by the health system as such individuals are at high risk of confidentiality breaches; or to respond to an individual request by a patient. Audits identify violators of policies as well as weaknesses in processes and technologies, involving Identification, Provisioning, Authentication, and Control. An identity management system is only as strong and complete as the processes in place to support the system and the staff who implement the policies. Recognizing that no identity management system is foolproof, audits provide a means of performing continuous quality monitoring of the identity management system in place and the compliance of the staff it governs. Because audits are retrospective, any transgression that is identified by an audit has already occurred and could be repeated if not addressed appropriately. Health systems should create policies and procedures to address identity management transgressions prior to performing audits and prior to initiating identity management programs. Such policies and procedures must comply with oversight regulations but also must be understood and supported by patients and staff. Lastly, the policies and procedures should be designed to support the care of patients by clinicians.

In what cases might audits be conducted? The nightly news reports on a subway accident and mentions a victim by name who is hospitalized at a local trauma center. Many clinicians and administrative staff appropriately access the patient's information during her course of treatment. The hospital's security department reviews a daily audit log and identifies an entire office group that has accessed the record without any professional need. Another example is when the pitcher for a nearby Major League baseball team, a recent patient at the hospital, requests a list of all hospital staff who have accessed his medical record. System audit logs report that only one nurse accessed the patient's ECG during a six hour stay in the Emergency Department, but the nurse reviewed the ECG 28 times and printed fifteen paper copies. The audit also reveals that this nurse is logged on to ECG system for six days continuously, despite only working three 12-hour shifts that week. Also, an audit would be performed when a new compliance policy requires that all information system accounts must be tracked in a database of health system personnel, both employed and affiliated. Annual audits will be required to assure that accounts are appropriately de-provisioned when individuals no longer are affiliated or employed with the health system.

HEALTHCARE DIFFERENTIATORS: PATIENTS, STAFF, WORKFLOW AND CULTURE

The Patients
The greatest differentiator for healthcare, when compared with other industries, is that in healthcare all standards, regulations, practices and policies are often put aside for the benefit of an individual patient. While such deviations of standard practice should only occur in extraordinary circumstances involving life and death situations, such circumstances occur on a regular basis in hospitals and emergency departments. A physician can often gain approval for a desired medication for a specific patient, regardless of cost; policies about the delivery of care, such as whether or not a procedure must be done in an operating room or at a patient's bedside, may be modified in cases of emergency. Similarly, identity management procedures may need to be disregarded

if there is an urgent need for an individual to gain access to a patient's record without the time to navigate policies and procedures. Such realities require that many policies and procedures in healthcare are crafted with flexibility and appropriate exceptions for emergent circumstances. Any audit results must be screened for transgressions that are actually work-arounds to care for patients appropriately. Policies and procedures should be created to address such circumstances in a manner that enables proper and timely patient care.

The Staff

Health systems depend on employed staff (e.g., nurses), affiliated staff (e.g., physicians), volunteers (e.g., transport staff) and others (e.g., students) for many tasks. Usually, multiple offices maintain independent databases to track these varied individuals, which impedes the monitoring of all persons who deliver care at a given health system. Additionally, some staff are only present occasionally (e.g., the physician who admits a patient to a hospital a few times each year), some staff may be transient (e.g., students and residents-in-training), and some staff may start on minimal notice (e.g., agency nurses). The continued flux of individuals adds another level of complexity to any identity management system. The existence of non-employed staff, whether affiliated or volunteer, often prevents the hospital from enforcing policies that create inefficiencies for such staff. An identity management system must be flexible enough to support the staffing requirements of health systems, easy enough to be used by transient staff, yet robust enough to be effective.

The Workflow

If James Carville were a medical informaticist advising an identity management project, as opposed to a political campaign manager, he would comment, "It's the workflow, stupid." The workflow in healthcare is fast and providers are frequently intolerant of even small delays and inefficiencies; patients do not wait to become sick, more complex, or even critical. To complicate technology deployments in healthcare, providers usually share computers that are distributed throughout a hospital or ambulatory care environment as opposed to having a personal device that is only used by one individual. For example, the description below illustrates how an individual computer might be used in a busy Emergency Department:

- 10:00 AM—Dr Branford checks a patient's laboratory test results
- 10:03 AM—Nurse Glick documents a patient's blood pressure reading
- 10:06 AM—Dr Maxfield orders a portable chest x-ray
- 10:10 AM—Dr Kent checks the status on a previously entered blood bank order
- 10:14 AM—Nurse Glick logs the administration of medication to a patient

In a hospital that has implemented an electronic medical record for clinical documentation, order entry and results reporting, each provider must sign on and sign off the computer and sign on and off various applications throughout the day in order to perform their professional tasks. In no other industry do so many different users share computers to the extent healthcare does; it is common in certain locations in hospitals for more than 50 individuals to use a single computer during a 24-hour period. "Fast user switching," or the ability for sequential users to quickly access a shared computer resource to perform individual tasks, is now a requirement for any identity management solution that is implemented in healthcare settings.

In addition to healthcare providers' need to rapidly access computers, signing on and off different computers throughout the delivery of care, these same providers must access multiple applications in order to review a patient's complete medical record. While most health systems select a core clinical information system to support the majority of information-based workflows, there are almost always additional self-standing information systems or applications. The reason for these self-standing applications is often that a unique workflow or environment, such as the provision of care in an ICU or the presentation of laboratory results or radiology studies, requires a specialized application for optimal efficiency and quality of care. Just as a physician reviews laboratory results, diagnosis lists, medication records, and other information in a paper chart prior to treating a patient, the physician needs to review the broad information available about a patient when the patient's record is computerized. However, signing on to multiple information systems, each of which usually have separate usernames and passwords and navigating multiple systems to review the information about a patient could require a clinician to spend several minutes every time a new computer is used. In order to save time, the busy clinician will often choose to use only a few applications, possibly omitting the review of important patient data, or to use an application that another clinician has already signed on to, disregarding the identity management policy violation that occurs.

"…[T]here is something about the ability of computers to disrupt rather than improve the work flow of people who are very busy," commented Dr Edward Shortliffe, Chair of Columbia University's Department of Biomedical Informatics, and an internationally renowned leader in the field of computers and medicine.[4] Physicians and nurses want fast access to information in an easy manner, not for the sake of reviewing the information, but rather to treat patients best. To complicate the healthcare workflows, within most healthcare settings exist different subworkflows—physicians in an ambulatory diabetes center use different workflows than physicians in an ICU and nurses in an Emergency Department use different workflows than nurses in a neurology service. Therefore, all healthcare identity management systems must maintain sufficient flexibility to function effectively if they are to be successfully deployed across a health system, with different technologies deployed in different settings.

The Culture

The focus on providing patient care and the close working relationships that develop between providers contribute to a culture of tolerance for 'shared access' to a patient's record. Physicians and nurses, as part of a care team, often feel comfortable sharing usernames and passwords for application accounts because they share the same information about the patient under normal circumstances. Additionally, people have difficulty remembering their multiple usernames and passwords needed for secure access to these information systems so sharing is viewed as the only means of accessing important patient information. The combination has produced an abundance of work-arounds to address forgetting a username or password at most health systems. Physicians and nurses write down their multiple usernames and passwords on cards, keyboards, monitors and other locations; additionally, they store them in PDAs or elsewhere. Recent regulations have required that health systems address this culture of information access sharing and even open information sharing; no identity management solution will be successfully implemented without the end users, including clinical staff, accepting that past practices about sharing patient information and access to patient information are no longer appropriate. The most successful identity management solutions will show end users that compliance with identity management policies and processes enables more efficient access to patient information and more effective care.

SOLUTIONS TO THE PROBLEMS OF IDENTITY MANAGEMENT

Technologies will continue to evolve and improve to meet the identity management challenges of healthcare, but several key solutions have matured and are being deployed widely. Examples include: single sign-on, strong authentication, password synchronization, single patient selection (or context management), system auditing and user provisioning. This section will review some of the more commonly deployed identity management technologies used in healthcare today.

Facilitating Access to Information

Username/Password Synchronization is the ability to standardize a single username and password across multiple information systems. Simply synchronizing usernames and passwords to require the same username and password of an individual across all information systems would be much easier for users and would dramatically streamline password management. Anecdotal information reports that several U.S. health systems have initiated password synchronization projects, but it is unknown if any health system has been able to standardize all usernames and passwords for an individual. Due to the unique username and password formats often required by different information systems, it is unlikely that this is achievable (i.e., alphanumeric requirements, number of characters, and symbol requirements vary across systems.) However, depending on an individual health system's needs, the information systems involved and resources available, password synchronization might offer sufficient value to justify the approach.

Single Sign-on (also known as simplified sign-on) is the ability to access any combination of applications as authorized by a secure credential repository with only one single set of credentials (i.e., one username/password used one time to access all appropriate applications.) Password management is streamlined as the user only has one set of credentials to maintain; workflow is streamlined as a user is only prompted one time to present credentials and afterwards simply accesses the information and information systems that are necessary. Single sign-on solutions leverage both technology standards and custom software adapters to sign-on an authenticated user to applications. Additionally, single sign-on applications single sign-off users from their applications. Proper sign-off of applications maintains smooth technical transitions between users and ensures that the next user of a computer does not have access to the prior user's patient information.

Strong Authentication requires a user to present a token (the "something you have") during the authentication process, often combined with requiring a user to present specific information (the "something you know"). The following technologies are being deployed in health systems with varying success:

Smart Cards have embedded chips that identify an individual and might include encrypted information about the individual's role in an organization; a physician or nurse could be required to swipe a smart card through a card reader and then input a password to authenticate that 'they are who they say they are' in order to access information systems.

RFID Proximity Cards, either active or passive, are used to identify an individual and are usually coupled with another form of authentication. Common examples of *passive* RFID proximity cards are the passes used in many industries to access employee-only parking lots. When a user places the card in front of a reader at the entrance to the parking lot, a small signal is stimulated and released from the card, identifying the user and opening the parking lot gate. Such an approach could also be used in a healthcare setting, but would still require another credential for effective security (otherwise anyone who picked up a dropped card could access patient information—again the "something you have and something you know"). *Active* proximity cards emit RFID signals that broadcast a user's location. As a physician wearing an active proximity RFID badge approaches a computer with an RFID reader, the physician is automatically identified to the device; a second authentication credential, such as a password or biometric identifier, would still be required for effective security ("something you have and something you know"). With active proximity RFID cards, when the physician walks away from the computer, the RFID reader informs the computer that the physician is out of range of use of the computer and a screen saver appears to shield patient data from being displayed; alternatively the physician could even be logged off of the device completely.

Number Generating Tokens: Tokens that generate and display changing numerical codes can be assigned to a specific individual and digital certificate. The nature of the changing codes, plus the addition of a password or other authenticating information, limits the ability for a shared or stolen code to be used by someone other than the assigned user. The most common use of such tokens in healthcare is for authentication to applications outside of an institution, whether for individual health systems or governmental programs.

▬ *Biometric Scanners*: Biometric scanners and readers verify that a presenting body part (e.g., fingerprint, iris, etc.) has the same features as a stored reference file previously identified as being that of a specified individual. While passwords and tokens can be shared, forgotten and lost, unique body parts are not as transferable between users. Many technologies have been developed to leverage the uniqueness of fingerprints, irises, retinas, ear pinnae and even pictures of a person's face. Fingerprint biometric readers appear to be the most commonly deployed in healthcare. Two main types of fingerprint readers exist—those that match a scanned fingerprint to an actual image of the user's fingerprint and those that perform minutia sampling and match a number of small points of a scanned fingerprint to a mathematical formula of the ridges of the user's fingerprint. In both cases, a reference database stores a file for comparison with that of the finger placed in the reader. New computers, both desktops and laptops, are incorporating fingerprint readers directly, making such technologies easier to deploy and better integrated.

Improving Navigation through Systems

Single Patient Selection (also known as Context Management) is the ability for a clinician or other computer user to select a patient in one information system and have all other applications synchronize on the same patient. Single Patient Selection is a navigational tool, decreasing the complexity of using multiple information systems to access a comprehensive view of a patient. If a physician prescribes a new medication for a patient with asthma, the following information systems might be needed:

- the EMR to electronically prescribe the medication
- the billing system to check that the medication is on the patient's insurance formulary
- the ECG system to screen the patient for pre-existing cardiac rhythm abnormalities

Just as single sign-on facilitates accessing these systems, single patient selection facilitates accessing one patient's information within these systems, enabling a clinician or other user to easily view an integrated medical record.

Single patient selection originated with the development of the HL7-CCOW standard (see following section on technology standards), but is now implemented with and without this standard at many health systems. Single patient selection technologies, like single sign-on solutions, function with information systems that are not compliant with the CCOW standard through software adapters custom built for each application. Combining single sign-on with single patient selection provides an effective visual integration tool for different information systems, while preserving the best-of-breed functionality that a specialty information system provides.

Knowing Who Reviewed the Patient's Information

Audit Reports: A complete audit report states who accessed which information from which patient, including the time, date and location (or computer) of access. Whether an audit is required for regulatory compliance, patient-centered customer care (i.e., a specific request by a patient for a report of who has viewed a patient's files) or another cause such as suspected transgression of a health system's security policy, the audit might require information to be gathered about information systems, technology hardware and even personnel. As health systems deploy more and more information systems, broader reaching audit systems that report activity in all potential information systems in a health system quickly and efficiently must be developed. Due to the number of information systems in healthcare, most health system IT staff will not have the time nor the capacity to review all information systems to determine if a patient's record has been accessed. Rather, it will require a global approach to review a patient's record and the access that occurred. Audit reports could be generated from individual information systems and then integrated into a single report or an integrated identity management solution can enable all information systems to be audited as one system. Such evolving auditing systems are becoming more appealing to health systems as the issues of patient confidentiality become a higher priority and the need to audit all information systems becomes more commonplace.

Creating, Maintaining, and Removing Access to Information

Provisioning Systems automate and streamline the creation and management of user identities and their corresponding application accounts. Advanced solutions use messaging systems, workflow engines, and customizable rules to automate and expedite the approval processes and workflows that accompany these tasks. Also, these processes must be able to be audited in an automated and efficient manner, just as the target information systems themselves. The decision process for awarding professional privileges and information access in healthcare is usually decentralized and delegated across multiple departments, possibly involving a credentialing office, human resources and even a clinical or academic division; provisioning solutions that streamline such processes and automate communications and escalations of each step in the creation of user accounts eliminate great inefficiencies and inaccuracies. Provisioning systems can provision, or deprovision, a user into an information system automatically with minimal manual data entry tasks, eliminating the potential for human error and, more importantly, decreasing the workload on all involved departments. In order to perform such tasks, these systems leverage technology standards for system integration, software connectors and adapters and messaging protocols. Provisioning system implementation projects have the potential to be extremely complex organizational change efforts, just as an enterprise resource planning (ERP) system or a CPOE system implementation. A large number and variety of human tasks usually exist in a health system to provision users into information systems and the individuals who perform these tasks are often located in different organizational departments and/or even different geographical locations. Automation of provisioning processes requires the transformation of these tasks and increases the accountability of all provisioning processes. Similar to the automation of ordering processes with CPOE or materials tracking processes for ERP, baseline provisioning practices cannot be, nor should they be, completely duplicated in an automated environment.

Visual Integration—a Workflow Solution and an IT Strategy

Visual integration of information systems uses single sign-on and single patient selection to present multiple information systems as one. Visual integration is not a replacement for integrated repositories of information, but rather a complementary solution to a related problem. Population-based reporting and analytics requires integrating patient information from multiple information systems on a single large database, but large databases are neither appropriate nor necessary for individual patient care. When a physician needs information about one patient, or needs to order medication for one patient, he requires fast transactions between his computer and the supporting application's database. Individual patient decisions by a provider do not require database integration from multiple applications either, if the information can be visually integrated and easily accessed. For example, a physician may want to review a patient's ECG prior to changing the patient's blood pressure medication; to do so the physician needs to review the patient's ECG and the existing medication list.

The physician performs the 'analytics' once the ECG and medication list is reviewed and prescribes a desired medication. The ECG and the medication list may be most effectively presented to the physician from individual, separate information systems that have been specifically designed for these tasks. Visual integration with single sign-on and single patient selection enable the physician to easily access this information in a seamless manner and to take advantage of the specialized design of the independent systems.

Visual integration enables a health system to present not only specialized information systems to users in an integrated manner, but also new and old systems. All hospitals today periodically replace information systems while trying to maximize value from existing legacy systems. Visual integration provides a platform upon which old systems and new ones can be integrated and continually changed, with the least amount of disruption to the end user experience. The physician signs on to all systems using single sign-on and navigates all systems using single patient selection; the only change remains that functionality within the applications.

TECHNOLOGY STANDARDS IN HEALTHCARE IDENTITY MANAGEMENT

Identity management technologies in healthcare often leverage existing standards for identity management, such as SAML (Security Assertion Markup Language) and SPML (Service Provisioning Markup Language) supported by OASIS (Organization for the Advancement of Structured Information Standards at www.oasis-open.org) or Integrated Windows Authentication (IWA) by Microsoft. However, due to the unique workflows of healthcare—such as the need for many clinicians to share a single computer and the need for single patient selection across multiple applications—the HL7 CMA (Context Management Architecture) was established. HL7 CMA is often referred to as CCOW, HL7 CCOW or Clinical Context Object Workgroup, the name of the workgroup within HL7 that maintains the HL7 CMA standard. The goal of HL7 CCOW is to "…facilitat[e]…the integration of applications at the point of use."[5] In doing so, CCOW defines standards that enable a software application to provide single sign-on and single patient selection to other applications that are compliant with the standard. Like other technology standards, CCOW decreases the complexity of linking information systems into a single patient record and maintaining the system integration because vendor applications are pre-built to function in compliance with the standard. Standards-based integration allows an information technology team to focus on application deployment, technology and platform support, user training, process redesign and other critical roles, without having to focus on achieving the technology integration. Because the security and patient selection protocols within CCOW are ratified by the HL7 CCOW committee, a highly expert level of scrutiny and open development minimize the risk to an individual health system that integrates systems using the standard.

SUCCESSFUL DEPLOYMENT STRATEGIES FOR HEALTHCARE IDENTITY MANAGEMENT SOLUTIONS

Implementing identity management solutions in healthcare is similar to implementing change and technology in other environments—the likelihood of success is directly related to the end user awareness of the problem with the original processes and workflows, as well as to the value perceived in the technology and new processes being introduced. Rogers, in his classic text *Diffusion of Innovation*, identified five key properties that determine how rapidly a new innovation is adopted by a social system:[6] relative advantage, compatibility, complexity, trialability and observability. Workflows and processes vary within a single health system that could affect each of the five key properties listed by Rogers. Non-modifiable circumstances such as the sterile environment of an operating room, the inability for a wireless network to be deployed in a particular building or the mobility requirements of respiratory therapists may affect these properties. A biometric fingerprint reader technology may work effectively in one environment, but a token with a changing numerical display might be better suited in another environment. Successful identity management solution implementations may vary in the specific technologies deployed, but the overall strategy of protecting the confidentiality of patient information while supporting an effective workflow for clinicians must remain. Pilot implementations that provide flexibility to identify and select different implementation strategies and technology solutions are best suited to health systems with a wide range of environments. Pilots can be used to demonstrate "relative advantage," prove workflow and cultural "compatibility," allow for full preparation to address issues of workflow and technology "complexity," provide opportunities for "trialability" of the new technologies and workflows and provide "observability" that the new approach will be successful in a specific health system.

THE FUTURE—CONNECTING COMMUNITIES AND THE NATIONAL HEALTH INFORMATION NETWORK (NHIN)

As the future of healthcare informatics is dependent on successfully connecting independent healthcare providers and exchanging patient information between them, the future of identity management will be to enable such exchanges to occur in a secure and efficient manner. Having the right information at the right place at the right time so that a person receives the right care also requires safeguarding the information from the wrong people. Health systems are just beginning to address identity management issues effectively within their own organizations. Policies, processes and technologies for identity management must develop further if we are to effectively protect patient information while making it available across an NHIN.

To accomplish this, standardized technologies and methodologies coupled with mandatory business practices are necessary to provide sufficient security systems that track user identities and only permit authorized access to health data for all NHIN-related and connected entities, including RHIOs. NHIN user identities must be tracked and maintained in a directory or database. Systems must be protected from unauthorized access. Data within systems must be protected from unauthorized modification and review.

…The backbone of achieving such protections is the ability to create electronic identities for all people known to the NHIN and to manage the set of inter-relationships and associated data access permissions that would be granted to each person. People include not only the clinical users of the NHIN, but the people about whom health information is exchanged. People also include friends and family who presently care for, or may someday be caring for, another person.[7]

As health systems become more sophisticated in identity management and technologies to support identity management continue to evolve, the driving issues of *security*, *privacy* and *efficiency* will remain critical to healthcare.

Acknowledgment: The author would like to thank Robert Seliger for his contributions to the content included in this chapter.

REFERENCES

1. The issue illustrated by Case #5 was first presented by Dr David Brailer, National Coordinator for the Office of Health Information Technology, during his keynote address to the American Medical Informatics Association Spring Congress 2005, Boston, MA. None of the other cases in this chapter were based specifically on individual occurrences, although all were influenced by true scenarios.

2. Council on Scientific Affairs, American Medical Association: Feasibility of ensuring confidentiality and security of computer-based patient records. *Archives of Family Medicine.* May;2(5):556–60.

3. Leiderman E. Association of Medical Directors of Information Systems Physician-Computer Symposium. July 2005. http://www.amdis.org/Liederman2005.pdf. Accessed November 24, 2006.

4. Austen I. For the doctor's touch, help in the hand. *The New York Times.* August 22, 2002:G:1.

5. Health Level 7 homepage. Available at: http://www.hl7.org/. Accessed on June 7, 2006.

6. Rogers E. *Diffusion of Innovation.* 5th ed. New York, NY: Simon and Schuster; 2003.

7. Hannet F, Hiscock J, Leviss J, and Seliger R. Development and Adoption of a National Health Information Network RFI Response. January, 2005. http://www.amdis.org/Leviss_Jaffe2005.pdf. Accessed November 25, 2006.

CHAPTER 4

Certification in Healthcare Information Technology

Abha Agrawal, MD, FACP
Mark Leavitt, MD, PhD, FHIMSS

Americans have enjoyed the benefits of tremendous advances in modern medicine over the last several decades. Physicians can now visualize internal body structures with astonishing clarity and speed, prescribe "miracle" pharmaceuticals that precisely target abnormal cells or molecules and perform surgery to repair and replace organs with minimal invasion. However, there remains an appalling gap between healthcare industry's adoption of modern technology pertaining to new diagnostics and therapeutics and its adoption of modern information technology pertaining to delivery and management of healthcare information.

According to recent estimates, only about 12% of the physicians in small offices and 19% of the physicians in large group practices or hospital outpatient settings utilize an electronic health record (EHR) for patient care.[1] Of the acute care hospitals, only approximately 18% have implemented EHRs.[2] Although slowly rising, healthcare information technology (HIT) adoption remains at a low level, as compared with other information-intense industries—despite an overwhelming evidence of the potential of HIT to deliver direct and indirect benefits for every aspect of healthcare. HIT has been shown to improve healthcare quality by reducing medical errors and improving clinical processes.[3,4] HIT can reduce the cost of healthcare for individual provider organizations and for the country as a whole,[5,6] and it can improve the efficiency of delivery and management of care.[7]

So, why should so many physicians and hospitals continue to do business using inefficient tools to provide care for their patients when there are over 200 types of EHR products readily available in the U.S. marketplace currently? This current situation of glaring discrepancy in the demand and supply of EHRs, despite the substantial evidence of its benefits, can be attributed to the following factors:

"RETURN" SEPARATED FROM THE "INVESTMENT"

Many research studies demonstrate positive return on investment (ROI) for EHR implementations; however, our American healthcare industry is unique in the sense that the "return" often is gained by a party other than the one making the "investment." In the current traditional methods of paying for healthcare, providers (physicians, healthcare facilities) get reimbursed for the performance of tangible services (such as a diagnostic CT scan or a surgical procedure) but they do not get reimbursed for the improvements in health outcome or efficiency resulting from using an EHR. Therefore, in the current situation, providers pay for EHR implementation but the benefits of the technology accrue to other parties such as payors of healthcare, insurers or patients.[8] This creates a fundamental deadlock of misaligned incentives that must be addressed before we can expect widespread adoption of HIT in the United States.

LACK OF INTEROPERABILITY

Current EHR systems are generally built using proprietary architectures and are not "interoperable." This means that a healthcare facility using one EHR can not easily exchange clinical information with another facility using another type of EHR. Further, because there currently is no single HIT product that can digitize the entire medical record for a patient, most large complex healthcare organizations are required to use several HIT systems for different components of patient care such as pharmacy, radiology, Computerized Practitioner Order Entry or CPOE, EKGs, billing and so on. Even within the same facility, various HIT systems can not communicate with each other to automatically exchange clinical information.

The lack of interoperability among various HIT systems negates many advantages of the technology. Patients often go to multiple physicians and hospitals and good clinical care requires access to comprehensive medical information from all sources. As a result, physicians may have to access multiple systems (generally requiring multiple logins) to access a patient's EKG, medications, discharge summary, radiological procedures and billing information. Patients have to fill in medical history forms repeatedly at different physicians' offices. Furthermore, in a medical emergency, missing or incomplete clinical data can result in sometimes fatal medical errors. Many physicians and patients are rightly dismayed at this current state of interoperability in HIT products and conclude that HIT is not "ready for prime time" yet.

The lack of interoperability arises from proprietary data formats and structures used by various HIT systems and the lack of uniform, consistent, implementable standards for clinical data such as prescriptions, medication history, patient care documentation and other medical vocabulary.

The issue of interoperability to enable clinical information exchange between systems must be addressed urgently if we hope to realize the full potential of HIT.

Security and Privacy

With "identity theft" and "privacy spills" appearing frequently in news, patients and providers alike are naturally concerned about protecting the privacy of health information. This issue needs to be addressed at three levels before physicians and patients will be able to place confidence in EHR systems. First, at the technical level, the architecture, the design and the implementation of EHRs and health information networks must ensure adequate privacy and security of clinical information. Second, consistent national policies and framework to support the privacy and security of health information should be developed. Third, physicians—and more importantly, patients—must be engaged in the discussion and decision making about privacy and security of clinical information.

THE NEED FOR CERTIFICATION IN HIT

In general, certification is a mechanism for enhancing the confidence, orderliness and transparency of a product or service in marketplace. Certification may encompass functionality, safety, compatibility or other aspects of products and services. The inspection and testing process performed when certifying products and services must be based on consensus-driven standards, unbiased inspection and testing, or both.

Certifying HIT products that meet a certain minimum standard of functionality, interoperability and security/reliability can address many of the aforementioned barriers to adoption and can become a catalyst for widespread HIT utilization.

First, certifying EHRs and the networks through interoperability can unlock the current deadlock between providers, payors/purchasers and the HIT vendors, as shown in Figure 4-1. With certified EHRs offering predictable, reliable and standardized functionality, providers will incur less risk in purchasing EHR systems and will be assured of their compatibility with other systems. At the same time, with EHRs delivering improved health outcomes and efficiencies, payors and purchasers of healthcare will be inclined to offer financial and/or other incentives for providers to install HIT products. With less risk and more incentives, providers will be more willing to purchase EHRs, creating a growing marketplace and faster sales cycles for HIT vendors. Vendors will be able to lower the cost of EHRs and develop a more robust product, further enabling HIT adoption.

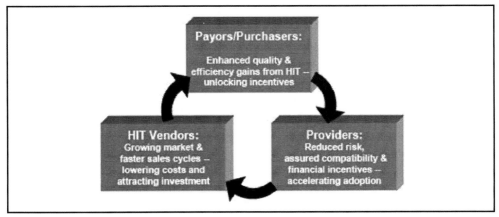

Figure 4-1: Certification as a Catalyst for HIT Adoption.

Second, the certification process incorporates the elements of interoperability both for EHR products and the health information network. Thus, certification ensures standards-based compatibility between various EHR products as well as the components of the health information network.

Third, certification ensures privacy of health information by enforcing security standards within EHR products and the network infrastructure.

CERTIFICATION IN THE NATIONAL HIT STRATEGY

Certification of HIT products has become a key component of the national HIT strategy over the last two years. In April 2004, President Bush announced a bold vision to provide most Americans with interoperable EHRs within the next ten years and this set in motion a chain of events that is leading to transformation of healthcare with information technology. Shortly thereafter, the Office of the National Coordinator for Health Information Technology (ONCHIT) was created under the Department of Health and Human Services (HHS) with Dr David Brailer, MD, PhD serving as its first National Coordinator. In July 2004, Dr Brailer released a *Framework for Strategic Action* outlining four goals and twelve corresponding strategies for improving healthcare. One of the key actions listed in the strategic framework was the private sector certification of HIT products to "develop minimal products standards for EHR functionality, interoperability and security."[9]

In response to this call for action, the Certification Commission for Healthcare Information Technology (CCHIT) was founded as the first organization in the United States with the goal to create credible certification mechanisms for various HIT products.

THE CERTIFICATION COMMISSION FOR HEALTHCARE INFORMATION TECHNOLOGY (CCHIT)

Origin and Mission

CCHIT[SM], an independent, voluntary, private sector initiative, is becoming the recognized certification authority for EHRs and the networks supporting them. Its mission is to accelerate the adoption of robust, interoperable HIT products throughout the U.S. healthcare system by creating an efficient, credible and sustainable mechanism for the certification of HIT products.

CCHIT was founded in July 2004, in response to the call for action embodied in the Strategic Framework of the ONCHIT, with the support of three leading industry associations in healthcare information management and technology: the American Health Information Management Association (AHIMA), the Healthcare Information and Management Systems Society (HIMSS) and the National Alliance for Health Information Technology (Alliance). In September 2005, CCHIT received the HHS award of a three-year, $7.5 million contract to develop and evaluate certification criteria and an inspection process for EHRs in three areas—ambulatory EHRs, inpatient EHRs and the network components through which they interoperate.

Organizational Structure

Figure 4-2 illustrates the organizational structure of CCHIT. CCHIT is governed by a nineteen member Board of Commissioners hailing from academic, private sector and governmental agencies. It is headed by the Chair of the Board. The Board oversees the work of CCHIT's professional staff and voluntary work groups. The roles of the Commissioners are to represent all stakeholders, provide strategic direction, ensure objectivity and credibility, provide guidance to and review the reports of the work groups and approve the final certification criteria and processes.

The Commission is made up of at least two representatives each from the provider, payor and vendor stakeholder groups and at least one from seven other stakeholder groups, including safety net providers, healthcare consumers, public health agencies, quality improvement organizations, clinical researchers, standards development and informatics experts and government agencies. The Commissioners serve staggered two-year terms.

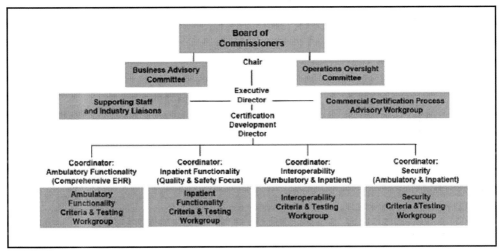

Figure 4-2: CCHIT's Organizational Structure.

The products of the Commission are created by its five volunteer work groups, each with two co-chairs from different stakeholder groups and approximately twelve to fourteen members representing the diversity of stakeholders. The work groups focus on developing the certification criteria (see below) and an inspection process by which products can be judged to be certified. The five workgroups include: ambulatory functionality, inpatient functionality, interoperability, security and commercial certification process advisory.

Stakeholders

Certified EHR products benefit many interested groups and individuals, including:

- Physicians, hospitals, health systems, safety net providers, public health agencies and other purchasers of HIT products, who seek quality, interoperability, data portability and security.
- Purchasers and payors—from government to the private sector—who are prepared to offer financial incentives for HIT adoption but need the assurance of having a mechanism in place to ensure that products deliver the expected benefits.
- Quality improvement organizations that seek out an efficient means of measuring that appropriate criteria have been assessed and met.
- Standards development and informatics experts that gain consensus on standards.

- Vendors who benefit from having to meet a single set of criteria and from having a voice in the process.
- Ultimately, and most importantly, consumers, who benefit from a reliable, accurate and secure record of their health.

CCHIT's organization and policies ensure adequate representation from each stakeholder group on the Board, as well as various workgroups.

CCHIT IN THE NATIONAL HIT FRAMEWORK

Certification is only one of several actions that are necessary to overcome the current barriers to HIT adoption. To achieve the larger vision for healthcare transformation through HIT, CCHIT works collaboratively with various other HHS contractors, with the American Health Information Community (AHIC) and with stakeholders throughout the public and private sectors, as illustrated in Figure 4-3.

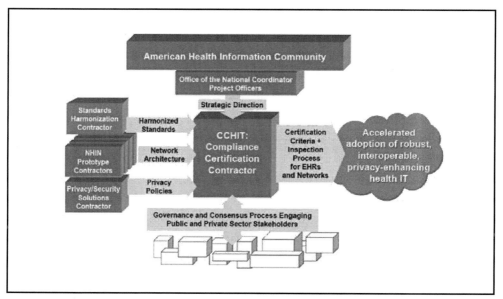

Figure 4-3: CCHIT's Role in the National HIT Strategy.

First, CCHIT depends on the standards harmonization contractor to develop and harmonize standards against which EHRs—and the infrastructure through which they interoperate—can be tested for compliance. CCHIT also provides feedback to the standards organizations and the ONCHIT regarding any gaps between the currently available HIT standards and the availability of compliant products in the marketplace, as well as the practicality of testing compliance to standards, thus facilitating the development and refinement of HIT standards.

Second, CCHIT collaborates with the National Health Information Network (NHIN) prototyping contractors who develop, demonstrate and document architectures for NHIN. It facilitates the development of appropriate certification criteria and test procedures to certify compliance of EHR networks with NHIN architecture.

Third, CCHIT also depends on the privacy and security solutions contractor to recommend standardized privacy and security policies against which CCHIT can test and certify the compliance of EHRs and their networks.

Finally, in order to develop an efficient and credible process that can be accepted by those who develop and invest in HIT, CCHIT engages with various public and private stakeholders throughout the healthcare industry.

Certification Criteria

CCHIT is developing certification criteria and processes for three types of products: ambulatory EHRs, inpatient EHRs and health information networks. For EHRs, the certification criteria are grouped into three categories: functionality, interoperability and security/reliability.

The functionality criteria specify a minimum set of features and functions in an EHR product. Some example of the functionality criteria for the 2006 certification of ambulatory EHRs include:
- Manage allergy/adverse reaction list
- Generate patient-specific instructions
- Drug-drug interaction checking
- Alerts for disease management, prevention and wellness
- Inter-provider communication

The interoperability criteria evaluate whether a product has the capability to perform standards-based data exchange with other sources of healthcare information. Some examples of the interoperability criteria for the 2006 certification of ambulatory EHRs include receiving laboratory results and sending electronic prescriptions. Other examples of the interoperability criteria on the 2007 certification roadmap for ambulatory EHRs include: receiving medication fulfillment history, referring or transferring care of patient and quality improvement reporting. Note that the criteria on the roadmap are dependent on the development by the standards harmonization group.

The security and reliability criteria test a product to ensure that it protects data privacy and is robust to prevent data loss. Some examples of the security/reliability criteria for the 2006 certification of ambulatory EHRs include:
- Control access to system
- Record audit trail of all events
- Provide for backup and recovery
- Documented procedures for installation, updating and protecting from viruses/ malware.

Criteria Development Process

Figure 4-4 shows the six-step standardized process that CCHIT has devised to develop various certification criteria and the actual certification. The documents and other publications produced by CCHIT are published for public comments at the end of steps A, B and D. These comments are discussed and addressed before moving onto the next step. At the time of this writing (April 2006), most of the steps for ambulatory EHRs have been completed and the process for inpatient EHRs is just getting underway at steps A and B. The process for certification of health information networks has not started yet.

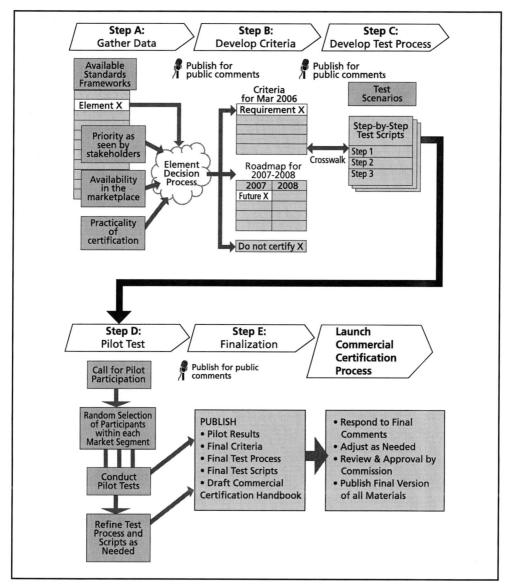

Figure 4-4: The CCHIT Certification Process.

Step A: Gather data. CCHIT evaluates commonly available standards and frameworks from various standards development organizations (SDOs), that develop voluntary local or national consensus on standards for a particular domain (e.g., healthcare), or a sub-domain (e.g., pharmacy, medical devices or imaging). If there are competing standards, CCHIT may reference several of them to support the recommended functionality. CCHIT also looks to the American National Standards Institute's Health Information Technology Standards Panel (ANSI-HITSP) to harmonize these standards as part of their charter from HHS.

Based on various standards and other considerations, potential elements for certification criteria are listed. These elements are subjected to a decision process incorporating factors such as stakeholders' priority, availability in the marketplace and practicality of certification. This work is then published for public comments.

Step B: Develop criteria. As a result of the element decision process and public comments, an element may get incorporated in the certification criteria, get placed on the future roadmap or may be found unsuitable for inclusion in the certification process. After various elements for each of the certification groups (functionality, interoperability and security/reliability) have been finalized and subjected to public comments, certification criteria are considered established for a specific group of HIT products (e.g., ambulatory EHRs).

Step C: Develop test process. This step involves the designing of simulated clinical scenarios and step-by-step test scripts for product testing. These scripts are developed to evaluate a product's compliance against various elements of certification criteria.

Step D: Pilot test. With the certification criteria and the test scripts ready, CCHIT proceeds to perform pilot testing of a select few EHR products. CCHIT announces a call to vendors for pilot participation and randomly selects EHR products within each market segment. Take ambulatory EHRs, for example; their market segments included enterprise, medium-size practice and small practice. The test processes and various test scripts are refined, if needed, during the pilot testing.

Step E: Finalization. After the completion of pilot tests, CCHIT makes the following available in the public domain for public comments: the results of pilot testing, the final certification criteria, the final test process, the final test scripts and eventually a commercial certification handbook. Based on the public comments, revisions are made, if needed, and after the review and approval by the Commission, the final certification criteria, test processes and test scripts are released.

Step F: Launch commercial certification process. In this final step, CCHIT announces its readiness for commercial certification testing. CCHIT started the commercial certification of ambulatory EHRs in May 2006.

DISCUSSION

CCHIT's certification criteria are derived from existing healthcare data standards. Because CCHIT itself is not a standards development organization (SDO), its work is linked to and dependent on the progress of SDOs and the standards harmonization contractor. Many functionality and security standards are just gaining consensus, while standards for interoperability are at an early stage of development. As new standards evolve, CCHIT must be prepared to refine its certification criteria in concert with the evolution of standards from year to year.

CCHIT does not test EHR products for usability that includes attributes such as friendliness of the user interface, ease of maintenance and the potential "down time" for a product in use. It is difficult to test and inspect the usability of a product. User-friendliness is a subjective and relatively non-specific attribute. Ease of maintenance and 'down time' of an EHR often relate to issues other than the product itself, such as the computer hardware, operating system and network installed at a facility. For provider organizations, however, the usability issues remain at least of as much concern as the functionality of EHR products.

Some hospitals and healthcare networks have already made considerable investments in HIT systems and have advanced EHR and other products already implemented. Some organizations, particularly early adopters, have implemented a "home-grown" EHR system over a period of many years. In these instances, the benefits of certification of a home-grown system or the potential adverse impact on healthcare delivery from using an uncertified home-grown product remain unclear.

CCHIT certification remains a voluntary process for HIT vendors in contrast to the mandatory requirement imposed on the makers of medical devices to get FDA approval before entering the market. One reason for this difference is that medical devices are considered to have a direct impact on patient safety. Therefore, they are subjected to mandatory approval by the FDA. However, if recent reports of the effects of technologies such as CPOE and bar-coding are any indication, it is becoming apparent that poorly developed or implemented HIT products can have a potentially adverse effect on patient safety as well.[4,5,6,10,11,12] It is expected that having a "CCHIT Certified" seal of approval will provide competitive advantage to a vendor. Market forces, rather than regulatory requirements, should drive their interest in CCHIT certification, especially in the current stage of the HIT industry. Ultimately, the real impact of CCHIT on the HIT marketplace will become clear only a few years after the certification process has been in operation.

Appendix 4-1: Helpful Links.

CCHIT http://www.cchit.org
Office of the National Coordinator for Health Information Technology (ONC) http://www.hhs.gov/healthit/
American Health Information Community (The Community) http://www.hhs.gov/healthit/ahic.html
Healthcare Information Technology Standards Panel (HITSP) http://www.ansi.org/standards_activities/standards_boards_panels/hisb/hitsp.aspx?menuid=3
The Leapfrog Group http://www.leapfroggroup.org/

Appendix 4-2: FAQs.

Is CCHIT a part of a government agency? No. CCHIT is an independent, voluntary, private sector initiative organized as a limited liability corporation.
Is CCHIT different from a Standards Development Organization (SDO) such as HL-7? CCHIT is not an SDO. It develops certification criteria based on standards developed by the SDOs.
How can I get a copy of the CCHIT's certification criteria and process? CCHIT's certification criteria, test scripts and test steps are in the public domain and can easily be accessed on its Web site.
How do I know whether a product is CCHIT certified? CCHIT publishes a list of CCHIT certified products on its Web site. Note that only the products that pass the certification are published.
I am a vendor. What happens if my product fails certification? CCHIT has established policies and procedures for retesting and appeal of the inspection process. If a product is not judged to meet the criteria, the vendor may correct the deficiencies and re-apply for certification.
What if I buy a CCHIT certified EHR and it doesn't do what the vendor or CCHIT said it does? A complaint procedure is in place to address this situation. If, after thorough investigation, the EHR product being sold does not perform as claimed during the inspection process, the vendor will be prohibited from advertising it as CCHIT certified and it will be removed from the certified products list.

REFERENCES

1. Gans D, Kralewski J, Hammons T, Dowd B. Medical groups' adoption of electronic health records and information systems. Practices are encountering greater-than-expected barriers to adopting an EHR system, but the adoption rate continues to rise. *Health Aff* (Millwood) 2005;24(5):1323–33.

2. Health Information and Management System Society. 16th annual HIMSS leadership survey; 2005. Available at: http://www.himss.org/2005survey/healthcareCIO_keytrends.asp. Accessed on November 8, 2006.

3. Bates DW, Leape LL, Cullen DJ, Laird N, Petersen LA, Teich JM, et al. Effect of computerized physician order entry and a team intervention on prevention of serious medication errors. *JAMA*. 1998;280(15):1311–6.

4. Tierney WM, Miller ME, McDonald CJ. The effect on test ordering of informing physicians of the charges for outpatient diagnostic tests. *NEJM*. 1990;322(21):1499–504.

5. Johnston D, Pan E, Walker J. The value of CPOE in ambulatory settings. *JHIM*. 2004;18(1):5–8.

6. Walker J, Pan E, Johnston D, Adler-Milstein J, Bates DW, Middleton B. The value of healthcare information exchange and interoperability. *Health Aff* (Millwood) 2005;(suppl)Web Exclusives:W5-10–W5-18.

7. Jha AK, Kuperman GJ, Rittenberg E, Teich JM, Bates DW. Identifying hospital admissions due to adverse drug events using a computer-based monitor. *Pharmacoepidemiol Drug Saf*. 2001:10(2):113–9.

8. Wang SJ, Middleton B, Prosser LA, Bardon CG, Spurr CD, Carchidi PJ, et al. A cost-benefit analysis of electronic medical records in primary care. *Am J Med*. 2003;114(5):397–403.

9. Framework for Strategic Action (http://www.hhs.gov/healthit/executivesummary.html)

10. Han YY, Carcillo JA, Venkataraman ST, Clark RS, Watson RS, Nguyen TC, et al. Unexpected increased mortality after implementation of a commercially sold computerized physician order entry system. *Pediatrics*. 2005;116(6):1506–12.

11. Koppel R, Metlay JP, Cohen A, Abaluck B, Localio AR, Kimmel SE, et al. Role of computerized physician order entry systems in facilitating medication errors. *JAMA*. 2005;293(10):1197–203.

12. McDonald CJ. Computerization can create safety hazards: a bar-coding near miss. *Ann Intern Med*. 2006;144(7):510–6.

CHAPTER 5

Ambulatory Electronic Health Record

Curtis L. Cole, MD

When looked at from the patient's perspective, the Ambulatory Electronic Health Record (AEHR) is probably closer to the patient's archetype of "my chart" than its acute care sibling. Nevertheless, the erstwhile second-class status of the AEHR stems from the socio-economic history of the EHR. The EHR was born in large, acute care institutions, largely to serve providers. Their view, as dictated by reimbursement methods, was encounter-based and focused on procedures and hospital stays. The notion of a single patient flowing through a series of complex encounters across providers over years was absent. So the hospital seemed bigger than the entire world outside it. This view was amusingly captured by Carter in a comparison to inpatient EMR implementations: "ambulatory care sites tend to be simpler."[1]

Fortunately, the world is changing. The HIMSS Ambulatory Care Initiative has identified two key trends that point to the centrality of the AEHR (See Figures 5-1 and 5-2).[2]

First, there is the growing massive imbalance in the scale of ambulatory encounters as compared to acute care encounters (1 billion versus 8 million, respectively, in 2003). Second, ambulatory healthcare expenditures have surpassed acute care expenditures and are growing faster. Despite this, the nation still spends about one-tenth as much on ambulatory information technology (IT) as it does on inpatient based systems.

In this chapter, we will explore how the AEHR differs from its inpatient counterpart by focusing on the key functions and workflows they support. We will examine key executive considerations such as cost, ROI and infrastructure. The chapter closes with a discussion of the status of the industry and where it looks to be headed in the future.

HIMSS defines the EHR as follows:

> The Electronic Health Record (EHR) is a secure, real-time, point-of-care, patient centric information resource for clinicians. The EHR aids clinicians' decision making by providing access to the patient health record information where and when they need it and by incorporating evidence-based decision

support. The EHR automates and streamlines the clinician's workflow, closing loops in communication and response that result in delays or gaps in care. The EHR also supports the collection of data for uses other than direct clinical care, such as billing, quality management, outcomes reporting, resource planning, and public health disease surveillance and reporting.[3]

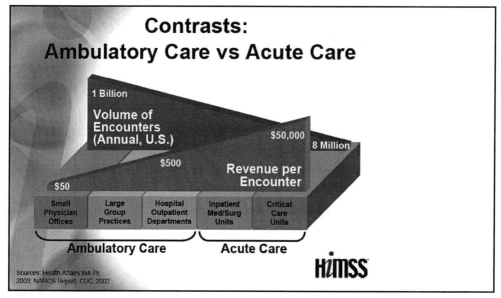

Figure 5-1: Key Trends in Comparing Ambulatory versus Acute Care—Contrasts: Ambulatory Care vs. Acute Care.

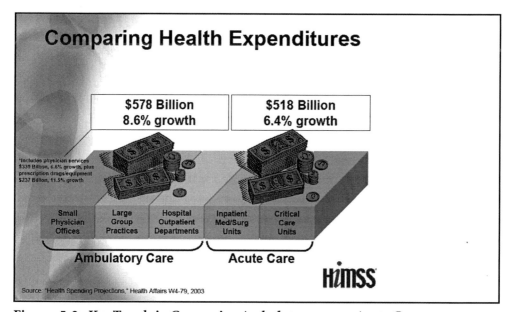

Figures 5-2: Key Trends in Comparing Ambulatory versus Acute Care—Comparing Health Expenditures.

While this academic description covers the waterfront, the marketplace boils it down to three categories of systems: Practice Management Systems, Clinical Systems and Biomedical Devices. We will examine each category as well as briefly consider

Infrastructure. We will start with Practice Management Systems because they are the first systems any practice should be implementing. The axiom, "no money, no mission," is certainly applicable in ambulatory medical practices. Clinical systems and biomedical devices are more glamorous and dynamic. Perhaps the least sexy of all is infrastructure. But, without it there can be none of the above, so we will also examine the fundamental infrastructure considerations that are critical in an ambulatory context.

PRACTICE MANAGEMENT SYSTEMS

Practice Management Systems (PMS) focus on two interrelated concepts: Patient Flow and the Revenue Cycle. These are the operational and financial sides of the same coin. They are the outpatient cousins to the ADT (Admit Discharge Transfer) and Patient Accounting systems.

Whether you view the PMS from an operations or a financial lens, the business begins with patient identification. And from this starting point, the divergence with inpatient systems begins. The concept of "registration" is very different between the inpatient and outpatient world. The conceptual difference is permanence. The ambulatory world treats registration as a persistent beginning to a lifetime record. Patients see their doctors over and over, but they only register once; they reasonably expect their doctor to remember them. In the inpatient world, registration is the beginning of a finite stay and is repeated with each admission.

From a systems perspective, the difference is the combination of three related functions: identification, registration and scheduling. Patient identification is increasingly the realm of specialized systems specific to this task known as the Electronic Master Patient Index (EMPI). These systems contain a database with a very small amount of data about every patient in their dominion. The job of the EMPI is to make sure that each patient has only one set of data even across multiple systems, specialties, locations and institutions.

Almost all PMSs have some EMPI functionality built in. Large PMSs tend to have more sophisticated functionality. A caveat for executives shopping for a PMS is to make sure this functionality is sophisticated enough to meet their needs *or* that the system is capable of taking direction from an external EMPI, which is increasingly the preference of large organizations. Too many PMSs are designed assuming they are in charge of patient identity. This can lead to significant sorrow when trying to integrate with other systems.

The details of patient identification can be mind numbing, particularly to those who fail to grasp their importance. But ignore them at your own peril as the ambulatory world can be deceptively simple in this regard. If you view each practice independently, it may be easy to keep a few thousand patients straight without a large number of duplicates. But when you combine practices, or try to combine data from patients across practices, you quickly realize that the ambulatory world is very large indeed. The lack of a single identifier makes matching logic more critical. And the well-documented failures and risks of using Social Security numbers make the task ahead look even more challenging.[4,5]

Once the patient is identified, the formal registration can begin. This is the collection of deeper patient demographics including insurance coverage information, emergency contacts, customer service information such as contact preferences, and similar non-clinical information. In the most sophisticated PMSs, insurance eligibility verification may occur at this step in an EDI (Electronic Data Interchange) transaction analogous to a retailer validating a credit card.

Scheduling

In the inpatient world, the process now moves to bed management. In the outpatient world, however, the next job is scheduling. Because patients are admitted to the hospital at a particular time and date, scheduling is inherent in the admission process. For the ambulatory patient, all future encounters will key off the original registration (with or without updates) and the schedule is the focus of new encounters.

Because the process of scheduling is so tightly linked to registration, it is not surprising that many clinical scheduling systems are integrated with registration systems within the PMS. There are a few key qualities of ambulatory scheduling that differentiate the various systems available on the market. Perhaps the most important is how they differ from non-clinical scheduling systems such as Microsoft Outlook™ or Oracle™ Calendar—that for clarity are referred to here as calendaring systems.

The main distinction between a scheduling system and a calendaring system is the linkage to the patient record. In a typical business calendaring system, the user cannot quickly locate a whole history of a given patient's appointments or sort them by type. This is routine in a scheduling system.

Clinical schedules are also linked to billing encounters. This is critical from the financial perspective. One of the first interventions in a typical revenue cycle enhancement program is to match charges against the schedule. This is possible manually with a calendaring system but can be made into an automated "missing charge report" in a clinical scheduling product. Another way of looking at this is that the schedule can define the encounter for the billing system.

Clinical scheduling systems typically support complex templates and rules to maximize patient flow and appointment availability. Concepts such as appointment type, bump lists, freeze and thaw, recurring visits and team care will have variable importance in different practices and specialties. For example, patients on specific chemotherapy protocols or physical therapy routines can be extremely complicated to schedule without software with the appropriate searching algorithms.

Resource linking is particularly critical in procedural areas. For example, in specialties with endoscopes, the availability of the scope itself and the time needed for sterilization must be accounted for by the scheduling system to maximize throughput. Linkage to materials management systems may also be important for inventory and cost controls.

In academic environments, there are complex supervision rules that must be accounted for to allow compliant billing. For example, the 1969 CMS IL372 regulations require that primary care supervisors oversee no more than four residents at a given time.[6] Without that ratio, the supervisor cannot bill for their supervision.

The most sophisticated practices use their scheduling systems to track all aspects of clinical workflow. Some systems can parse a variety of wait times such as time-to-room, time-in-room, time-with-RN and time-with-MD. When used well, these tools fulfill the data manager's need to optimize patient flow, maximize resource utilization, and improve patient satisfaction.

Billing

The core of most PMSs is the financial component. The tools needed to manage billing and accounts receivable are enormously varied due to the wide variety of reimbursement rules and methods through the country. The key difference with inpatient systems is the focus on professional fee billing rather than facilities fee. One important, and possibly counter-intuitive, feature this may imply is the need for the *ambulatory* PMS to support *inpatient* professional billing. Some physicians who see inpatients do not bill "globally" or through the hospital; they send their bills from their office. Therefore, certain types of integration with the inpatient system, such as an ADT interface, may be desirable.

Executives attuned to the current regulatory environment will note the need to synchronize the facility and the professional fee bills in terms of procedure and diagnosis. Given that two staffs, with two different managers, following two sets of rules, using two different systems are responsible for this suggests this will be fraught with peril. And it gets worse when you consider the multiple specialists that may be billing for the same case (e.g., surgery and anesthesia) and that different coding systems may be required (e.g., HCPCS and CPT). At this point, few of the systems on the market today are facile at this kind of cross-provider billing reconciliation.

Today's financial systems put increasing emphasis on capturing data as early in the encounter as possible. The shift from back office to front desk is a major component of revenue cycle enhancement projects. Many systems now automate charge capture at the point-of-care. There are significant opportunities for both revenue enhancement and cost control by automating this step. Costs fall if you can eliminate charge entry clerks. And revenue goes up if the computer can help you optimally code clean claims that speed out the door.

There is an important architectural decision point here. Should the "encounter form" data (a.k.a. super-bill) be entered into a clinical system or a practice management system? The IT manager who is blind to the actual workflow will generally prefer direct entry into the PMS. Entry into the clinical system will require an interface into the PMS, unless they are the same system. Understanding the workflow is the key to resolving this question. Most physicians will have little or no need to use the PMS. Therefore, if you want the provider to capture the billing data, it may make more sense to capture it from within the clinical system. Ideally, the billing codes fall out of the documentation, in which case the issue is moot. As discussed below, this remains an ideal more than a reality.

A relatively new entrant into the marketplace is the PDA-based (Personal Digital Assistant) charge capture system. These systems may be stand-alone or integrated with a PMS or clinical system. Regardless of the platform, these systems offer another way to eliminate paper encounter forms and capture data more accurately and directly into the billing system.

ROI from these systems stems from the reduction in lost charges and reduced service due to posting lag. As such, their value is largely based on the relative inefficiency of whatever paper-based system is in place. Executives need to be cautious when evaluating such systems. Their value is only in capturing revenue that was otherwise never captured, or on the time-value of money that was captured late. In some cases, that may be quite large. But it may be fairly modest where paper systems work well.

In many environments where part-time clinical employment is the norm (e.g., academia), the value may be further mitigated by vendor fees that do not acknowledge the less than full-time use of the system. Conversely, in consultation-rich specialties, such systems can be a godsend of convenience to physicians, particularly if they practice in multiple locations.

Another nuance executives need to be aware of is the definition of the encounter itself. As with registration, terminology here is imprecise and can be confusing. My preference is to refer to the billable event as the encounter and the face to face meeting with the patient as the visit. But the increasing prevalence of phone, Web and other virtual "visits" makes this topic inherently fluid. Regardless of how you refer to the event, the system must know the rules for the definitions. These are generally determined by the payor and may or may not make sense to the clinician. For example, a nine month pregnancy may be a single encounter with multiple visits. Similarly, a visit to a doctor's office that results in referral to the emergency room may be combined as a single encounter (the "72-hour rule"). A visit to multiple different doctors on a single day may be considered a single encounter. The billing system needs to understand these rules. Again, cross-institutional reconciliation may be necessary to ensure complete accuracy in some scenarios.

Managed Care

The most fundamental distinction among practice management systems is support for the various forms of managed care. Practices that take on capitation without a PMS that is fully capable of tracking expenses and supporting risk management are almost certain to fail. Such systems are complex to properly set up and maintain, even when backed by billion dollar insurance companies. This goes a long way toward explaining the falling popularity of this form of reimbursement.

While traditional fee-for-service still exists in some form in most markets, some permutation of managed care is the norm in most areas. While the technology to support managed care exists, it is still very poorly implemented by many PMS vendors. This is, no doubt, in part because few insurance companies support the technology either.

The key technologies to support managed care are EDI and robust master file management. The diversity of payor rules, the frequency of changes to the rules and the frequency that patients change payors essentially require that providers check eligibility and authorization prior to any service. Despite federal pressure to support EDI, this remains far from ubiquitous.

Many PMS vendors partner with EDI clearinghouse vendors to simplify their own EDI communication. The concept is that providers only need to communicate with one company and they communicate with all the payors for you. Conversely, as payor, you only need to communicate with one clearinghouse rather than thousands of providers. The intermediary is therefore more important to the payor than the provider, particularly if your PMS strictly adheres to the transaction protocols.

Internet standards should allow for direct payor-provider communication. Particularly for large providers, the clearinghouse should not be necessary. Similarly, for small providers who purchase PMS services from a larger entity such as an ASP (Application Service Provider), the clearinghouse should be optional, particularly in the increasing number of markets with very few payors. Payors often mandate the use of a clearinghouse. Further, many vendors charge large transaction fees cutting in to already slim margins. This practice has not been tested in court and certainly violates the spirit of laws intended to simplify healthcare communications. But absent stronger regulatory enforcement, cheap disintermediation will be resisted by the clearinghouses. Therefore, executives should pay attention to this issue going forward as significant efficiencies will be won or lost depending on how the issue of clearinghouses develops.

Claims Editing and Submission

Once the encounter is captured, the next layer of system functionality is charge editing. In many instances, charges may be clean at the point of entry and can quickly flow to the payor. In many other settings charges must be analyzed for exceptions, discounts, consistency with other claims, the addition of modifiers or other interventions management may want to make before sending the claim. In some systems, these edits can be done in real time and advise the provider or charge entry staff to make changes immediately. In others, the claims are batched and analyzed in bulk. A list of exceptions is created and worked over time.

The goal of editing is to ensure that every claim that is sent to the payor is a clean claim. Sophisticated PMS vendors provide tools that mimic the adjudication rules used by payors and alert the provider to impending rejections before the claim even goes out the door. Clean claims mean no rejections, faster payment and reduced re-processing costs. Not surprisingly, claim editing is another frequent focus of revenue enhancement efforts.

It is worth pausing here to note a potential pitfall in the ROI analysis of Practice Management Systems or system add-ons. Note that I mentioned that revenue can be enhanced by automating charge entry and also by editing charges. When analyzing the financial return from these efforts, it is important to consider who will be making the charge edits. This is not to imply that these two efficiencies are necessarily either/or. But individual workflows need to be well understood before assuming cost reductions. Revenue enhancement may not cut costs and vice versa.

Ready or not, the claim is now sent out. The ability to print a paper claim remains a requirement of any PMS—if for no other reason than downtime at an intermediary. But most claims today are sent electronically. This may be via a clearinghouse or directly. In either event, logs of the transactions are essential to avoid disputes over lost claims.

The payor now adjudicates the claims and if a flaw is found, the claim is rejected. Here again, there is an opportunity for efficiency if the payor communicates the rejection electronically. Most companies still send rejections via paper. Well-managed practices key these rejections into the PMS with their often obscure rejection codes so that practice administrators can track the reasons for rejection over time and correct any systematic problems that emerge.

Master File Management

This brings us to the second key technology for supporting managed care, strong master file management. All information systems use a variety of tables and dictionaries to drive the lists and other user interface elements customized to your location or practice. For example, a list of physicians you commonly refer to (or are sent referrals from) is one such provider dictionary. In the world of managed care, keeping track of who is "in plan" and "out of plan" is a major problem. Any provider who has dropped out of plan can tell you that it may take months or even years for their name to disappear from the payor's list, particularly if they are in a shortage specialty.

IT managers are vexed by the need to provide users with accurate data without good sources for the data. Many vendors offer portions of these data for sale. But their accuracy may be suspect and they often lack key information needed to match existing data. States may have good data, but refuse to provide it in a usable form. And if you can the get data, unless your PMS can manage adds, changes and deletes well, updates may be an all or nothing proposition that can wreak havoc on existing record references and makes mixing data from multiple sources impossible. This specific problem may get better or worse when a national provider identifier is approved depending on how it is implemented.

This issue is relevant to claims adjudication because of the many nuances of billing that require accurate look-up tables. For example, specialists may need to indicate the license number of a referring physician on the claim or it will be rejected. Therefore, the easiest path to clean claims would be a clean dictionary of referring providers.

Payment Posting and Contract Management

Of course, most claims are not rejected. The next challenge for the PMS is payment posting. Here again, efficiency would demand electronic payment posting. The reality is far different. The details of payment posting vary considerably—some providers use bank lock-boxes and other services that simplify or complicate the process—but the basics are the same.

The payor sends a payment with an EOB (Explanation of Benefits), typically for many claims at once. The job of payment posting is interpreting the EOB and assigning the correct amount of money to each claim. In large practices with manual payment posting, this may take many FTEs. The procedure is also error prone, making this whole process a ripe target for automation. Bar coding, optical character recognition and a variety of other technologies have been applied to try to clean up payment posting with varied degrees of success. Rich EDI is probably the most promising solution, short of adopting a single payor insurance plan.

Once posted, there are two more problems the PMS must contend with: overpayment and underpayment. Overpayment most commonly occurs when both the patient and the payor send the provider a payment. This requires a method for refunding that, in many practices, requires a link to a separate Accounts Payable system.

In today's world of managed care conglomerates, underpayment is the more serious problem. Even within one company, claims may be processed by multiple different systems that may not all have the current contract and payment policies loaded. Therefore, inappropriate rejections and underpayments are common and often appear to be idiosyncratic. Further, in many states, there is little accountability by regulators. In a study performed at Weill Cornell and Emory between 3–8% of all reimbursements from managed care companies were underpaid as compared to contract. While this represents tens of millions of dollars to providers, annually payors are only fined a small fraction of this amount by regulators; this leaves enforcement of the contract up to the prowess of the providers' management and information technology.[7]

Contract management systems, whether integrated or added on to the PMS, are the provider's defense against these errors. If the PMS knows how much the payor is supposed to reimburse for a given procedure, it can alert the provider to underpayments, either individually or systematically. Underpayments of a few dollars are the most insidious, as the cost of reprocessing the claim will exceed the difference collected. This is why tracking underpayments over time is essential, allowing for underpayments to be addressed in bulk.

Full-featured practice management systems provide many more features and functions. Some provide scanning and document management capabilities. Some manage paper charts in ways analogous to a hospital HIM system. And some have sophisticated materials management capabilities that are particularly important in specialties where expensive medications or equipment are used.

One final critical feature to any PMS is reporting. The biggest payoff to any information system comes from the ability to extract and manipulate data that has been entered during the routine course of business. Cheaper systems come with pre-configured reports and few tools to manipulate them. More sophisticated systems provide myriad options for extracting data and configuring reports.

Clinical Systems and Biomedical Devices

The distinction between clinical systems and biomedical devices is becoming both difficult to make and less important. Traditionally, the line between them was apparent—devices were typically electro-mechanical, diagnostic and procedure oriented. From an IT perspective, they were data sources. Perhaps the most important distinction was that biomedical devices were regulated by the FDA. Any changes to their function required recertification. Conversely, information systems were electronic, transaction and documentation-oriented and unregulated in their plasticity.

While some of these distinctions still hold today, their importance is increasingly moot. Clinically, it is completely natural that the systems a cardiologist or radiologist use to make a diagnosis should be fully integrated with the systems they use to report their findings. Similarly, from a patient's perspective, the test report is no less part of their medical chart than the note of the physician who ordered the test or procedure.

It is not surprising, therefore, that the marketplace for these once separate entities is now merging. The leading manufacturers of biomedical devices like GE and Siemens are now also leading vendors of electronic medical records.

That said, this chapter will not examine further traditional, "know one when I see one," biomedical devices like EKG and x-ray machines, regardless of how proximal they may have become to clinical systems. One reason for this is that they are still purchased and managed differently in most institutions. But more important, biomedical devices do not fit as cleanly into the major thesis of this section. That is, clinical systems are the essential *workflow* managers of ambulatory medicine—or, at least, they should be.

The reason to emphasize workflow is that it is the key to success for executives who need to purchase, implement and manage these systems. A brief history of clinical systems shows that this was not always the case. Many, if not most, clinical systems on the market today reveal a *modular* orientation that reflects how their development was funded similar to any well thought-out technical architecture.

A VERY BRIEF HISTORY OF THE AEHR

The first attempts to build electronic medical records were largely in the outpatient arena. Barnett's landmark work in the 1960 with COSTAR[8] emphasized increasing the availability and organization of medical records. Separate modules for registration, scheduling and the actual clinical encounter form were implemented.

In the 1970s, McDonald at Regenstrief, as well as Stead and Hammond at Duke, developed outpatient medical record systems.[9,10] The Regenstrief system also used encounter form data input similar to COSTAR, but pioneered the emphasis on automated reminders. Stead and Hammond's "TMR" system actually attempted to go paperless, using clerks to enter data.

Throughout the 1970s and 1980s, technology became more affordable and adequate to the task of building medical records. Computers moved from mainframes to mini-computers in the 1970s, and from mini-computers to micro-computers in the 1980s. At this time, you may recall, most medical centers were organized in a very decentralized manner. Outside the institutions, independent practitioners and small groups were still the norm. Therefore it is not surprising that the medical record systems that developed reflected this departmental and practice-oriented organization. When graphical programming and database management tools became ubiquitous in the 1990s, these forces of "dis-integration" were even more profound. Commercial systems were specialty-focused, procedure-oriented and doctor-centric.

Large institutions were installing more centralized systems in hospitals but, even there, the industry was moving toward decentralized client-server designs. The sales teams advocated "best-of-breed"—as much a justification for the way things were as for any nobler architectural reason.

What resulted is the situation most institutions and practices are in right now. Every business unit or clinically-distinct entity has (or wants) their own information system that meets their needs. There are significant merits to this approach. Many niche systems do, in fact, meet the workflow requirements of any given specialty much better than general purpose systems that are "customized" for their environment. The needs of a cardiology practice offering echocardiography and cardiac graphics are quite distinct from gastroenterologists offering in-office endoscopy—though both are sub-specialties of Internal Medicine. Venture into radiation oncology, physiatry, ophthalmology or almost any other common outpatient medical specialty and you will find radically different functional requirements, workflows and expectations.

ORDER ENTRY AND RESULTS REPORTING

This challenge of sub-specialization exemplifies perhaps the most fundamental strategic IT choice facing an executive who manages clinical systems—the choice between an aggregation of interfaced best-of-breed systems versus a monolithic system. If each subspecialty can have a better system for themselves if they purchase separately, is the total greater or less than the sum of the parts? Does a unified platform offer economies of scale and degrees of interoperability not feasible with multiple interfaced systems? Interestingly, it is the very same debate managers faced ten to twenty years ago, but at an even less granular level. Time was when order entry and results reporting systems were separate. And in many ambulatory practices, this remains true today.

The earliest and most basic clinical systems were result reporting systems that allowed viewing of the output of laboratory and other biomedical devices. Lab data are typically numeric and *relatively* easy to categorize and display. Textual results, such as pathology and radiology results, were also fairly analogous to other data routinely managed by early business computers. Graphical results and images arrived later with the more powerful hardware and software required to support these modalities.

Typically absent from simple result reporting systems is any facility for data *entry*. The user interface characteristics required for data entry and data display are radically different, the former being far more challenging. Early "monolithic" systems had a relatively modest goal of unifying all the entered data into a single repository, while specialized data entry systems were permitted in departmental silos.[11]

More recently, due to the economic power of the physician's pen, many hospitals have focused on order entry systems as the centerpiece of their clinical systems efforts.[12,13] In the ambulatory world, order entry can be a small or insignificant component of the workflow in some specialties. Further, the economic imperatives are very different in the outpatient world and the return on investment from an order entry system may be harder to realize than at a hospital. That said, ambulatory order entry is still a big business. Many laboratories will give physicians a results reporting system if they will use their on-line order entry system. The laboratory gains efficiencies, but they still have to give the physician an incentive to use a potentially less convenient system than paper. In large institutions and practices, order entry systems can be very helpful in controlling the flow of referrals. Order entry systems are all but essential in ambulatory practices under capitation in order to control utilization.

Evidence suggests that ambulatory CPOE can be time neutral to physicians, but not all order entry systems are created equal.[14] The minimal systems, some of which are now free, just write prescriptions. For specialists that prescribe a lot of medications, comprehensive support for refills including aging and reminders can be a major time saver and are frequently the first clinical systems installed. Prescriptions are different from inpatient orders in several respects. The ability to print prescriptions in locally mandated formats is not to be assumed. Inpatient systems also generally have limited formularies, whereas outpatient systems generally need all available drugs. Worse still, in managed care environments, ambulatory systems often have to maintain multiple formularies and distinguish between drugs that are on and off plan. Medicare Part D has made this function almost essential, and yet almost universally unsupported as of this writing.

Inpatient systems tend to be more focused on drips and compound preparations. These exist in the outpatient world (e.g., in oncology infusion centers). Such sites need the full medication administration record (MAR) functionality common to inpatient systems. But they are certainly less common and typically less complex than in the inpatient setting. Conversely, ambulatory centers that do dispense drugs often do so without a pharmacist as intermediary. This means that the system must support the functions pharmacists provide. For example, when a sample is given, the system must produce a label with instructions for the patient and log the lot number of the drugs dispensed.

E-prescribing, the transmission of prescriptions electronically, is getting a great deal of attention lately. As of this writing, such systems are more demonstration projects than mainstream practice. Most pharmacies still lack either the systems to support receiving such prescriptions or the systems have not been modified to reliably process the prescription when it arrives. To really work well, such systems require bi-directional communication that requires reconciliation of currently incompatible standards between pharmacy and physician systems. As a result, some systems resort to faxing behind the scenes—a procedure that is fraught with security and privacy problems. Still, this is clearly the wave of the future and executives would be remiss in not planning for this capability.

Similarly, prescription fill information is becoming available electronically from payors. This technology has the potential to dramatically alter physicians' ability to influence patient compliance. However, because ambulatory patients administer their own individual doses and may not submit claims for every prescription filled, the reconciliation of fill data with the original prescription is problematic at best. The potential of this capability to improve care is large.

For laboratory orders, key features in an ambulatory environment again differ from the inpatient world. Most hospitals send all their lab specimens to one laboratory. This may be desirable in the outpatient world, but managed care contracts often mandate the use of a particular lab. The ability to control default routing rules based on contracts is a vital revenue control point for sites that maintain their own laboratory.

True integration with multiple laboratories is technically very challenging but it is also very desirable for many reasons. If the outbound order and the incoming result are linked, known in jargon as "loop closure," then there is more potential for sophisticated features like alerts and reports. For example, a common cause of malpractice claims is the failure to note an abnormal Pap result. Systems with loop closure can alert a physician both to the arrival of an abnormal result and the *failure* of any result to return after a specified time, diminishing the risk of lost data.

The most difficult aspect of linking to multiple labs is reconciling the coding systems for the orders and the results. As of this writing, there is no satisfactory coding system for either orders or results; those that do exist are poorly cross-mapped. CPT® is often used when placing orders, but it is too imprecise and incomplete to be used exclusively. Similarly, LOINC® is emerging as a standard for coding results, but it is also very incomplete and idiosyncratically applied. Certain areas, such as microbiology and transfusion medicine, remain particularly problematic. The National Library of Medicine is presently funding an effort to map CPT and LOINC. While this will help, the fact remains that operations managers faced with multiple laboratories need to commit considerable resources to mapping if they want results to line up across reporting agencies and want to pursue perfect loop closure.

The ability to configure order sets in ambulatory systems is not dissimilar to inpatient order entry systems. Likewise, clinical decision support rules have similar value in both settings. In the outpatient world, there is the additional uncertainty of knowing all medications a patient is taking. This is a topic of considerable conflict in organizations with shared charts. Some specialists object to seeing the full list of medications in their chart fearing responsibility for drugs they do not prescribe. Of course, this is an issue of legal liability, not medical care. But it can require system managers to jump configuration hurdles before specialists will buy in to a common EHR.

Regulatory agencies have jumped into this debate with recent mandates for "medication reconciliation." The Joint Commission on Accreditation of Healthcare Organizations (JCAHO) made this one of its national patient safety goals in 2005.[15] They require that at transitions of care, providers exchange a complete list of the patient's medications. They explicitly include discharge to ambulatory settings. A shared electronic medical record should make this process easier, if not automatic, with the record itself. But the pass-off between EHRs will require a substantial improvement in the state-of-art interfacing technologies. While technically feasible, few systems support this kind of automated reconciliation today. JCAHO based their recommendation on staffing and process models from the inpatient world[16] and the practicality of implementing their ideas outside of hospitals was obviously not considered given the aggressive timetable of their goals and the state of the AEHR.

Analogous to DRG reimbursement in inpatient settings, one of the more complex features in ambulatory order entry is "medical necessity" checking. The quotation marks here are to emphasize that the definition of medical necessity is an insurance construct, not a clinical assessment, per se. The primary impetus for this requirement comes from Medicare. Through a process called National and Local Coverage Determinations (NCD/LCD—previously called Local Medical Review Policies or LMRP), Medicare will only reimburse for tests that it deems medically necessary.[17] Because these rules frequently do not meet the needs of individual patients, physicians need to be alerted when they are ordering a test that is not covered. For example, I recently had a patient with cancer who needed heart tests prior to taking a cardiotoxic drug. It would be clinical malpractice *not* to perform the test but it was not considered "medically necessary" from a financial standpoint.

There are two major reasons to generate NCD/LCD alerts. The first is the intended effect of the regulation: to draw attention to the physician that the test or drug may not be clinically indicated and an alternative should be sought. The second reason is to alert both patient and provider that charges will go unpaid by the carrier. For providers, particularly laboratory and radiology facilities, this can be a key source of uncollected debt. The ordering provider should give the patient an ABN (Advanced Beneficiary

Notice) that alerts the patient how much they are likely to be charged for what the payor may deem unnecessary.

The process for documenting medical necessity is fairly crude. The diagnostic code (typically ICD-9) the physician associates with the order (typically coded by CPT®) either matches an approved list designed by the NCD/LCD or not. Practices that are very focused on downstream revenue may seek even more sophisticated alerts to question providers who order tests with codes that they may incorrectly be using as "rule outs," rather than using symptom codes. This is presently at the boundary of commercial system functionality.

The last major category of order entry functionality is referrals. These are similar to inpatient consult orders but are a great deal more complex due to third party reimbursement rules and geographic variation inherent to outpatient care. In many managed care plans, the ordering provider is supposed to solicit an eligibility and pre-approval code before sending a patient to another specialist. Some systems automate this process to an extent, but the rules and documentation requirements are quite variable making it potentially difficult for any system to fully automate this process. If providers find themselves or their staff spending hours soliciting these approvals, executives would be wise to spend as much time re-negotiating contracts to simplify and standardize these procedures versus trying to get the IT staff to automate a chaotic process.

In an ideal patient experience, the referrals can be linked to the scheduling process. This is quite plausible if the order entry system is integrated with the scheduling system and the payor rules allow for such simplification. In reality, this kind of service is most likely to be found only in highly-integrated care delivery systems, regardless of their IT infrastructure.

DOCUMENTATION

While results reporting and order entry remain the core of many electronic medical records, the key to the ambulatory medical record is documentation, particularly from physicians. This is the most technically difficult challenge for any medical record system for several reasons. The major challenges in medical informatics generally come together in physician documentation. User interface design, workflow management, structured vocabulary, database performance and hardware limitations are all major limiting factors to what we can practically deliver to support the most elemental component of medical care—the doctor-patient interaction.

As with results reporting and order entry efforts already discussed, the first efforts to automate physician documentation were modular. Specific attempts to capture a progress note, a procedure note, a Subjective-Objective-Assessment-Plan (SOAP) note or a flow sheet have all had varying degrees of success. The simplicity of scribbling pen on paper exceeds any EHR, though an EHR can provide legibility, standardized practice, ubiquitous access, and clinical decision support.

There is a profound and complex number of nuanced features that need to be added together to build a fully functioning ambulatory documentation system. Not all of these features are needed for every practice or every specialty. Nevertheless, they may be essential to even a single physician in a group; failure to accommodate the requirement may eliminate the ability to automate that physician in the EMR. This is a key point that is lost on many IT managers and is worth exploring.

There is a difference between essential and non-essential "customization." Detailing the many essential and optional functionality offerings in ambulatory systems is beyond the scope of this chapter. More comprehensive lists are readily available elsewhere.[18,19]

Some of the features that illustrate the difference between critical and extraneous customization vary by specialty or setting: Drawing is a basic element of some physician documentation (e.g., ophthalmology) that is completely absent in some specialties. Similarly photography is essential in plastic surgery but optional in most general internal medicine practices. Flow sheets are the primary method of documenting in some specialties, particularly those with repeated visits over a finite period of time (e.g., obstetrics) or in practices focused on a particular disease or procedure (e.g., diabetes or dialysis.) Many "disease management" systems focus on this kind of documentation. Some practices have extensive forms completion requirements (e.g., general pediatrics or practices with heavy managed care oversight like cognitive psychology.) Similarly, specialists who do procedures have very different documentation requirements than those doing evaluation and management. In academia, the ability to extract data generated at the point-of-care into research databases is critical to the research mission over and above immediate clinical needs. Consultation-heavy practices require robust correspondence support. Any practice with a wide referral base outside the EHR user base will require a scanning system to handle paper brought into the office; practices that are completely self-contained will have little need for this feature. Practices using physician extenders or supervising residents and students will have complex co-signature requirements.

These kinds of features differentiate systems that can succeed in particular practices and specialties from those that might actually harm productivity by forcing the implementation of a parallel system that works around the oversights. The challenge for the executive is to differentiate these essential business functions from optional features that may slow down implementation and run up costs.

The key to understanding which features provide value and which do not is to examine workflow. This is where systems that deliver functionality in modules reach their limits. All the features in the world can be present in a system. If they do not hang together for the users in a manner that flows logically within real world use, then the system may cause more harm than good. The Certification Commission for Healthcare Information and Technology (CCHIT) has published certification requirements that detail the functionality and AEHR should achieve.[20] But these requirements say nothing about how the functions work together to achieve a manageable workflow. The Apple Newton introduced amazing new functionality, but was practically unusable so it failed in the marketplace. The unwritten requirement is that all these functions must work for the physician without slowing him or her down or compromising his or her sanity.

EMR enthusiasts try to sell these inherently inefficient modular systems by emphasizing the myriad benefits that occur downstream once the initial penalty is paid. These downstream benefits are real and profound. They start with simple legibility, simplified filing and access, and the ability to use one data entry point for multiple purposes, such as a progress note and a consultation letter.

These benefits are the essential foundation upon which most present office automation efforts are currently justified. But executives looking for ambulatory solutions today need not stop there. The greatest potential of these systems comes when they can predict where the user will go next and lead the provider through the visit. This is exactly the opposite of a modular system where the provider may have to disrupt the workflow to search for different functions.

This is beyond the current state of the art in commercial clinical systems. Still, it is where today's executive should be looking when deciding what is needed.[21] Workflow analysis quickly leads to the recognition that system integration is required to make sure data flows in a coordinated manner to work.

Through the examination of workflow, four key functions of clinical systems that go beyond any individual module are revealed as essential to the system architecture; messaging, interfaces, decision support and patient data entry.

MESSAGING

Messaging could, perhaps, be viewed as a module itself. Indeed, if a practice had limited funding, the cheapest and easiest system to implement to increase efficiency would be an instant messaging system. But within a full featured EMR, clinical messaging can become the central task management tool of a practice. The key difference is the ability to route a message within the context of a patient's chart. This context extends the physician's capacity to utilize support staff freeing the physician for more productive work. Leading products categorize messages into multiple queues such as new results, orders awaiting co-signature, messages from colleagues and even personal notes about tee times. Messages can go to multiple staff at once, work down a queue or be rerouted during vacations or for on-call coverage.

Some systems clearly separate messaging from Task Management. In larger practices, this is probably wise. As the physician workflow progresses along the patient encounter, a variety of tasks queue for the ancillary staff such as rooming and taking vitals, drawing blood and processing referrals. How elegantly these processes are integrated with the system will dictate the success of managing the entire practice workflow rather than just isolated pieces of it.

Secure messaging is generally inherent within a given EHR. Communicating between EHRs and over the Internet generally requires different technology that is lacking from most existing systems. This is likely to become more integrated given the HIPPA mandate all providers face.

INTERFACES

Interfaces are the glue between modules of non-integrated systems and the mechanism for sharing data across entirely dissimilar systems. The richness and complexity of interfaces is more than enough of a topic for a whole book in itself. But the key points executives need to understand about interfaces in ambulatory systems relate to what interfaces can and cannot accomplish.

A purely stand-alone system requires no interfaces. Such systems are not uncommon in a small ambulatory setting, though they are quite limited in functionality. We have already reviewed the key administrative interfaces required for practice management. Electronic linkages to insurance companies are mandated by HIPAA so the era of stand-alone systems is clearly coming to a close.

Early efforts at interfaces were so-called point-to-point custom interfaces that required coding far too extensive for all but the largest ambulatory providers. In 1979, the American National Standards Institute (ANSI) charted the Accredited Standards Committee (ASC) X12 "to develop uniform standards for inter-industry electronic interchange of business transactions – electronic data interface (EDI)." In the past 25 years, that body has developed more that 300 business-to-business transaction sets.[2]

In the late 1980s, healthcare joined the EDI standardization process with the creation of HL7 (Health Level 7), a set of semantic standards for exchanging data between healthcare information systems. HL7 was accredited by ANSI in 1994.[23] These standards define many of the key transactions that are necessary to implement clinical and practice management systems. Besides the basic insurance transactions, ambulatory systems are not practical in most instances without laboratory and radiology results feeds, and typically, ADT/Registration, scheduling, orders, transcriptions and pharmacy interfaces. Other common interfaces include a wide variety of diagnostic devices such as endoscopes, spirometers, EKG systems and similar equipment associated to individual specialties.

Anyone attending to practice workflow quickly realizes that more and better interfaces are critical to physician efficiency.[24] And, just as quickly, the deficiencies of current interface standards are revealed. The problems are not dissimilar from those faced in inpatient settings, but the emphasis is typically different.

The first problem is the need for multiple interfaces itself. Interfaces are rarely "plug and play" and even once implemented, they generate error queues and exceptions that require policies, procedures, and staff resources to handle. In a large healthcare system, an interface group may be dedicated to these issues. In a small ambulatory practice, this is often impossible and the errors either will go uncorrected or the interface is eliminated.

Ambulatory practices within larger institutions face a related problem of scale. While large IT shops may have the staff to handle implementation and error queues, the priorities of integrating a single obscure medical device may be quite low compared to a new laboratory feed for the whole hospital. But without that device, the single physician or practice cannot do their job. For example, it may be easier for a whole hospital to do without an interface to a spirometer than for an allergist or pulmonologist in their private office.

The problem rests in the interfaces themselves. As mentioned above, HL7 is primarily a *semantic* standard. It dictates what the message means, not how it is said. There are two problems left unsolved. First, the semantic standards are quite limited. HL7 covers the basics only, and even there, enormous flexibility remains such that two vendor systems can both be "compliant" and not be able to understand one another. Second, HL7 does not standardize how messages are sent. This is called *syntax*. Luckily, a new day is rapidly emerging due to the advent of a widespread syntactic standard called, XML, which HL7 is integrating into its new standards.[25]

Presently, a debate is raging about the best way to combine semantic and syntactic standards. This has tremendous relevance to executives interested in ambulatory systems. The key argument is between advocates of comprehensive detail versus ubiquitous simplicity. It is not completely unfair to characterize this as a battle between the haves and the have-nots.

Those who have wide-ranging systems with rich feature sets need comprehensive standards to move data between systems. Some of the features lay people desire or even expect from clinical systems require extremely advanced interfacing techniques. Consider the perfectly reasonable expectation that a patient's laboratory results or medication list should be able to move from physician to physician. To do this without any loss of information would require that we agree to use far more sophisticated semantic standards that include vocabularies for lab tests and medications. As mentioned above, vocabularies like LOINC® and RxNorm system are not comprehensive or adaptable enough for use in all settings. Even if they were widely adopted, local customizations would be the norm adding even more complexity to the interfaces.[26]

Those who have fewer resources or are just trying to get into the game are willing to settle for far simpler standards. For example, the ASTM CCR[27] (Continuity of Care Record) which has been embraced by the American Academy of Family Physicians, takes a "snapshot" of patients at transitions of care in an XML document standard. Semantic details are optional allowing for the basic transmission of information that advocates call good enough and critics view as the lowest common denominator. AAFP's first criterion for EHR-related activities is "affordability." They are also articulate in advocating plug and play compatibility and avoiding "vendor lock."[28] This is largely in reaction to what many perceive as the opposite tendency in the HL7 standard. Ironically, while some consider HL7's complexity specifically designed to serve vendor interests, many vendors themselves set up their own advocacy group separate of HL7 in 2004; their group, the HIMSS Electronic Health Record Vendor Association (EHRVA) was set up with promotion of "extensibility to other document types and discrete data" as an explicit goal.[29]

This debate has serious long term importance to any executives overseeing ambulatory systems in the coming decade. Support for CCR is very easy to achieve, but most vendors have not given their support as they haven't been asked to give it. Most vendors do support various aspects of HL7; exactly which aspects—and whether or not they will meet individual needs—requires fairly close scrutiny.

A relatively new HL7 standard, called the Clinical Context Object Workgroup or CCOW, has significant promise for ambulatory centers in that it can help avoid other costly interfaces altogether. CCOW is a standard for flipping between different applications without requiring a new logon and even carrying the existing patient context. Therefore, a user can move from a laboratory results reporting system to a documentation or order entry system with a few clicks. The actual data stays in each system and cannot flow between them without building specific interfaces. But for sites that lack the resources to deal with all the complexity just described, CCOW may offer enough of the illusion of integration that physicians can still get their work done.

DECISION SUPPORT

Most modern clinical systems have some form of rules and alerts engine to improve quality, revenue and compliance. The extent to which data flows across modules dictates the sophistication possible in the delivery of alerts. The simplest systems are passive and post-hoc. They take data already created and analyze it in batch form, generating reports or messages to be responded to after the fact. Such systems remain important today as we will always want to look backwards or across encounters for such diverse reasons as drug recalls or auditing.

Modern systems also allow for real time alerts that can actively modify how care is delivered. A modest amount of research has demonstrated or suggested the efficacy of computerized alerts in improving a variety of quality measures such as vaccination and screening tests,[30,31] reducing over-utilization,[32,33] and avoiding adverse events.[34,35] Serious issues remain, however, that executives need to resolve as this technology is pursued in the future. For example, overwhelming physicians with too many alerts can be counter productive.[36] Too little research has been done on the relevancy of alerts in sub-specialties and in patients with complex co-morbidities. And the maintenance of the knowledge base that drives complex alerts is costly and potentially dangerous if not done correctly.[37]

For ambulatory systems managers, a good starting point is whatever alerts can be purchased in a subscription form so that the knowledge base is easy to maintain. Drug interactions, medical necessity rules and formulary lists are some examples of commercially available rule sets. Even some of these will require configuration resources to work optimally. For example, drug-disease interactions will require that problems and lab results are coded in a particular way that the rules engine can detect.

Another area to investigate is whatever pay-for-performance guidelines providers are subject to in your practice. Another chapter in this book expands on quality issues in greater detail. A few points regarding ambulatory systems are worth reiterating here. First, payors are evaluating "performance" primarily based on claims data. These data are fraught with peril.

In two recent samples at our institution, data from the payors was found to be incorrect for more than 90% of the patients. Because payors are cutting reimbursements and tiering physicians based on these data, the ability to analyze your actual performance may become critical to maintaining revenue. Such analyses can be quite difficult unless you have highly structured data and excellent documentation compliance from your providers.

Consider the following typical ambulatory quality metrics:

1. Percentage of patients with congestive heart failure currently taking an angiotensin converting enzyme inhibitor (ACEI) or angiotensin receptor blocker (ARB).
2. Percentage of diabetics with a glycohemoglobin measurement within the past six months.
3. Percentage of hypertensive patients with an ophthalmology exam within the past year.
4. Patients over the age of sixty-five with pneumococcal vaccination.

Performance on all four metrics could be improved with an alert to the provider at the point-of-care. Further, it is not at all unlikely that one patient could trigger all four alerts so making it easier for the provider to comply rather than to ignore the alert is a real issue. This presents the system manager several technical challenges. First, all the diagnoses need to be coded with sufficient specificity that the correct patients are identified. Second, the laboratory, medication, vaccination and ordering data need to be available in a form that includes and excludes the correct patients. Do you want providers to have to slow down and explain to the computer why a particular patient with a particular potassium or renal condition should not get an ARB? If the insurance company is going to make the physician say so then it is probably worth the effort. If not, it is probably worth coding this out of the alert. Does your system capture enough data from events outside your practice to reliably know if a patient did or did not see the ophthalmologist?

In many instances, payors have access to a broader set of data than the physician caring for the patient. They also may be missing data that doctors would like to know is missing—such as the failure to fill the prescription for the ARB or breaking the ophthalmology appointment.

At this time, few systems can respond to all the issues raised by pay for performance and quality management initiatives. So, once again, the best the executive can do is learn about the technical issues involved and plan for the optimal combination of solutions for your practice.

PATIENT DATA ENTRY

The final workflow optimizing technology to discuss is patient data entry (PDE). Here again, separate modules may exist to give patients questionnaires, allow them to sign consents and authorizations online, or even conduct clinical interviews. But once this technology is integrated into the full EHR the power to radically alter physician workflow becomes apparent.

If a patient can fill out their complaints, family, social and past medical history, and review of systems online prior to meeting with the physician, several positive consequences will result. Computerized interviews provide more data, allow for the asking of more sensitive questions, give patients more time to answer, can be adapted for language, hearing impairments and education level, and when fed into the EMR, it can lower the amount of time physicians spend documenting.[38] Further, by obtaining structured data before the patient is seen, these systems provide clues the computer needs to present physicians with the most appropriate content and structure for their own workflow.

While these systems are still at the bleeding edge of clinical computing today, the very first computer applications for medicine, a half century ago, were patient interviewing tools.[39,40] Clearly the goals of those systems remain compelling. Today's managers, however, still need to decide individually when the technology will be developed enough to add value ready for their practice.

INFRASTRUCTURE

The infrastructure issues for ambulatory systems are also similar to inpatient systems, but different in emphasis. The scale of ambulatory systems varies from single physician offices to large multi-state groups with thousands of providers. Obviously very different technologies are needed to serve these different constituencies.

Regardless of size, one of the most fundamental questions that needs to be answered early is the degree that integration is desired in technology and content. Some vendors provide a centralized platform from which huge numbers of users can share a common chart over large geographical distances. Others distribute the systems often replicating the chart in multiple locations if content needs to be shared. Smart, well-intentioned people can argue the pros and cons of this and a thousand other architectural differences. The key to getting the right solution for your organization is, once again, workflow.

If you know how your organization works (or should work,) you can find the right system. If you share a medical record number across disparate sites, then chances are you need some kind of centralized system for keeping them in sync. If not, then you do not need to solve this problem, unless you want to share other data. If you have a lot of remote rural sites with variable networking infrastructures, then a system that relies on high bandwidth connectivity is off the table. Conversely, if you are in an urban environment with immense radio interference issues, a system that relies on a crowded wireless network band may not be advisable. If workstation conflicts, horsepower and management are issues, a thin client architecture may be appealing. In settings without the necessary IT staff, however, this may add complexity rather than reduce it.

Supportability and reliability are other key issues that differ in the ambulatory world. Ask yourself the impact of the loss of a single computer to a busy outpatient center without technical support for 24 or 48 hours. Is that acceptable? Can you afford a shorter time frame? Downtime happens, by accident or design. Does your system provide you with the back-up tools to get by for an hour, a day, a week?

Conversely, diffuse geography may put you at the mercy of an unreliable Internet provider or ASP. In that case, your workflow may be forced to accommodate idiosyncratic infrastructure rather than vice versa.

Interoperability with inpatient records varies in importance by practice and specialty. Security and privacy issues similarly may differ according to the interoperability of the workflow both locally (e.g., nurse and doctor charting on the same patient in the same room) and regionally (e.g., sub-specialty referrals across a multi-entity organization).

Earlier, the monolithic versus best-of-breed decision was referenced as well as repository-based architectures. A related dimension to consider is the segregation of transactional and reporting systems. The system that supports day-to-day operations needs to be oriented toward high speed, single patient transactions. Reporting systems generally look across patients and do not require sub-second response times. Therefore, these jobs are often separated into two separate systems.

A detailed discussion of infrastructure is beyond the scope of this chapter. But one rule of thumb to keep in mind is that while it may seem expensive, infrastructure is rarely a good place to skimp. Hardware is often the cheapest way to hide the inadequacies of software. But this is only true if you focus on the real bottlenecks as opposed to technical fashion. A final example illustrates this point. A good manager will push back on a simultaneous request for "wireless networks" and "100G to the desktop." If real work can be done at wireless speeds, why do you also need wired speeds two orders of magnitude faster? When selecting infrastructure components, plan for the future but be realistic about the speed of change your institution can handle so you do not waste money on capacity you will not use before it is obsolete.

COSTS AND RETURN ON INVESTMENT

While data is spotty and inconsistent, it is generally accepted that most physician practices now have some form of information technology but that very few have even close to a full EHR.[41,42] Not surprisingly, practice management systems have far greater market penetration than purely clinical systems. As discussed above, PMSs provide a direct impact on revenue and cost control. The value of purely clinical ambulatory systems is often more abstract or delayed. Chismar and colleagues have presented an economic model of EMR adoption that illustrates how larger entities like payors and hospitals gain more quickly from EHRs than small providers.[43] Scrutiny of other models that show benefit from EMRs also reveal that system benefits are greater than those to the individual physician.[44,45] That doesn't mean the value is not present, but given the large start up costs, physicians are poorly incented to adopt systems that benefit others more than themselves yet cost them more than the prime beneficiaries.

At a very high level, the value of the EHR to society is potentially huge.[46] Enhanced quality, better outcomes, an improved patient experience, and lower total costs are all great. But should the individual doctor or practice foot the bill? There are plenty of other barriers to adoption of EMRs, including physician resistance to change, concerns about productivity, the complexity of installation and conversion of existing paper medical records (see Figure 5-3).[47,48]

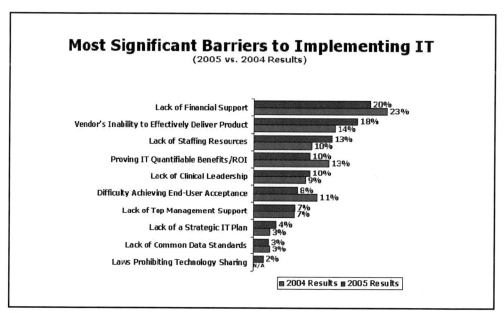

Figure 5-3: Most Significant Barriers to Implementing IT.

Recent proposals to address the financial concerns would still leave other barriers that should be considered by more thorough ROI analyses.[49] Doctors care about money. They also care about quality, time, convenience, regulatory compliance and a host of other issues that must all be taken into account to truly calculate ROI. This is, of course, not feasible and the inadequacy of the literature to date reflects that point.

For example, some studies show ROI by reducing duplicate orders.[33] Under capitation that is valid, but your revenue might fall under fee-for-service. At our center, we recovered millions of dollars of revenue that was going to outside providers that our EHR very gently pointed back inside. The cost was borne by our doctors and the benefit accrued by our hospital. From a business perspective, this is a big win for the medical center but it will not show up in academic studies of ROI. This is because from society's perspective, this was just a cost shift, not a real reduction in the total cost of healthcare.

Other studies have shown return from up-coding and the converse is also touted as a benefit by improving regulatory compliance.[50] Other financial benefits include reduced transcription costs, reduced chart pulls, decreased charge posting costs, pay for performance and various other efficiencies.

Critics of these studies abound.[51] It is difficult to accurately account for the costs of implementation. Once live, there are hidden costs rarely accounted for in any analysis. Dealing with temporary employees is far more complex in an automated environment where training is more complicated and less intuitive than in the paper world. Conversely, benefits like integrated access to reference materials or sophisticated reporting capabilities are extremely difficult to assign value to in a finite period of time. Even the cost of the software itself is hard to standardize and is almost always overemphasized as a cost relative to the much higher intangible costs such as disruption, morale effects and functional losses from system deficiencies.

Ultimately the value of the EHR needs to be judged like that of an elevator in a skyscraper; it has become an essential tool of the trade.[52] Too few ROI analyses ask what the ROI is of the analysis itself. Like the word processor and the typewriter, e-mail and the fax machine, or cars and horses, the EHR will come and will transform ambulatory care. Today's executives need to manage the change, not predict it.

That said, predicting the future direction of the ambulatory EHR industry is relevant. Vendors still rapidly come and go. The technology is evolving rapidly. What you buy today will be obsolete soon. Expect it and plan accordingly. Assume your vendor will change so protect your data and your investment in the knowledge it took to automate your practice. As a rule of thumb, only 20% of an implementation costs are vendor fees. Not all of the remaining 80% is lost if you need to change vendors. Wise process redesign will deliver value now and in the future with one system and the next. The delayed returns from automation will also translate from one system to the next as they come from the EHR technology itself, and not from any given brand.

The current round of vendor consolidation is marketed as a chance to increase interoperability, particularly with the biomedical devices made by the large conglomerates buying EHR vendors. But we may also see dramatic reductions in serviceability if these vendors oversimplify and cut the wrong costs. Will their size and oligopoly power destroy innovation? Consider the conflicting incentives facing just one vendor with multiple product lines and seemingly competing interests. Will a vendor that sells MRIs and EHRs support an EHR to help reduce the over-utilization of expensive MRIs, a business with far more profit than software? Large HIT software vendors are also employers who need to control medical insurance costs. Interoperability with competitors would reduce healthcare expenditures but might cause loss of market share. How large HIT vendors balance their own internal conflicts could have as much an impact on the future of the industry as technology itself.

The technology is also hard to predict. The big problems facing informatics for the past 30 years have not fundamentally changed. The nature of the human-machine interface, the physical limits of hardware, and the complexity of medical vocabulary are still problems today. The expansion of the EHR outside academia only adds new problems of scale, configurability, flexibility, complexity, control and ever lower fault tolerance.

The next generation EHR, evolving today, is focused on integration, standards, ubiquity, mobility, reliability, quality, outcomes and of course, workflow. Dangers to look out for include over simplification, information overload, alert fatigue, over dependence and depersonalization. The next generation of ambulatory care is also emerging today full of potential opportunities and dangers. And as a key part of that future, the ambulatory electronic health record is surely both an opportunity and a danger.

FREQUENTLY ASKED QUESTIONS

Q: *My consultants and vendor advise me to "keep it vanilla" to stay on time and under budget, but my doctors all demand customizations that sound clinically reasonable. How do I balance these conflicting demands?*

A: Customization is often the most difficult management challenge of an implementation. If you want a single EHR to span diverse specialties, then you will have to customize to some extent—unless you are comfortable having ophthalmologists and cardiologists reduced to a lowest common denominator, which is unlikely to result in high quality care. Conversely, yielding completely to subspecialty customization can defeat the purpose of unifying the patient record and indulge wasteful, often dangerous intra-specialty variation that high quality institutions are trying to reduce. There is no easy answer and the answer will change as both computer technology and medical expertise advance.

Q: *We can't afford to build custom templates for every sub-specialty workflow. The doctors currently dictate but some of the ROI for the EHR is supposed to come from eliminating transcription costs. Can we use voice recognition instead?*

A: Voice Recognition (VR) is perpetually three years away. Consider how the following sentence written silently might sound to a patient if it were spoken to VR instead: "The unkempt, malodorous, obese patient, appearing older than her stated age, complained of an old liver." Do you want to say this in front of her? Didn't she really complain of a cold shiver?

Even if accuracy was improved, voice recognition is still expensive and time consuming to set up, slow to navigate and requires time-consuming proofreading. In terms of long range ROI, it produces text, not structured documentation; the value of the data is lower, particularly in systems that otherwise offer advanced features like alerts, coding assistance and complex reporting. Still, many physicians are accustomed to dictating their notes and, for physicians who cannot type, this can be a tempting intermediate step toward a more complete EHR. Doctors who are not facile with computers will struggle just as much with voice recognition as they would a conventional

EHR. So the applications are still limited. For users with upper extremity disabilities, this technology may be essential.

REFERENCES

1. Carter JH, ed. *Electronic Health Records: A guide for clinicians and administrators.* American College of Physicians – American Society of Internal Medicine. Philadelphia; 2001.

2. Leavitt M. *Ambulatory Care: IT's Emerging and Growing Fast.* Dallas, TX: HIMSS Annual Conference; Feb 14, 2005. Available at: http://www.himss.org/content/files/2005proceedings/sessions/edu007.pdf. Accessed March 19, 2006.

3. Health Information and Management Systems Society Electronic Health Record Committee. HIMSS electronic health record definitional model version 1.1. Available at: http://www.himss.org/content/files/EHRAttributes.pdf. Accessed March 19, 2006.

4. Carpenter PC, Chute CG. *The Universal Patient Identifier: a Discussion and proposal: Proceedings of the Annual Symposium on Computer Applications in Medical Care*; 1993:49–53.

5. Electronic Privacy Information Center. Social security numbers. September 2004. Available at: www.epic.org/privacy/ssn. Accessed March 19, 2006.

6. Association of American Medical Colleges. Physicians at teaching hospitals audits. Available at: www.aamc.org /advocacy/library/ teachingphys/phys0040.htm Accessed March 12, 2006.

7. Zall RJ. The truth about managed care: the silent provider discount. *Managed Care Quarterly.* 2004;Winter;12(1):11–5.

8. Grossman JH , Barnett GO, Koespell TD. An automated medical record system. *JAMA.* 1973;263: 1114–20.

9. McDonald CJ, Overhage JM, Tierney WM, et al. The Regenstrief medical record system: a quarter century experience. *Int J Med Inf.* 1999;54:225–253.

10. Stead WW, Brame RG, Hammond WE, et al. A computerized obstetric medical record. *Obstet Gynecol.* 1977;April;49(4):502–9.

11. Clayton PD, Sideli RV, Sengupta S. Open architecture and integrated information at Columbia-Presbyterian Medical Center. *MD Computing.* 1992;September–October;9(5):297–303.

12. Ash JS, Gorman PN, Seshardri V, et al. Computerized physician order entry in U.S. hospitals: results of a 2002 survey. *J Am Med Inform Assoc.* 2004;11:95–99.

13. Cutler DM, Feldman NE & Horwitz JR. US adoption of computerized physician order entry systems. *Health Affairs.* 2005; November–December;24(6):1654–1663.

14. Overhage M, Perkins S, Tierney WM, McDonald CJ. Controlled trial of direct physician order entry: effects on physicians' time utilization in ambulatory primary care internal medicine practices. *J Am Med Inform Assoc.* 2001;8(4):361–371.

15. Joint Commission on Accreditation of Healthcare Organizations. 2007 national patient safety goals. Available at: http://www.jointcommission.org/PatientSafety/NationalPatientSafetyGoals. Accessed May 14, 2006.

16. Rozich JD Standardization as a mechanism to improve safety in health care. *JCJQS.* 2004;January;30(1): 5–14.

17. Centers for Medicare and Medicaid Services. Medicare Coverage Center. Available at: http://www.cms.hhs.gov/center/coverage.asp. Accessed March 18, 2006.

18. U.S. Department of Health and Human Services, Health Resources and Services Administration, Bureau of Primary Health Care. Functional requirements for electronic medical records and disease management systems. Available at: ftp://ftp.hrsa.gov/bphc/docs/2001pals/2001-13.pdf. Accessed November 25, 2006.

19. Drury B. Ambulatory EHR functionality: a comparison of functionality lists. *JHIM.* 2006;Winter;20(1): 61–70.

20. Certification Commission for Healthcare Information Technology. CCHIT final criteria: functionality for 2006 certification of ambulatory EHRs. Effective May 1, 2006. Available at: www.cchit.org. Accessed November 8, 2006.

21. East TD. The EHR paradox. *Frontiers of Health Series Management.* 2005;22(2):33-5.

22. Schrotter FE ASC X12 25th birthday celebration: 25 years of business to business accomplishments. Keynote Address; June 7, 2004; Chicago, Ill. http://public.ansi.org/ansionline/Documents/News%20and%20Publications/Speeches/X12-25th%20 Birthday%20Keynote%20-%20FINAL.pdf. Accessed March 19, 2006.

23. Health Level 7 Homepage. Available at: www.HL7.org. Accessed November 8, 2006.

24. Walker J, Pan E, Johnston D, et al. The Value of Health Care Information Exchange and Interoperability. *Health Affairs Web Exclusive,* January 19, 2005. Available at: http://content.healthaffairs.org/cgi/content/abstract/hlthaff.w5.10 Accessed March 18, 2006.

25. Mead CN. Data interchange standards in healthcare IT – computable semantic interoperability: now possible but still difficult. Do we really need a better mousetrap? *JHIM.* 2006;Winter;20(1):71–78.

26. National Library of Medicine. Unified medical language system. Available at: http://www.nlm.nih.gov/research/umls/rxnorm_main.html. Accessed March 18, 2006.

27. ASTM International. ASTM Committee E31 on Healthcare Informatics. Available at: http://www.astm.org/cgi-bin/SoftCart.exe/COMMIT/COMMITTEE/E31.htm?L+mystore+kprv3048. Accessed March 19, 2006.

28. AAFP Center for Health Information and Technology homepage. Available at: http://www.centerforhit.org/x174.xml. Accessed March 19, 2006.

29. Health Information and Management Systems Society. HIMSS electronic health record vendor association statements and positions. Available at: http://www.himssehrva.org/ASP/statements.asp. Accessed March 19, 2006.

30. McDonald CJ, Hui SL, Tierney WM. Effects of computer reminders for influenza vaccination on morbidity during influenza epidemics. *MD Computing.* 1992; 9:304–312.

31. Shea S, DuMouchel W, Bahamonde L. A meta-analysis of 16 randomized controlled trials to evaluate computer-based clinical reminder systems for preventive care in the ambulatory setting. *J AM Med Inform Assoc.* 1996;3(6):399–409.

32. Bates DW, Kuperman GJ, Rittenberg E, et al. A randomized trial of a computer-based intervention to reduce utilization of redundant laboratory tests. *Am J Med.*1999;106:144–150.

33. Harpole LH, Khorasani R, Fiskio J, et al. Automated evidence-based critiquing of orders for abdominal radiographs: impact on utilization and appropriateness. *J Am Med Inform Assoc.* 1997;4:511–521.

34. Gandhi TK, et al. Adverse drug events in ambulatory care. *NEJM.* 2003;April 17;348:1556–1564.

35. Gurwitz JH, et al. Incidence and preventability of adverse drug events among older persons in the ambulatory setting. *JAMA.* 2003;May 5;289:1107–1116.

36. Weingart SN, et al. Physicians' decisions to override computerized drug alerts in primary care. *Archives of Internal Medicine.* 2003;November 24;163:2625–2631.

37. Koppel R, Metlay JP, Abigail Cohen, et al. Role of computerized physician order entry systems in facilitating medication errors. *JAMA.* 2005; March 9;293:1197–1203.

38. Bachman JW. The patient-computer interview: a neglected tool that can aid the clinician. *Mayo Clin Proc.* 2003;January;78(1):67–78.

39. Brodman K, van Woerkom AK, Erdmann AJ Jr, Goldstein LS. Interpretation of symptoms with a data-processing machine. *Archives of Internal Medicine* 1959; May;103:776–782.

40. Brodman K, Erdmann AJ Jr, Lorge I, Wolff HG. The Cornell Medical Index; an adjunct to medical interview. *JAMA*. 1949; June 11;140:530–534.

41. Reed MC and Grossman TM. Limited information technology for patient care in physician offices. Center for Studying Health System Change. Issue in Brief: 89;2004;September.

42. Health Information Management and Systems Society. 16th annual HIMSS leadership survey. Sponsored by Superior Consultant Company/ACS Healthcare Solutions. Available at: http://www.himss.org/2005survey/healthcareCIO_keytrends.asp. Accessed on March 19, 2006.

43. Chismar WG, Thomas SM. The economics of integrated electronic medical record systems. *Medinfo*. 2004;11(Pt 1):592-6.

44. Wang SJ, Middleton B, Prosser LA, et al. A cost-benefit analysis of electronic medical records in primary care. *Am J Med*. 2003;114: 397–403.

45. Miller RH, West C, Brown TM, et al. The value of electronic health records in solo or small group practices. *Health Affairs*. 2005;September–October;24(5):1127–1137.

46. Hillestad R, et al. Can electronic medical record systems transform health care? Potential health benefits, savings, and costs. *Health Affairs*. 2005;September–October;24 (5):1103–1117.

47. Gans D, Kralewski J, Hammons T, Dowd B. Medical groups' adoption of electronic health records and information systems. *Health Affairs*. 2005;September–October;24(5):1323–1333.

48. Miller RH. Sim I. Physicians' use of electronic medical records: barriers and solutions. *Health Affairs*. 2004;March–April; 23(2):116–126.

49. Rosenfeld S, Bernasek C, Medelson D. Medicare's next voyage: encouraging physicians to adopt information technology. *Health Affairs*. 2005;September–October; 29(4):1138–1146.

50. Barlow S, Johnson J, Steck J. The economic effect of implementing an EMR in an outpatient clinical setting. *JHIM*.2004;Winter;18(1):5–8.

51. Walker JM. Electronic medical records and health care transformation: EMR supported health care transformation is too immature for credible estimates of its costs or benefits. *Health Affairs*. 2005;September–October;24(5):1118–1120.

52. Goodman C. Savings in electronic medical record systems? Do it for the quality. *Health Affairs*. 2005;September–October;24(5):1124–1126.

ADDITIONAL READING:

Markle Foundation. *Linking Health Care Information: Proposed Methods For Improving Care and Protecting Privacy*. February 2005. Available at:
www.connectingforhealth.org/assets/reports/linking_report_2_2005.pdf. Accessed on November 8, 2006.

Woodcock E. *Mastering Patient Flow: More Ideas to Increase Efficiency and Earnings*. Medical Group Management Association (MGMA); October 2003.

CHAPTER 6

Return on Investment

Dov Rothman, PhD

Healthcare information technology has attracted much attention from private and public sector practitioners and policymakers. Many hope that healthcare IT will lead to reductions in medical errors, improvements in quality of care and reductions in costs.[1]

The optimism of healthcare IT advocates notwithstanding, there are two fairly obvious reasons why it is important for decision makers to pay attention to the financial implications of healthcare IT investments. First, healthcare IT systems are expensive.

The cost of implementing a computerized practitioner order entry system (CPOE) at a 500-bed hospital—in the absence of major network upgrades—has been estimated to be about $8 million, with ongoing maintenance costs of $1.35 million per year.[2] Second, given most healthcare providers' current financial conditions, large-scale investments that do not promise positive financial returns—even when they promise attractive benefits such as reductions in medical errors and improvements in quality of care—are difficult to justify.

This chapter describes standard techniques that healthcare executives can use to estimate the financial impact of investment in healthcare IT. The standard metric by which financial impact is assessed is return on investment (ROI). The following pages describe the steps of a ROI analysis. To illustrate, a ROI analysis of a hypothetical electronic medical record is then presented.

RETURN ON INVESTMENT

The return on investment (ROI) is the expected contribution to profitability from a project or an investment. ROI can be measured in terms of dollars or as a percentage rate of return.

ROI Measured in Dollars

Figure 6-1 shows a formula for determining a project's net present value (NPV), a form of ROI dollar measurement.

A project's ROI is the net present value of the project's returns (net benefits), that is, in turn, the sum of the returns (net benefits) discounted by the project's cost of capital:

$$\text{Net Present Value} = \frac{NB_1}{(1+r)^1} + \frac{NB_2}{(1+r)^2} + \frac{NB_3}{(1+r)^3} + \dots + \frac{NB_n}{(1+r)^n} = \sum_{t=1}^{n}\left[\frac{NB_t}{(1+r)^t}\right],$$

where NB_k is the return during period k, and r is the project cost of capital.

Figure 6-1: Net Present Value.

Constructing an estimate of a project's ROI requires estimates of: (1) the expected benefits and costs that are incremental to the project; (2) the timing of these incremental benefits and costs; and, (3) the project's perceived risk relative to the average risk of the institution's other investments. These components are discussed below.

Expected Benefits and Costs

The expected stream of current and future benefits and costs relevant to a ROI analysis are only those that are expected to result if and only if a project is implemented. Such expected benefits and costs are said to be incremental to the project under consideration, and are typically referred to as incremental benefits and costs. One can think about estimating incremental benefits and costs in terms of two discrete steps: identification of the types of benefits and costs potentially incremental to the project and their quantification.

Identifying the types of benefits and costs potentially incremental to a project requires the use of counterfactual logic. For each possible benefit and cost, one must consider whether it would have been realized absent the project. If the answer is yes, then that benefit or cost is not considered incremental, and should not be considered in the ROI analysis.

Identifying what benefits and costs are incremental to a project is typically context-dependent. Consider a project that would require implementation help from technical support. If technical help would need to hire more technicians or if existing technicians would need to work additional hours to provide such support, then the associated costs are incremental and should be included in the ROI analysis. However, if technical support would be able to provide implementation help without hiring more technicians or increasing the number of technician hours while continuing to do all the work it was doing before, then the costs associated with implementation help are not considered incremental and should not be included in the ROI analysis.

Quantification is the second step in estimating incremental benefits and costs. In a ROI analysis, each potential benefit and cost is a random variable and the expected NPV of the project is estimated using the expected values of each incremental benefit and cost. For present purposes, one can think of the expected value of a random variable as the random variable's most likely value.[A] As such, quantifying the expected incremental benefits and costs involves identifying a range of values that each benefit and cost could take and choosing the values within these ranges that are deemed to be most likely.

Expected Timing of Incremental Benefits and Costs

The time-value of money concept states that the value of a dollar received today is worth more than the value of a dollar to be received tomorrow. This implies that, all other factors being equal, a project that offers a relatively immediate return is more attractive (financially) than a project that offers a relatively delayed return. Consequently, the timing of the expected stream of incremental benefits and expenses should be considered. It is not enough to predict the incremental revenues and expenses expected from a project over a given time period. This time-value of money consideration can be especially relevant for projects that require large initial capital outlays and that are not expected to generate net benefits for several years.[B]

Perceived Project Risk

Risk assessment is an integral part of ROI analysis. A project's perceived risk relative to the risk of an organization's average project is necessary to determine the project's cost of capital.[C] A project's cost of capital is the interest that could have been earned by investing the capital required for the project in an alternative investment of similar risk. As such, a project that is relatively risky should be assigned a relatively high cost of capital. The reason is that the capital used to finance a relatively risky project could have been invested in a relatively risky stock market portfolio, and relatively risky stock market portfolios yield relatively higher expected returns.[D]

Project risk is measured by the dispersion of a project's possible returns; the more highly dispersed the possible returns, the riskier the project. The reason is that the greater the dispersion of a project's possible returns, the higher the probability that a project's realized return will be significantly lower than expected.

Recall that in a ROI analysis each potential incremental benefit and cost is a random variable. Some of these so-called random variables are known with a high degree of certainty. For example, the initial cost of hardware necessary for a given IT system can be estimated relatively precisely. Other random variables are known with less certainty. For example, the incremental benefits or implementation costs of an IT system likely depend on factors that are difficult to forecast; depending on future developments, the incremental benefits and/or implementation costs can turn out to be much larger or much smaller than expected.

Two projects can have the same expected net present value but one can be riskier than the other if its incremental benefits and costs are more uncertain (i.e., if the possible values that its incremental benefits and costs can take are more dispersed.) For example, an investment that pays $0 with a probability of .50 and pays $10 with a probability of .50 has the same expected value ($5) as an investment that pays $5 with a probability of one. The two investments yield the same return on average, but the first investment is clearly more risky than the second.

Thus, to assess a project's risk, one must consider the uncertainty regarding the estimated NPV. A project's discount factor can then be approximated by adjusting an institution's overall cost of capital up or down. Because an institution's overall cost of capital reflects the risk of an institution's average investment, whether the adjustment is up or down depends on whether the project under consideration is more or less risky than the institution's average investment.

Summary of Dollar-Denominated ROI

The steps associated with a ROI analysis are easily summarized by a series of questions:

1. What are the expected incremental benefits associated with the project under consideration?
2. What is the expected timing of these incremental benefits?
3. What are the expected incremental expenses associated with the project under consideration?
4. What is the expected timing of these incremental expenses?
5. How risky is this project relative to the institution's average investment? What is the appropriate project cost of capital?

ROI Measured as a Percentage Rate of Return

The ROI of a project can also be assessed by a metric called the internal rate of return (IRR). This is a measure of a project's expected percentage profitability. Technically, the IRR is the discount rate at which the present value of a project's expected incremental benefits equals the present value of a project's expected incremental expenses. Given a stream of expected incremental benefits and expenses, the IRR of a project is found by solving for the discount rate that makes the NPV of the project zero.[E] Practically, if a project's predicted IRR is greater than the project's cost of capital, then the project's predicted NPV is greater than zero. Conversely, if a project's predicted IRR is less than the project's cost of capital, then the project's predicted NPV is less than zero. This is intuitive. The project's cost of capital reflects the return that could have been earned by investing the resources required for the project in an alternative investment of similar risk. As such, if the IRR is less than the project's cost of capital, then investing the resources required for the project in an alternative investment of similar risk would earn a higher expected return than the project. This suggests that the project should not be undertaken. Put somewhat colloquially, an IRR that is less than the project's cost of capital suggests that the project's required resources can be better spent elsewhere.

Time Payback

The payback period of a project is the expected number of years or months required to recover the project's investment. Payback is estimated by computing the discounted cumulative net cash flows and is said to occur when these discounted cumulative net cash flows become positive.

Time payback can provide useful information about a project's liquidity and risk. The shorter a project's payback time, the sooner a project is expected to generate positive cash flows. Also, the shorter a project's payback time, the less risky the project since cash flows expected far into the future are inherently more uncertain.

Assessing Risk

Risk assessments are done primarily via scenario analyses. The basic purpose of the scenario analysis is to measure the variability of NPV as the factors that determine a project's net present value—the incremental benefits and costs—take on different values. Two such methods are Monte Carlo Simulation and Scenario Analysis. Sensitivity analysis is another technique that can complement the latter.

Monte Carlo Simulation

A Monte Carlo simulation is the more sophisticated type of scenario analysis. The simulation is implemented using a spreadsheet application such as Microsoft Excel.[F] One first specifies a probability distribution for each uncertain variable; these probability distributions effectively describe the possible values that each variable can take and the probabilities that each variable takes these possible values.[G] The simulation program then draws a value of each uncertain variable from its probability distribution. These draws are then used to compute the net present value of the investment. Repeating this process over and over, perhaps 10,000 times, results in a distribution of net present values. The standard deviation of this distribution measures the investment's risk.

From the practitioner's perspective, specifying probability distributions for uncertain variables is the most challenging aspect of a Monte Carlo simulation. A practical approach is to assume that each uncertain variable follows a triangular distribution. The advantage of using the triangular distribution is that the distribution of a random variable that is triangularly distributed is completely described by the lowest, most likely and highest possible values that the random variable can take. As such, under the assumption that a random variable follows a triangular distribution, one need only specify the lowest, most likely and highest value that the variable can take to specify its distribution.

The steps are easily summarized:
1. Specify a probability distribution for each uncertain variable.
2. Draw a value of each uncertain variable from its probability distribution.
3. Compute and record the NPV of the project using these draws.
4. Repeat this process 10,000 times.
5. Calculate the standard deviation of the distribution of NPVs obtained from these simulations.

Worst-Case, Most-Likely Case, Best-Case Scenario Analysis

A simpler way to implement a scenario analysis than a Monte Carlo simulation is to define a worst-case scenario, a most-likely scenario, and a best-case scenario; the worst-case scenario is the worst possible combination of values that the uncertain variables can take, while the best-case scenario is the best possible combination of values that the uncertain variables can take.[H] One then computes the net present value in each scenario, and then computes the standard deviation of the distribution of these net present values.

The steps are as follows:

1. Define a worst-case, most-likely and best-case scenario.
2. Define the probabilities that the worst-case, most-likely and best-case scenarios can occur.[1]
3. Compute the net present value of each scenario.
4. Compute the standard deviation of the NPVs.

Coefficient of Variation ≈ RISK

The coefficient of variation is the risk per unit of return. It is considered a better measure of comparative risk than the standard deviation when projects have widely differing NPVs.[3] Following a scenario analysis, it is easily computed by using the formula in Figure 6-2.

$$CV = \frac{SD[NPV]}{E[NPV]}$$

where SD[NPV] is the standard deviation of NPVs, and E[NPV] is the expected value of NPVs.

Figure 6-2: The Coefficient of Variation.

Sensitivity Analysis

A sensitivity analysis measures how the predicted NPV of an investment varies when one potential incremental or cost changes. Sensitivity analyses are less realistic than scenario analyses because they effectively hold all other variables constant. However, they can be useful in identifying which benefits and/or costs are most important to a project's success.

A CASE STUDY

This section describes a ROI analysis of an electronic medical record system. The data are from a study, "A Cost-Benefit Analysis of Electronic Medical Records in Primary Care," written by Wang et al and published in The American Journal of Medicine.[4] The purpose here is not to describe every detail of the study, but to use it to illustrate how a ROI analysis can be implemented in practice.

Wang et al consider the costs and benefits of electronic medical record usage by primary care physicians in an ambulatory-care setting, and estimate the net financial benefit per physician of switching physicians from a traditional paper-based medical record to an electronic medical record.

Costs

Drawing from various sources, Wang et al identify and estimate the following costs:

- Purchase (or lease) of necessary software ($1,600 per provider per annum licensing fee)[J]
- Purchase (or lease) of necessary hardware ($6,600 per provider every three years)[K]
- Implementation and training ($3,400 per provider in the first year)

- Ongoing maintenance and support ($1,500 per provider per annum)
- Temporary lost productivity associated with switching systems ($11,200 per provider in the first year)[L]

These estimates are reproduced in Table 6-1. The key figure is the present value of total costs, $42,900. This is the present value of the expected cost per physician of switching to an electronic medical record.

Table 6-1: Estimated Costs.

	Initial Cost	Year 1	Year 2	Year 3	Year 4	Year 5	Total
Costs							
Software license (annual)	$1,600	$1,600	$1,600	$1,600	$1,600	$1,600	
Implementation	$3,400						
Support	$1,500	$1,500	$1,500	$1,500	$1,500	$1,500	
Hardware (refresh every 3 years)	$6,600			$6,600			
Productivity loss		$11,200					
Annual costs	$13,100	$14,300	$3,100	$9,700	$3,100	$3,100	$46,400
Present value of annual costs*	$13,100	$13,619	$2,812	$8,379	$2,550	$2,429	$42,900

* Assumes a 5% discount rate

(From "A Cost-Benefit Analysis of Electronic Medical Records in Primary Care," The American Journal of Medicine, April 1, 2003, Volume 114, pp.397–403.)

Notice the difference between the present value of total costs and the simple sum of total costs. The present value is smaller since it takes into account the fact that not all costs are incurred immediately. This difference illustrates the importance of considering the timing of expected costs.

Benefits

Drawing from various sources, Wang et al identify and estimate the following benefits:
- Cost savings from reduced chart pulls ($3,000 per provider per annum)[M]
- Cost savings from reduced transcription costs ($2,700)[N]
- Avoided costs due to reductions in adverse drug events ($2,200), reductions in drug utilization ($16,400), reductions in laboratory utilization ($2,400) and reductions in radiology utilization ($8,300)[O]
- Increases in revenues due to charge capture improvement ($7,700) and decreases in billing errors ($7,600)[P]

These estimates are presented in Table 6-2. The key figure is the present value of total incremental benefits, $129,300; this is the present value of the expected (gross) benefit per physician of switching to an electronic medical record. Again, notice the difference between the present value of total benefits and the simple sum of benefits. The present value is smaller since it accounts for the fact that not all benefits are realized immediately. This difference illustrates the importance of considering the timing of expected benefits; one would over-estimate the gross benefits of the electronic medical record by about $25,000 per physician (assuming a 5% discount rate) by ignoring the timing of expected benefits.

Table 6-2: Estimated Benefits.

	Year 1	Year 2	Year 3	Year 4	Year 5	Total
Benefits						
Chart pull savings	$3,000	$3,000	$3,000	$3,000	$3,000	
Transcription savings	$2,700	$2,700	$2,700	$2,700	$2,700	
Prevention of adverse drug events		$2,200	$2,200	$2,200	$2,200	
Drug savings		$16,400	$16,400	$16,400	$16,400	
Laboratory savings				$2,400	$2,400	
Radiology savings				$8,300	$8,300	
Charge capture improvement				$7,700	$7,700	
Billing error decrease				$7,600	$7,600	
Annual benefits	$5,700	$24,300	$24,300	$50,300	$50,300	$154,900
Present value of annual benefits*	$5,429	$22,041	$20,991	$41,382	$39,411	$129,300

* Assumes a 5% discount rate

(From "A Cost-Benefit Analysis of Electronic Medical Records in Primary Care," The American Journal of Medicine, *April 1, 2003, Volume 114, pp.397–403.)*

Net Present Value and Internal Rate of Return

The net present value of expected benefits is computed as the present value of expected (gross) benefits less expected costs. Given the estimated values of benefits and costs described above, the net present value of the electronic medical record system is predicted to be $86,400 per provider.

The internal rate of return is estimated using the future values of net benefits (gross benefits less costs). Recall that the internal rate of return is the discount rate at which the present value of expected incremental benefits equals the present value of expected incremental expenses. Using Microsoft Excel's internal rate of return function, the estimated internal rate of return is 73%. This is significantly larger than the assumed discount rate of 5%.[Q] Table 6-3 shows the estimated net benefits from the case study.

Table 6-3: Estimated Net Benefits.

	Initial Cost	Year 1	Year 2	Year 3	Year 4	Year 5	Total
Net benefit	($13,100)	($8,600)	$21,200	$14,600	$47,200	$47,200	$108,500
Present value net benefit*	($13,100)	($8,190)	$19,229	$12,612	$38,832	$36,982	$86,400

* Assumes a 5% interest rate

(From "A Cost-Benefit Analysis of Electronic Medical Records in Primary Care," The American Journal of Medicine, *April 1, 2003, Volume 114, pp.397–403.)*

Time Payback

The cumulative net cash flows are presented in Table 6-4. The first row presents the non-discounted cumulative net cash flows. The second row presents the discounted cumulative net cash flows. Both show that the electronic medical record is expected to have "paid for itself" by the beginning of the third year.

Table 6-4: Time Payback.

	Initial Cost	Year 1	Year 2	Year 3	Year 4	Year 5
Cumulative net benefits (1)	($13,100)	($21,700)	($500)	$27,200	$61,300	$108,500
Cumulative net benefits (2)	($13,100)	($21,290)	($2061)	$23,651	$49,383	$86,400

* Assumes a 5% interest rate

(From "A Cost-Benefit Analysis of Electronic Medical Records in Primary Care," The American Journal of Medicine, *April 1, 2003, Volume 114, pp.397-403.)*

RISK ASSESSMENT

Scenario Analysis

One can implement a simple scenario analysis by defining a worst-case, most-likely-case, and a best-case using ranges of values provided by Wang et al. The ranges for all variables are reproduced in Table 6-5.

Table 6-5: Scenarios.

	Worst-Case	Most-Likely-Case	Best-Case
Costs			
Software	$3,200	$1,600	$800
Implementation	$3,400	$3,400	$3,400
Support and maintenance	$3,000	$1,500	$750
Hardware	$9,900	$6,600	$3,300
Temporary productivity loss	$16,500	$11,200	$5,500
Benefits			
Reduced chart pulls	300	600	1200
Reduced transcription costs	20%	28%	100%
Reduced adverse drug events	10%	34%	70%
Reduced drug utilization	5%	15%	25%
Reduced laboratory utilization	0%	8.8%	13%
Reduced radiology utilization	5%	14%	20%
Increased charge capture	1.50%	2%	5%
Reduced billing errors	35%	78%	95%

Plugging these values into Tables 6-1 and 6-2, one can compute the net present value of the electronic medical record for each scenario and then use this distribution of net present values to compute the standard deviation of the net present values and the coefficient of variation (see Table 6-6).

Table 6-6: Variability of NPV.

	Worst-Case	Most- Likely-Case	Best-Case	E[NPV]	SD[NPV]	Coefficient of variation
NPV	($15,772)	$86,400	$222,200	$94,807	$84,554	.89

Note: Because Wang et al did not provide estimates of each scenario's likelihood, I somewhat arbitrarily assumed that the probability of the worst-case was .25, the probability of the most-likely-case was .50, and the probability of the best-case was .25.

According to these estimates, under the most pessimistic assumptions, the electronic medical record would result in a loss of $15,772 per provider, while under the most optimistic assumptions the electronic medical record would result in a profit of $222,200 per provider.

Recall that the purpose of the scenario analysis is to assess the investment's risk, and that the reason why the investment's risk matters is that it determines the appropriate discount factor ("project cost of capital"). Thus, if the standard deviation and/or coefficient of variation estimated above were deemed high relative to an organization's other projects, the discount factor used to estimate the net present value should be adjusted upward. Conversely, if the standard deviation and/or coefficient of variation estimated below were deemed low relative to an organization's other projects, the discount factor should be adjusted downward.

Sensitivity Analysis

One can also examine the sensitivity of the predicted net present value to changes in individual variables. For example, the most likely scenario assumes a 15% reduction in drug costs. When the cost avoidance associated with reduced drug costs is assumed to be zero, the predicted NPV falls to about $31,000 per provider. When the cost avoidance associated with prevention of adverse drug events, drug savings, laboratory savings and radiology savings is assumed to be zero, the predicted NPV falls to about $6,000 per provider. While three variables are changed here, one can think of this last exercise as an assessment of the sensitivity of predicted NPV to changes in quality of care related incremental benefits. When the expected benefits associated with process improvements (reduced charts, reduced transcription costs, charge capture improvement and reduced billing errors) are assumed to be zero, the predicted NPV is about $37,000 per provider.

These last analyses reveal how sensitive the predicted NPV of the electronic medical record is to assumptions about incremental quality of care benefits. This could be particularly relevant to a healthcare provider considering adopting an electronic medical record who does not expect to internalize the quality of care related benefits. For example, depending on other factors, the benefits associated with reductions in drug costs could be appropriated by payors rather than providers.

SUMMARY

This chapter has described standard techniques for predicting the ROI of potential healthcare IT investments. In practice, these techniques are likely to be used in different ways depending on the context. For some types of IT investments, the tools described in this chapter are directly applicable. In other contexts, these tools might not be directly applicable, but still can serve as a useful template. Whether or not one can quantify the expected ROI of an IT investment, it is worth asking the questions that would need to be answered to do so.

FREQUENTLY ASKED QUESTIONS

Q: *How do costs previously incurred but associated with a potential IT investment figure into a ROI analysis?*

A: Costs previously incurred are considered sunk and, by definition, are not incremental, even when they are directly associated with a potential IT investment. For example, consider a hospital that is considering a computerized practitioner order entry system (CPOE) and who previously paid $20,000 to a consultant to conduct a feasibility study. In a ROI analysis, the money paid to the consultant last year is a sunk cost and should not be considered in the ROI analysis; the consultant's fee has been spent whether or not the CPOE system is adopted. However, if adopting the CPOE system would necessarily entail hiring the consultant again, perhaps for implementation assistance, then the consultant's fee for the implementation assistance is incremental and should be considered in the ROI analysis.

Q: *How are opportunity costs considered in a ROI analysis?*

A: It depends. The opportunity cost associated with using capital to finance an investment is accounted for by the discount factor used to compute the present value of incremental cash flows. Consequently, the opportunity cost of capital should not be included as an incremental cost in a ROI analysis. To do so would constitute double counting. However, non-financial opportunity costs should be considered incremental expenses. For example, consider an IT system that requires a dedicated room to store a server. Suppose also that the only available room to store this server is currently being used as a gift shop. The foregone profits associated with closing the gift shop to house the server are relevant opportunity costs.

Q: *Does project risk affect go-no-go decisions differently when measuring ROI in terms of NPV versus IRR?*

A: Not really. When measuring ROI in terms of NPV, project risk affects go-no-go decisions by affecting the predicted NPV, which affects the go-no-go decision. When measuring ROI in terms of IRR, project risk affects go-no-go decisions by determining the threshold IRR necessary for a project's expected return to be greater than the opportunity cost of capital.

Q: *How does the time payback method account for returns that occur after the breakeven point?*

A: It does not. This is a significant limitation of the time payback method. For example, two projects could have the same expected time payback even though one project's returns declined after the breakeven point and the other project's returns increased after the breakeven point.

Q: *Many of the theoretical benefits of health IT systems are "soft" and difficult to quantify. How do standard ROI analyses incorporate such intangible benefits?*

A: There is not a well-defined methodology for dealing with these types of benefits (Fisher et al, 2004).[5] In many situations, it is probably imprudent to try quantifying intangible benefits. This, however, does not mean that the mode of reasoning involved in a ROI analysis is not useful. Whether one can or cannot quantify all potential benefits and costs, one should ask the types of questions involved in a ROI analysis.

REFERENCES

1. Pricewaterhouse Coopers LLP. *Reactive to adaptive: transforming hospitals with digital technology*. Global Technology Centre: Health Research Institute; May 2005.

2. Kuperman G, Gibson R. Computer physician order entry: benefits, costs and issues, improving patient care. *Annals of Internal Medicine*. 1 July 2003;139(1):31–39.

3. Gapenski L. *Healthcare Finance: An Introduction to Accounting and Financial Management*. Aupha Press; 3rd edition (September 2004). Washington, D.C.

4. Wang S, Middleton B, Prosser L, Bardon C, Spurr C, Carchidi P, et al. A cost-benefit analysis of electronic medical records in primary care. *Am J Med*. 2003;114(5): 397–403.

5. Fisher J, Shell C, Troiano D, Pricewaterhouse Coopers LLP. *Measuring the costs and benefits of healthcare information technology: six case studies*. Prepared for the California Healthcare Foundation; September 2004.

NOTES

A. Technically, an expected value is a probability weighted average, $\sum_{i=1}^{n} p_i x_i$, where pi is the probability that the random variable x equals xi, and n indexes the number of different realizations of the random variable x.

B. The time value of money concept is easily explained: a dollar received today can be invested at a given interest rate. As such, receiving a dollar tomorrow rather than today means foregoing the interest that could have been earned on that dollar. Therefore, a dollar received today is worth more than a dollar to be received tomorrow.

C. The cost of capital is the discount factor used in the net present value calculation.

D. In the context of an ROI analysis, one can think about a project's opportunity cost as the return that could have been earned by taking the capital used for the project and investing it in a stock market portfolio of similar risk.

E. Financial calculators and spreadsheets have built-in functions that perform these calculations.

F. The capability is an add-in in Microsoft Excel.

G. One can specify correlations between different variables to capture the possibility that when one set of incremental benefits and/or costs are higher than expected, other incremental benefits and/or costs will tend to be higher or lower than expected.

H. One can think of the worst-case as the scenario where everything goes wrong and the best-case as the scenario where everything goes right.

I. While in reality, many outcomes other than the worst, most-likely and best can occur, in this simple scenario analysis, the probabilities that the worst-, most-likely and best-case scenarios occur should sum to one.

J. This figure was based on the per provider per year costs of the electronic medical record system at the authors' institution, Partners HealthCare. They note that license fees for commercially available software have been estimated at between $2,500–$3,500 per provider for the initial software purchase, plus annual maintenance fees of 12–18%.

K. They assume that hardware will be replaced every three years and implicitly assume that the resale value of the hardware is zero.

L. They assume initial productivity losses of 20% in the first month, 10% in the second month and 5% in the third month.

M. The average cost of a chart pull at their institution is $5 and the expected reduction in chart pulls is 600. This latter figure was based on the reduction at one Partners HealthCare clinic.

N. Average transcription costs at their institution were $9,600 per provider per year. They assumed a 28% reduction.

O. These estimated savings were computed using estimates from a seven-member expert panel. Note that these benefits are only realized under capitation.

P. These benefits are expected to be realized beginning only in year four since the analysis assumes that advanced decision support features of the electronic medical record would not be implemented immediately.

Q. One can also verify that the present value of net benefits equals zero at a discount factor of .73.

ADDITIONAL READING

Computerized Physician Order Entry: Costs, Benefits and Challenges – A Case Study Approach. Authored by FCG for the American Hospital Association and the American Federation of Hospitals. January 2003.

Evans RS, Pestotnik SL, Classen DC, Clemmer TP, Weaver LK, Orme JF Jr, Lloyd JF, Burke JP. A computer-assisted management program for antibiotics and other anti-infective agents. *N Engl J Med*. 1998;January 22;338(4):232-8.

PricewaterhouseCoopers. Measuring the costs and benefits of health care information technology: six case studies. September 2004. Available at: http://www.chcf.org/topics/hospitals/index.cfm?itemID=105676. Accessed May 14, 2006.

Mullen R, Donnelly JT. Keeping it real—building an ROI model for an ambulatory EMR initiative that the physician practices espouse. *J Healthc Inf Manag*. 2006;Winter;20(1):42–52.

CHAPTER 7

Health Information Exchange

Mark Lipton, MD

MRS. JONES

Version One

Mrs. Jones, a fifty-seven-year-old female, was brought to the emergency department with painful swelling of her left leg. A deep vein thrombosis, or clot in her leg vein, is evident upon examination. The patient was given *Lovenox*, a potent anticoagulant, at usual doses. Unknown to the treating physicians, Mrs. Jones had moderately severe kidney impairment that can cause excessive buildup of drugs such as *Lovenox*.

Late the following day, the patient became confused and exhibited left-sided arm and leg weakness. Neurologic workup revealed the presence of a cerebral bleed. The patient ultimately recovered from the bleed, but not without a prolonged and expensive hospitalization and rehabilitation.

Version Two

Mrs. Jones, a fifty-seven-year-old female, was brought to the emergency department with painful swelling of her left leg. On registration of the patient, an automated search was initiated in the regional data exchange. A recent blood test was located at another institution, revealing the presence of moderately severe kidney impairment.

On examination, a deep vein thrombosis is evident, and the patient was given *Lovenox* at a dose appropriate to the level of kidney impairment. Mrs. Jones had an uncomplicated and brief hospital stay after effective treatment for her thrombosis.

Perhaps the best understanding of the value of health information exchange can be gained by examining the "use case" depicted by the two versions above. In this example, the timely availability of pertinent clinical information allowed Mrs. Jones' treating physician to avert a potentially lethal cerebral bleed in version 2. Effective medical decision-making is vitally dependent on the treating clinician having adequate information at the point-of-care. Key information that guides clinicians include medical problems, medication lists, allergy lists, contact information for family and treating physicians and results of diagnostic tests. Such information is commonly absent in both primary care[1] and hospital emergency rooms,[2] and has been linked to medical error and adverse outcomes. Many times, this information does exist outside the reach of the treating clinician, but access is unavailable due to missing charts, lack of electronic access to data residing outside of the point-of-care or problems ascertaining that such data is available.

THE QUALITY ISSUE

In 1999, the Institute of Medicine (IOM) published a scathing report on medical errors in American healthcare. It reported that 98,000 deaths annually are attributed to preventable medical errors.[3] Among the safety issues raised were lack of access to clinical information and lack of information systems to share such information. A follow-up series of recommendations by the IOM was published in 2001.[4] That report underscored the importance of utilizing information technology to automate the medical record, enable automatic clinical decision support at the point-of-care, and create a national health information infrastructure to enable effective communication of patient clinical information between organizational boundaries.

Healthcare quality improvement has been well-substantiated for the case of electronic medical records, computerized practitioner order entry (CPOE), and computerized clinical decision support in both the inpatient and ambulatory healthcare venues. In the inpatient realm, real-time computerized decision support and practitioner order entry resulted in a 55% decline in serious medication errors.[5] In the outpatient realm, computerized health records have been demonstrated to improve healthcare quality, particularly by improving preventive care through automated reminders, reducing prescription errors resulting from illegibly written prescriptions and by reducing the frequency of healthcare being given without access to the patient's records.

Inasmuch as electronic health records and decision support can improve the safety and quality of healthcare delivered at a single location of care, the fact is that a patient's healthcare almost always involves multiple healthcare providers at multiple locations. These include physician office/clinic, hospital, emergency department, nursing facility and diagnostic centers. The movement of patients among these healthcare locations has been associates with an increased risk of adverse events—a healthcare system vulnerability particularly suitable for improvement by Healthcare Information Exchange (HIE).

ECONOMIC BENEFITS

The potential benefits from clinical data exchange are not limited to quality and safety improvement. By allowing a clinician to access clinical information obtained at other healthcare venues, cost savings would be expected to result. Three principal economic effects of clinical data exchange would be:

- Discovering prior diagnostic workup would reduce or eliminate duplication of tests and procedures. This would save the payor both the technical and professional components of the diagnostic procedure cost.
- In the ED, prior information can better inform the decision about hospital admission. For example, a prior electrocardiogram tracing, when compared to the current one, may obviate the need for admission if no change is detected in a low-risk patient presenting with presumed non-cardiac chest pain. As a result, an expensive and inappropriate hospital admission would be averted.
- Reduction of adverse drug events due to drug-drug interactions or to drug-allergy conflict would decrease treatment costs for those events, and likely reduce frequency of hospital admission.

Although the cost reduction of healthcare are under intense study in a variety of extant Regional Health Information Organizations (RHIOs), no comprehensive understanding of these savings has been achieved. In Indiana, the IHIE RHIO has been reported to result in a cost savings of about $26 dollars per ED visit,[6] but actual cost savings to the other participants of the healthcare economy and to the healthcare system as a whole has yet to be determined.

The economic impact of HIE will largely depend on the unique characteristics of each clinical data exchange implementation, and will be influenced by such factors as the scope of different types of healthcare entities enrolled, the "penetration" into each type of healthcare facility (e.g., the percentage of regional hospitals enrolled), the specific suite of clinical data elements included in the exchange and other regionally specific factors including population health characteristics.

INTRA- VS. INTER-ORGANIZATIONAL SOLUTIONS

Within healthcare organizations, such information needs have been addressed by data electronic medical records (EMRs) that collect information from the various clinical and laboratory departments in those organizations. Although creating these EMRs is by no means a trivial technical or financial undertaking, they have been demonstrated to be an invaluable clinical tool that reduces medical error and improves quality of care.[7] Furthermore, when combined with automated alerting systems, significant benefits have been demonstrated in avoiding adverse drug events and other adverse patient outcomes. While the development/purchase and deployment of electronic medical records is an expensive project, the business issues and concerns surrounding patient privacy are relatively straightforward within an organization; local clinical and financial factors are taken into account, and the data never leaves the confines of the organization that is regarded as a single entity under HIPAA.

The scenario described involving Mrs. Jones involves clinical information passing instantly from one healthcare entity to another. This entails disparate organizations (usually competitors in a local healthcare marketplace) cooperating in a venture to provide confidential information to one another. Such HIE has been envisioned to address the fact that the patient healthcare experience does not usually occur under the umbrella of a single provider organization. In fact, patients commonly transition from their primary care to other venues including hospital, skilled nursing facilities and ambulatory surgery centers. This ongoing transition in care venue introduces additional opportunities for adverse medical events; numerous studies have substantiated that the patient is particularly vulnerable to such events at the time of such transitions in care.[8]

Unfortunately, despite the perceived benefits to patient care that HIE can provide, the barriers to establish such an infrastructure remain high. Such barriers include apportioning the cost among participants, special patient confidentiality issues that apply when information is transmitted from one institution to another, organizational issues in a highly competitive regional healthcare market and others. These issues will be discussed more fully in the "Challenges and Issues" section of this chapter.

HISTORICAL PERSPECTIVE

The American pioneers of HIE were the community health information networks (CHINs) that were started around 1990. The early 1990s saw the growth of managed care, with a responsive consolidation of healthcare provider organizations into integrated health delivery networks (IDNs). The IDNs needed a means of managing the clinical process through collection and exchange of clinical data within its boundaries, and CHINs arose as a collaborative investment by the IDNs to facilitate such data exchange. Lorenzi[9] details the rise and fall of CHINs, attributing their ultimate failure to multiple factors including competition, conflicting missions, poorly conceived objectives by CHIN members, financing issues and technical features that included less sophisticated technology of the time not supporting an efficient centralized community-wide data repository.

Despite the demise of the CHIN, the need to share clinical data was no less compelling. The patient safety and quality literature was rife with examples of quality lapses due to healthcare transitions, as well as the opportunities for improvement in healthcare quality through the use of automated clinical decision support systems[10] based on access to electronic patient data.

The next generation of HIE efforts were focused on improvement in patient outcomes, and included efforts in Indianapolis, Santa Barbara, Massachusetts and Tennessee. These collaborative efforts became known as Regional Health Information Organizations (RHIOs). The RHIO was a largely clinical initiative, with most coming into existence based on the growing evidence that medical care was safer, more effective and more efficient when the treating clinician had the appropriate information at the point-of-care. Many of these projects took shape with the active participations of physicians, and were sponsored by health provider organizations or not-for-profit collaboratives. There are presently over 100 RHIO projects at various stages of maturity. The projects were generally started through grant funding, with later development requiring more sustainable funding.[11]

REGIONAL VS. NATIONAL HIE

The benefits of having electronic health records (EHRs) that can participate in health information exchange (termed "interoperable" health records) has caught the attention of local and national government leaders, who envision leveraging HIE on a national scope. In 2004, Dr David Brailer was appointed the National Coordinator For Healthcare Information Technology by President Bush. Among Dr Brailer's stated priorities are providing clinicians with electronic health records and automated clinical decision support, as well as connecting disparate electronic health records.

The federal agenda in promoting interoperable electronic health records and health information exchange is to address the runaway costs of medical care and uncertain value and effectiveness, as well as the safety of care given to its citizens.[12] There is a firm conviction at the highest levels of government leadership that many of these problems are remediable through development of healthcare IT, but there is also an equal conviction that the funding for the bulk of this development should be the marketplace. Several pilot initiatives have been funded through Agency for Health Research and Quality (AHRQ) to establish regional data exchange projects and grants have been announced by the Department of Health and Human Services (HHS) to coalitions of healthcare IT vendors to address the issues of standards adoption, software certification and privacy protection.[13] Despite these grants, the bulk of the funding for interoperable medical records—and the regional infrastructures to connect them—is expected to derive from the cost-savings and other value delivered to healthcare payors, providers and other participants in the healthcare economy.

The vision of widespread HIE has been expanded to one of nationwide infrastructure (national health information infrastructure or "NHII"). It is clear that such a national infrastructure can only be realized through the aggregation of local HIE efforts ("local health information infrastructures" or "LHIIs"—essentially synonymous with RHIOs). The challenges of creating the NHII are multiple, not the least of which is our citizens' distaste for perceived intrusions into their personal matters by government. The lack of agreed-upon standards in electronic communication and the way health data is stored and represented is another challenge for both the LHII and NHII efforts. Furthermore, coordination among the many extant and planned RHIOs will be essential for the NHII to succeed.[14] The nomenclature of health information exchange (also called clinical data exchange) has become so complicated that a glossary is needed. Table 7-1 is a list of such terms.

Table 7-1: HIE Glossary.

CDE	Clinical Data Exchange – similar to HIE
CHIN	Community Health Information Network – precursor to RHIOs
HIE	Health Information Exchange
LHII	Local Health Information Infrastructure – essentially a RHIO
MPI	Master Patient Index – an directory of patient demographic data
NHII	National Health Information Infrastructure
RHIO	Regional Health Information Organization
RLS	Record Locator Service – a MPI for RHIOs
SNO	Subnetwork Organization – an LHII that connects to the NHII

CURRENT RHIOS

The list of RHIOs in operation is growing, with about 106 such projects in various phases of planning or operation nationwide at the time of this writing. Most started with clinical data exchange in the ED, although some projects have been outgrowths of existing administrative and financial health data exchanges. Several regional health data exchanges stand out in terms of maturity and functional status.

Indiana Health Information Exchange

The Indiana Health Information Exchange (IHIE) was incorporated February 2004 as a not-for-profit organization, although data exchange has been occurring for about ten years. It was conceived and planned by several members of the Riegenstrief Institute, a renowned informatics center,[15] and connects all five major hospital systems, four homeless care organizations, eighty-five primary care providers, as well as county and state public health agencies in Indianapolis. It has a formal board structure with representation from major healthcare providers and payors, public health agencies, governmental representatives (mayor's office) and the University of Indiana.

IHIE was started with grant funding amounting to about $9 million from Biocrossroads, a regional not for profit dedicated to advancing healthcare in Indiana. In addition, it received some start-up funding from participating organizations. Ongoing funding derives from a unique value-added service that it provides—IHIE electronically transmits lab reports from regional clinical laboratories to physicians' offices for about $.40 per report, about half the non-electronic cost to the laboratories with paper report transmission and postage. This method of funding, involving "value-added services" has distinguished IHIE as a standout among RHIOs in developing a robust ongoing business model.

IHIE has statewide reach for transfer of population health statistics such as vaccination data, but the most extensive clinical data exchange occurs within Indianapolis. The clinical data includes hospital pathology, laboratory and radiology results, hospitalizations, ED visits, medication, vaccination and certain ambulatory care data. The technical model for IHIE is a central repository model (i.e., all data is stored in—and accessed from—a central database.)

Santa Barbara County Care Data Exchange (SBCCDE)

The SBCCDE started in 1999 with a $10 million grant from the California Healthcare Foundation. It later received another $5 million from its technical development partner[16] and is currently in the early stages of widespread deployment after a challenging piloting phase.

The governance of SBCCDE follows a divisional structure with a coordinating Care Data Exchange Council consisting of senior representatives of the anchor organizations and public health agencies. Care Data Alliances (data exchange participants with common data exchange needs and interactions) and a Technical Advisory Committee and a Clinical Advisory Committee report[17] to the Council.

The technical model is a peer-to-peer model where clinical data transacted in the exchange is housed in the originating organization. It has a central record locator service and security management service.

As the first large-scale data exchange in the U.S., SBCCDE has been cited as an ambitious undertaking that has faced significant challenges on several fronts.[18] Technology issues prevailed until late 2005 when a robust technical solution to the performance issues of their peer-to-peer model were worked out. Due to the long delay in implementation, many clinicians lost interest in the project. In addition, contractual and legal concerns with the vendor and among the participants presented additional challenges to the RHIO. Despite this inauspicious start, the SBCCDE is hoping to regain momentum and become financially self-sufficient later in 2006.

Massachusetts Simplifying Healthcare Among Regional Entities (MA-SHARE)

MA-SHARE was an outgrowth of an existing administrative and claims data exchange in Massachusetts called the Massachusetts Health Data Consortium (MHDC), which has been in operation for over 25 years. In 2003, MA-SHARE was started to foster clinical data exchange projects within the state.[19] The first clinical project was the Medsinfo-ED project, which allows hospital ED-based physicians to access medication history though Rx-HUB® prescription database. This project only has recently started and is being evaluated for delivered value as well as being used as a platform for other data exchange projects.

The governance structure of the MA-SHARE organization (a not-for-profit "arms-length" spin-off from MHDC) consists of an Advisory Committee and Executive Subcommittee under the leadership of the Chairman of the Board of MHDC.[20] Other members include three representatives each from the hospitals, physicians, payors, healthcare organizations, state government, academic institutions, community organizations and five representatives from an array of constituencies including academic, civic and other organizations.

The stated aim of MA-SHARE is to become economically self-sufficient within five years of operation. It is anticipated by the planners that most of the ongoing funding will derive from user subscription fees.[21]

HIE CHALLENGES

The barriers to HIE adoption have been high, a lesson learned from the failed CHIN era. In the United States, only a tiny minority of patients receive their care in an environment that includes a clinical data exchange. The high bar to launching a RHIO is due to factors such as competitive concerns, privacy and security issues, technical challenges and financial issues.

Competitive and Organizational Concerns

Most regional healthcare economies are composed of competing healthcare providers and payors who are likely to be disinclined to enter into a data-sharing agreement, particularly given the value that such data has in terms of strategic planning and marketing. Because most patients receive the bulk of their care from primary care ambulatory clinics and practices, most data is expected to reside in such practices. The concept of sharing one's practice information with local hospitals (some of whom vie for the same patient base as the community physicians) presents a challenge that requires extraordinary trust building.

Another organizational challenge relates to the "who" question. In building the partnership that will give rise to the RHIO, the temptation is to limit leadership involvement to few forward-thinking organizations that would seem to produce the greatest momentum to achieving the exchange's goals. This expediency must be balanced against the larger consensus that will be gained by including other potential stakeholders in the process. It is common for a few lead organizations to collaborate to form the initial RHIO entity. Once more mature and [hopefully] initially funded, they then invite other organizations to join the effort.[22]

A prerequisite to building the consensus necessary to create a RHIO is trust building. Oftentimes, RHIO development is catalyzed by a trusted neutral third party whose interests do not conflict with the participants. The concept of "shared gain" must be developed and championed, but this oftentimes requires sponsorship by a cadre of respected and trusted clinicians. The most successful efforts have indeed been led by physicians whose active advocacy of patients' well-being serves to mitigate these competitive issues.

Business and Financial Challenges

There are compelling opportunities to leverage HIE to reduce costs of healthcare, but there are relatively few studies that have systematically defined the magnitude of this benefit or the parties to whom the benefit accrues. There has been some modeling of the healthcare economic benefits of HIE based on assumptions about admissions averted, reduced duplicate testing and reduced adverse medical events. One such study calculated that the annual cost savings of a fully implemented national healthcare information exchange would amount to $78 billion.[23] Despite overwhelming modeling evidence as well as limited studies and reports of cost savings by RHIO participants, the cost savings arguments have proven difficult to transform into business plans that convince RHIO participants and benefactors that ongoing financial support is a good financial decision.

In addition to the problem that the cost savings of HIE have not been rigorously proven, the question arises of who the beneficiary is of these savings. Our healthcare economy is frequently a paradigm of misaligned incentives—endeavors that might save the payor money (like reduced hospital admissions) penalizes the hospital and physicians. Conversely, the cost savings due to reduced testing that HIE might bring to a hospital in a capitated contract would be meaningless to the payor. Clearly, a schema in which the costs of the information exchange are fairly assigned to the participants based on proportionate benefits is an important goal of the RHIO business plan.

The costs of initial implementation of most RHIOs are too large (commonly in the $10 million range) to be borne by the healthcare providers or any single non-dominant healthcare payor. Most RHIOs have derived their initial funding from federal (e.g., AHRQ) or state grants, or from healthcare philanthropic organizations. While some RHIOs have obtained grant funding for the first few years of operational expenses, the development of a robust sustainability model has eluded many efforts. Some approaches use subscription fees that are paid by all participants in the data exchange; others exploit value-add services such as transmission of claims or laboratory data. In fact, some efforts (Massachusetts, Indiana) developed clinical data exchange as an outgrowth of existing administrative and financial data exchange infrastructures.

For health data exchange to maximize its true potential, it must cover patients through the continuum of care.

Technical Issues

The technical issues involved in establishing a RHIO are quite considerable and transcend the provision of a communication mechanism among healthcare entities. One of the key design decisions faced by RHIO implementers is whether the data exchange will follow a repository or a peer-to-peer (or commonly a hybrid peer-to-peer) model.

The repository model specifies that all data obtained from the myriad contributors to the RHIO is persistently stored in a central repository; information queries, authentication management and record storage are being handled by the central service. The advantage of this model is performance and relative simplicity compared to the other models at the expense of raising issues of data ownership, since the data now resides in persistent form in a central location. Figure 7-1 illustrates the simplest representation of a central scheme.

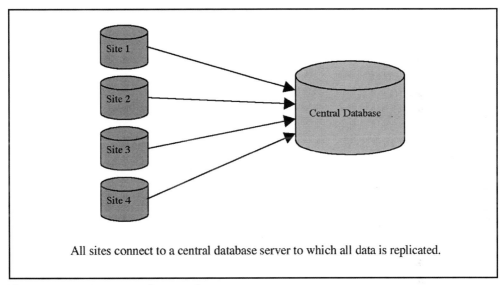

All sites connect to a central database server to which all data is replicated.

Figure 7-1: **Schematic of Central Repository.**

The peer-to-peer model (often tokenized as P2P) is a network of data storage sites that are "equals" on the network. Data remains local to each site (or with each health data provider as in the case of the RHIO) and a data query by one peer is executed against the other peers. The drawback to this model is the performance hit that such queries may incur on the databases of each peer, as well as the increase time each query may take to fully execute. The peer-to-peer model is illustrated in Figure 7-2.

The pure peer-to-peer model usually is modified to a hybrid model among those RHIOs that do not use a repository schema. In the hybrid model, the infrastructure is largely peer-to-peer in that no *clinical* data is stored centrally. However, it is reliant on some centrally-located services, such as a directory service (or in HIE parlance, a "record locator service," or RLS) or authentication and security services. Finally, the databases at each site (which are usually in continual use for the thousands of daily transactions required for clinical care) are commonly connected to an "edge server" that has a replica of the data that the RHIO has specified in its data exchange data elements. This tends to reduce the performance sacrifice that a simple peer-to-peer model entails. The hybrid model is illustrated in Figure 7-3.

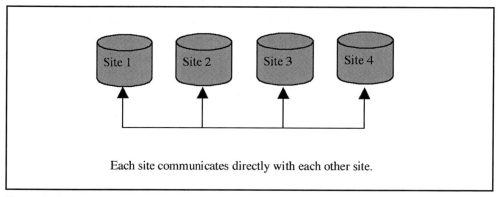

Each site communicates directly with each other site.

Figure 7-2: Peer-to-Peer Model.

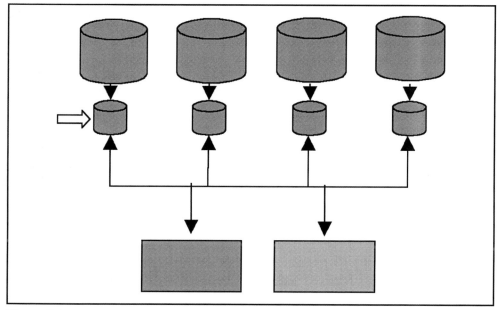

Figure 7-3: Hybrid Model with Central Record Locator and Security Services.

The technical issues go further than overall model definitions. One of the more important technical challenges entails the record locator service. Hospitals commonly use a master patient index (MPI) to unambiguously identify patients. The necessity of the MPI is apparent when one considers that many departmental systems (such as clinical lab and EKG) use unique identifiers that are generated by the lab or EKG system. The MPI collects these numbers, and maps them to the single hospital-wide patient identification number. This enables lookup of a patient's longitudinal data across all departments. The MPI is also used for determining whether a record exists for a specific patient.

For instance, when a patient presents for registration prior to admission, the registrar checks the MPI for the patient's prior records based on demographic information such as name, zip code, social security number and/or other parameters. Armed with this data, the registrar can determine whether the patient requires a new enrollment process and new patient identification number or whether an existing identification number is to be used. Furthermore, the MPI can apply probabilistic logic to determine the likelihood of a match between candidate demographics. The software to accomplish this task is complex and must be "tuned" to the particular demographic complexion of the local market (for example, how best to handle last name similarities). This RLS can be used in a MPI that spans organizations. The RLS must contend not only with the challenges inherent in local patient matching, but must also resolve patient identification problems across an entire region. This task is made no easier by the fact that there is significant disinclination to utilize social security numbers for fear of identity theft and efforts to establish a national patient identifier have languished.

Standards Issues

One issue that plagues designers of medical information systems is that of standards. In essence, data is captured at the source (such as lab systems, EKG systems and hospital admission-discharge-transfer systems) in a variety of formats. For a RHIO to be feasible, the data must be standardized across organizations such that all data relevant to a patient will be presented in a consistent and comparable format. The approach to this issue among healthcare IT vendors has been the promotion of industry-wide standards of data representation and transmission. Some of these standards have gotten considerable momentum, such as the ICD-9 standard for representing diagnostic codes, the CPT-9 standard for medical procedures, SNOMED for pathologic diagnostic codes, LOINC for clinical laboratory results and the HL-7 standard for coding medical transactions.

Nevertheless, there has not been universal adoption of even these standards. Many IT vendors still cling to proprietary schemas of data representation. This is in part due to supporting legacy systems deployed prior to standards availability, in part to make the customer more dependent on sourcing their IT needs to the vendor due to interfacing issues and in part due to the fact that, in some cases, there has not been a clear consensus about which standard will emerge as the appropriate choice. The issue of discordant data and messaging standards has led to the current emphasis on "interoperability."

Privacy and Security Issues

One of the thorniest issues designing a clinical data exchange is that of ensuring patient privacy and security. Under the HIPAA statutes, there is a federal guideline about both privacy constraints on transmission of electronic protected health information (EPHI) as well as general recommendations on security practices. In addition to this federal legislation, state statutes commonly apply to such information practices. Such state legislation often places even more constraints on EPHI transmission.

HIPAA does provide for the transmission of EPHI as required for treatment, payment or operations (such as quality assurance). The transmission of patient health information through a RHIO is indeed for treatment, but all the healthcare entities involved—the hospital or ambulatory site that is the data provider/user and the RHIO— must execute a business associate agreement ("BA") that delineates the privacy responsibilities of each party. All patients must be given a copy of each entity's HIPAA policies that must include an opt-out that has to be honored. Finally, the handling of substance abuse records and mental health records is treated specially in several states.

They require special consent procedures not covered under the treatment, payment and operations exemptions.

Information security represents another challenge that has two dimensions—technical and policy. The technical infrastructure of the clinical data exchange must allow for encrypted transmission of information, technically enforce a standard for authentication and permissions, and allow auditing of all access. The ever-present challenge to security that affects all manner of e-commerce is the "hack"—a malicious breach of safeguards that can result in the exposure of confidential information. No site can plausibly assert that it is immune to such attacks. Given the highly sensitive nature of the information involved, however, it behooves the systems designer to ensure that the data exchange is as resistant as possible to them.

From a policy standpoint, standards must be set for password strength (how easy it would be to guess a password), password expiration time, assignment of access privileges and audit policies. These issues are indeed faced by any healthcare organization with Internet access, but are increased in scale in the instance of a RHIO by the sheer number of patients involved. A security breach has the potential to expose thousands of records to the nefarious eye of the perpetrator. Therefore, it is vital to maintain a very high standard of security awareness and vigilance by all participants, with continual review of technology and security policies.

Liability Issues

The issues of liability, particularly medical malpractice, figure among the concerns of RHIO participants. Several perceived factors contribute to the specific risk of RHIO implementation:

- There is a concern that the presence of RHIO-related information will increase the community standard of practice such that the expectation will be that all providers will have considered the information from other sources before making diagnostic or therapeutic decisions. Should suspect information be dismissed or should available information be overlooked by the treating physician, then departure from this standard may be claimed.

- Should information be erroneous (due to the error of the originator of the information or patient misidentification by the RLS) then the decisions made by the treating physician could result in a malpractice suit. Further, the discovery process preparatory to a medical malpractice proceeding might now involve numerous organizations involved in the RHIO, with a combined explosion in documentation overhead and legal defense effort.

- The RHIO itself might be subject to liability claim in the event that the wrong information was delivered to a participant that purportedly contributed to patient injury.

At the time of this writing, the case law has little light to shed on the concern about RHIO-associate increases in medical malpractice liability exposure,[24] largely due to the newness of the RHIO care paradigm. Hopefully, the improved quality of care that the clinical data exchange will enable will, in the long term, *reduce* malpractice litigation.

NYCLIX – A CASE STUDY

One of the best ways of understanding the complexities inherent in health information exchange is to review the case study of such an effort. The greater New York metropolitan region consists of the five boroughs of New York City, as well as the counties of Nassau, Suffolk and Westchester. The 2005 population was 11.8 million in 2003, with 1.6 million hospital admissions in over ninety facilities, 4.6 million ED visits, and 22.6 million clinic visits[25] in that year.

The New York Clinical Information Exchange (NYCLIX) project started in the summer of 2004 under the stewardship of the Greater New York Hospital Association (GNYHA), a trade organization representing over 250 regional hospitals, long term care and other not-for-profit healthcare entities in the region. The Information Technology Steering Committee of GNYHA was formed to discuss possible collaborative IT projects that delivered value to its sponsoring organizations. Based on efforts launched in other areas of the country, the IT Steering Committee members concluded that the most compelling project would be to create a regional health information exchange with an initial focus on emergency department care. Also based on the experience of other regional health information exchange efforts, it was clear that a neutral third party was necessary to convene the project. Because the GNYHA is a trade organization of hospitals in the metropolitan area with a membership that includes most of the major healthcare providers in the region, it made a good choice as a convener of this effort.

Similar to many other HIE efforts, the emergency department was chosen as the initial choice of "use case" since it seemed to be the locale where information exchange would most positively impact patient care quality and safety. Furthermore, the high-value of information exchange in this clinical venue seemed to override competitive concerns among organizations, and a high degree of buy-in among the Strategic IT Committee members resulted. The roster of healthcare organizations involved in the initial planning phase is listed in Table 7-2.

In December 2004, funding sources were considered. NYCLIX successfully applied for a NIH-National Library of Medicine planning grant, with one of the member institutions (NYU Medical Center) serving as a sponsoring organization and the author as principal investigator. In March 2006, a two-year planning grant award was announced. It serves as the initial funding source to complete planning for the exchange. Concomitant with this, an application was made to the New York State Department of Health for additional funding to support the costs of implementation of the information exchange. Results of this application were forthcoming as of the time of this writing.

In October 2005, the Department of Health of New York made a much-anticipated announcement of a grant program ("HEAL-NY") to fund healthcare IT projects that promoted HIE or EMR dissemination. Accordingly, the NYCLIX workgroup submitted an application one month later to the state for funds to implement NYCLIX. In June 2006, the NY State Department of Health announced a $2.36 million grant award, a portion of the $9.8 million requested. These monies serve as the initial funding for the implementation of NYCLIX.

Table 7-2: NYCLIX Roster.

Name	Organization Type
NYU Medical Center	Hospital System
Catholic Health Services of Long Island	Hospital System
Continuum Health Partners	Hospital System
Group Health Incorporated (GHI)	Payor
Greater New York Hospital Association	Industry Association
Health Quest	IT Vendor
Island Peer Review Organization (IPRO)	Peer Review Organization
Kingsbrook Jewish Medical Center	Hospital System
Lenox Hill Hospital	Hospital System
Maimonides Medical Center	Hospital System
Medical Society of the State of New York	Professional Society
Memorial Sloan-Kettering Cancer Center	Hospital System
Montefiore Medical Center	Hospital System
The Mount Sinai Hospital	Hospital System
New York City Department of Health and Mental Hygiene	Government Health Agency
New York City Health and Hospitals Corporation	Hospital System
New York-Presbyterian Hospital	Hospital System
Saint Vincent Catholic Medical Centers	Hospital System
United Hospital Fund	Healthcare Charitable Organization
Visiting Nurse Service of New York	Home Health Agency

Around the time of the June 2005 submission of the NIH grant, actual planning activities for the NYCLIX data exchange started, and the immense task of providing the organizational infrastructure began. The main planning body—termed the "NYCLIX Workgroup—originally included thirteen healthcare organizations as well as representatives from Group Health Incorporated (a major regional healthcare payor), the United Hospital Fund, the NY State Department of Health, and the Island Peer Review Organization (a Quality Improvement Organization under contract by CMS). The Workgroup sanctioned the establishment of a subcommittee structure as listed in the Table 7-3.

Table 7-3: NYCLIX Subcommittees.

Subcommittee	Responsibility
Governance	Create a governance structure for the nascent NYCLIX RHIO
Technical	Design the technical architecture of the RHIO
Evaluation	Devise an evaluation plan to demonstrate the quality and economic impact of NYCLIX
Business	Create a business sustainability model that will ultimately fund NYCLIX past the inception phase
Communications	Handle internal and external communications. Also has primary responsibility for grant-writing.
Legal	Review HIPAA and liability issues. Prepare participation documents. Coordinate with legal staff of participants.
Clinical Advisory	Serve as the "voice of the clinician." Helps define functional requirements and interface specification.

These subcommittees have been meeting about once monthly and are following the basic work plan laid out in the NIH-IAIMS grant.

These subcommittees have been meeting about once monthly and are following the basic work plan laid out in the NIH-IAIMS grant.

Governance

The NYCLIX Steering Committee realized that in order to apply for startup grant funding, it would be necessary to have a single "neutral" organization assume the position of the applicant entry. Initial discussions among NYCLIX leadership proposed that one of the organizations on which the Chairman or Vice Chairman of the Steering Committee served as faculty (NYU or Columbia) would become the applicant organization for further grant support. This consideration was rejected due to both competitive concerns as well as the additional fiduciary responsibilities that the applicant organization would shoulder under the terms of the Healthcare Efficiency and Affordability Law for New Yorkers (HEAL NY; or, other subsequent implementation grant) requirements. It was decided that an independent not-for-profit entity would best serve the needs and a 501-c corporation was established—NYCLIX, Inc.

At the time of incorporation (February 2006), the Board of Directors was comprised of thirteen healthcare provider organizations that would actually contribute and use the clinical data in the exchange, plus the NYC Department of Health and Mental Health. In addition, a separate class of non-voting board members was created. This consisted of public and private organizations whose input would be deemed valuable for the Board to consider in its planning and decision-making. The reasoning behind the one-provider organization, one-voting board seat structure was that in the perceived high-risk earliest stages of this groundbreaking effort, each organization would need the comfort of direct voting representation on important issues. Furthermore, NYCLIX was small enough to accommodate a representative from each organization while allowing for efficient board functioning. An additional healthcare organization joined the NYCLIX effort (Columbia Faculty Practice Organization), bringing the total number of healthcare provider organizations to fourteen. The governance structure as submitted in the HEAL-NY application is shown in Figure 7-4.

In June 2006, the NYCLIX Board appointed an Executive Committee of three officers, three other Board Members and the Chair of the Technical Subcommittee. The Executive Committee is charged with setting agenda for Board meetings and making decisions not requiring full Board approval. The Steering Committee, comprised of all subcommittee chairs, does most of the work involved in coordinating efforts among the subcommittees and assisting each subcommittee in determining priorities and overcoming barriers.

Planning activities as of the date of this writing have yielded a governance structure, a not-for-profit organization, a preliminary clinical and financial evaluation work plan and significant progress in defining a technical architecture based on the clinical data exchange elements defined by the Clinical Advisory Subcommittee. The data elements selected in order of priority of importance to an emergency physician were EKG images, discharge summaries, medication list, laboratory data, radiology reports, problem lists, provider identification information, text reports of cardiology studies and allergies.

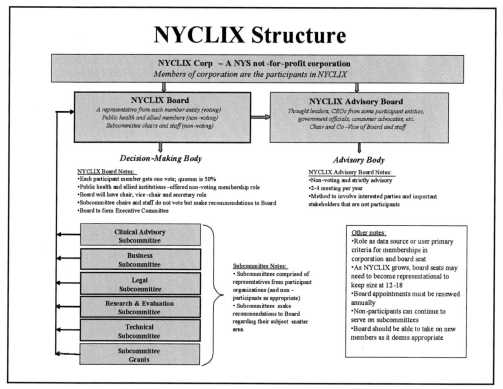

Figure 7-4: NYCLIX Governance Structure.

The principal challenges currently facing NYCLIX include: (1) completing technical planning and implement the clinical data exchange with less funding than initially contemplated; (2) formulating a robust business plan; and, (3) obtaining sufficient capital to expand the data exchange to other care venues and participant organizations. Given the broad commitment and involvement of the participant healthcare organizations, the current momentum that health information exchange has in our healthcare ecology and the initial successful funding efforts, the outlook for NYCLIX is cautiously optimistic.

REFERENCES

1. Smith PC, Araya-Guerra R, Bublitz C, Parnes B, Dickinson LM, Van Vorst R, Westfall JM, Pace WD. Missing clinical information during primary care visits. *JAMA*. 2005 Feb 2;293(5):565–71.

2. Stiell A, Forster AJ, Stiell IG, van Walraven C. Prevalence of information gaps in the emergency department and the effect on patient outcomes. *CMAJ*. 2003;169(10):1023–1028.

3. Institute of Medicine. *To Err is Human: Building a Safer Health System*. Washington DC: National Academy Press, 2000.

4. Institute of Medicine. *Crossing the Quality Chasm: A New Health System for the 21st Century*. Washington DC: National Academy Press, 2001.

5. Bates DW, Leape LL, Cullen DJ, et al. Effect of a computerized physician order entry and a team intervention on prevention of serious medication errors. *JAMA* 1998;280:1311–6.

6. Overhage JM. Dexter PR. Perkins SM. Cordell WH. McGoff J. McGrath R. McDonald CJ. A randomized, controlled trial of clinical information shared from another institution. *Annals of Emergency Medicine*. 2002; January; 39(1):14–23.

7. Bates DW and Gawande AA. Improving safety with information technology. *NEJM*. 2003;348:25 26–34.

8. Patterson E.S., et al.: Hand-off strategies in settings with high consequences for failure: lessons for health care operations. *Int J Qual Health Care*. 2004;April;16:125–132.

9. Lorenzi, N.M. Strategies for creating successful local health information infrastructure initiatives. Available at http://aspe.hhs.gov/sp/NHII/LHII-Lorenzi-12.16.03.pdf. Accessed April 13, 2006.

10. Kuperman GJ, Teich JM, Gandhi TK, Bates DW. Patient safety and computerized medication ordering at Brigham and Women's Hospital. *Joint Comm J Qual Improv*. 2001;October;27(10):509–21.

11. Bartschat W, Burrington-Brown J, Carey S, Chen J, Deming S, Durkin S, et al. Surveying the RHIO landscape. A description of current RHIO models, with a focus on patient identification. *Journal of AHIMA*. 2006;January;77(1):64A–64D.

12. U.S. Department of Health and Human Services. Statement by David J. Brailer, M.D., Ph.D., National Coordinator for Health Information Technology, U.S. Department of Health and Human Services, before U.S. House of Representatives, Committee on Government Reform Hearing on Healthcare and the IT Revolution. Available at: http://www.hhs.gov/healthit/t050929.html. Accessed April 13, 2006.

13. U.S. Department of Health and Human Services. HHS awards contracts to advance nationwide interoperable health information technology. Available at: http://www.hhs.gov/news/press/2005pres/20051006a.html. Accessed April 13, 2006.

14. Halamka J. Overhage JM. Ricciardi L. Rishel W. Shirky C. Diamond C. Exchanging health information: local distribution, national coordination. As more communities develop information-sharing networks, a coordinated approach is essential for linking these networks. *Health Affairs*. 2005;September–October; 24(5):1170–9.

15. Indiana Health Information Exchange. Available at: http://www.ihie.com/origins.htm. Accessed April 16, 2006.

16. Colorado Health Institute. The promise of healthcare information technology: improving the quality and cost-effectiveness of healthcare in Colorado. Available at: http://www.coloradohealthinstitute.org/publications/HIT_White_Paper.pdf. Last accessed April 18, 2006.

17. California Healthcare Foundation. Moving toward electronic health information exchange: interim report on the Santa Barbara County data exchange. Available at: http://www.chcf.org/documents/ihealth/SBCCDEInterimReport.pdf. Accessed April 29, 2006.

18. eHealthInitiative. Community profiles: Santa Barbara County data exchange. Available at: http://ccbh.ehealthinitiative.org/profiles/SBCCDE.mspx. Accessed April 23, 2006.

19. MA-SHARE. Medinfo-ED final report August 2005. Available at: http://www.mahealthdata.org/ma-share/projects/medsinfo/20050825_MedsInfo-ED_FinalRpt.pdf. Accessed May 4, 2006.

20. Massachusetts Health Data Consortium. Leadership and staff. Available at: http://www.mahealthdata.org/ma-share/leadership.html. Accessed on May 4, 2006.

21. Glaser J. Regional health data exchange—the Massachusetts experience. Available at: http://www.health.state.mn.us/e-health/summit/glaser.pdf. Accessed May 4, 2006.

22. Ross D, et al. NHII 2004 governance track background paper. Available at: http://www.healthpolicyohio.org/OHHIT/NHII_2004/governance_paper.pdf. Accessed April 18, 2006.

23. Walker J, Pan E, Johnston D, Adler-Milstein J, Bates DW, Middleton B. The value of health care information exchange and interoperability. *Health Aff* (Millwood). 2005 Jan–Jun; Suppl Web Exclusives: W5-10–W5-18.

24. Brian Wyatt, in personal communication.

25. Greater New York Hospital Association. Health Care Statistics 2005.

CHAPTER 8

Nursing Informatics: Perspectives for Healthcare Executives

Leanne M. Currie, RN, DNSc

Nursing informatics is defined as the intersection between nursing science, information science and computer science.[1] Staggers and Thompson (2002) provide a more descriptive definition, as follows:

> Nursing informatics is a specialty that integrates nursing science, computer science, and information science to manage and communicate data, information, and knowledge in nursing practice. Nursing informatics facilitates the integration of data, information, and knowledge to support patients, nurses, and other providers in their decision making in all roles and settings. This support is accomplished through the use of information structures, information processes, and information technology.[2]

These definitions have several implications. First, as each field is transformed (nursing science, information science and computer science), the field of nursing informatics may be transformed as well. Second, synergies between and amongst the fields may impact the overall field of nursing informatics. Third, the nurse informaticist functions as a translator between clinicians and computer systems developers to ensure that information structures, information processes, and information technology support clinical decision making. And fourth, not only can nursing knowledge guide the design of computer systems, but the data derived from such systems can also inform nursing practice. This last point is an important consideration for those interested in nursing quality and nursing research because a well-designed computer system will have data that can be trusted and thus re-used for purposes across the care continuum.

Nursing informatics has been in formal existence for over 30 years. It focuses not only on hospital systems, but also on other areas of nursing including, long-term care, home care, public health nursing, community nursing, ambulatory care, telehealth and nursing administration. The nurse informaticist can have several types of training and education, and may subsequently assume different roles in a given organization. Increasingly, organizations are seeing the benefit of formally trained nurse informaticists assuming mid-level and senior leadership roles, including those with titles such as manager of clinical informatics, director of nursing informatics (DNI) and chief information officer (CIO).[3]

It is well-recognized that as the largest professional group in healthcare organizations, nurses are critical to the success or failure of a clinical information system implementation. Despite the trend to move towards nurse informaticists in leadership roles, the degree to which nurses participate in clinical information system development remains minimal. In a recent Web-based survey by the HIMSS nursing informatics task force, just over a third (36%) of respondents indicated that they have actively participated in selection or implementation of information systems at their hospital or healthcare network. Another 27% indicated that they had participated at a moderate level, but 37% reported that they have never participated in CIS implementation or development.[4] A reported potential bias with this survey was that because it was Web-based, it is likely that the respondents were more technologically savvy than non-respondents. Therefore, the level of participation may be higher in this study than in reality. This is important because nurses are often critical in the success or failure of system implementations and these data suggest that the positive impact that nurses can make on an IT project has not yet been harnessed. Executives need to understand the scope, practice and potential for nursing informatics in all levels of organizations. The following chapter provides an overview of nursing informatics and identifies strategies that executives might use to maximize the potential of nursing informatics in different healthcare settings.

ROLES OF NURSE INFORMATICISTS

The role of the nurse informaticist is wide ranging and can include educator, project manager, consultant, analyst, researcher, manager, director and senior executive. In 1994, the American Nurses Association (ANA) outlined the standards and scope of practice of the *Informatics Specialist*. This description recognizes an informatics specialist as a person with at least a master's degree in nursing or clinical informatics. Because development, implementation and management of information systems is a very complex process, there are a wide variety of titles and job descriptions given to nurse informaticists. Indeed, the roles have been so varied that the Nursing Informatics Working Group of the American Medical Informatics Association (AMIA-NIWG) has posted a Web page for individuals to post nursing informatics job descriptions and titles to help in clarifying the scope of practice and roles.[3,5]

Some titles used for nurse informaticists refer to roles for system implementation or development team group members (e.g., clinical systems analyst, informatics nurse, nursing analyst and systems administrator). An individual with a systems administrator title typically does not perform tasks related to programming, but will participate in determination of functional and design requirements (i.e., defining what the system *should do* and how the system *should look*). In addition, system analysts may participate in standardized terminology development, system implementation or system refinement. It should be noted that individuals in the role of nursing system development analyst need not always be nurses; many formally trained biomedical informaticists possess the skills to understand the domain of nursing and associated nursing activities and, while not ideal, individuals with information systems training and no clinical training have often learned about nursing workflow from on-the-job experience. Titles that reflect the clinical information systems training role include clinical informatics educator or informatics nurse trainer. This is a common role, and will likely continue to be a nurse informaticist role particularly because nursing has been a leader in clinician and patient education in many healthcare organizations.

Increasingly, organizations are seeing the need for nurse informaticists in leadership roles such as IS clinical project leader, clinical informatics manager, director of nursing informatics or chief information officer. The increase in the number of organizations defining these roles derives not only from organizational need, but also from a recent increase in the availability of formally trained nurse informaticists, particularly those with doctoral education. Senior nurse informaticist executives will oversee wide-ranging development efforts, with a team of nurse analysts reporting to them.[3] Leadership at this level will promote communication with other executive leaders to ensure that an organization's objectives are realistic and that the information system is in alignment with the organization's objectives.

In general, the role of the nurse informaticist will largely depend on the type of educational preparation and related work experience for the individual; however, deep knowledge of and exposure to the environment in which the system will be implemented is beneficial to those in all of the roles, and formal training can provide a solid foundation for individuals in these roles.

HUMAN FACTORS

One of the main reasons to be prudent about information system development is patient safety. In the past decade, several Institute of Medicine (IOM) reports have highlighted the potential for information technology to improve patient care.[6,7] From a nursing perspective, one of the most important reports, *Keeping Patients Safe: Transforming the Work Environment of Nurses*, asserts that well-designed systems can facilitate the work of the nurse and that developers must be mindful about the impact of such technologies on the work of the clinician. As with other high-risk industries like the airline industry, information systems in healthcare that increase distractions (e.g., via interruptions) can negatively impact quality.[8]

Indeed, a group of recent publications that highlight the negative impact of information systems on patient outcomes have sparked a debate about the usefulness of information technology.[9,10] These reports identified several situations in which patient outcomes were negatively impacted by information systems such as an increase in medication errors facilitated by the poor design of a Computerized Practitioner Order Entry (CPOE) system.[11] These reports also documented that, in the face of an inefficient or confusing information system, clinicians use *workarounds*, i.e., alternate strategies to "get the job done" that are not supported by the clinical information system and that can facilitate medical errors. For example, Rogers and colleagues reported that rather than using a preformatted pick list, medication orders were entered using free text within a Nursing Communication function. The effect of this workaround was to by-pass the clinical information system's drug-drug interaction screening increasing the risk for medication errors. Proponents of well-designed information systems and formal informatics departments pointed out that the systems described in these reports were older systems in place in organizations that did not have robust informatics infrastructure.[12] They also noted that situations such as these described often derive from poor implementation practices including those that neglect human factors considerations.[13] As part of an informatics team, the nurse informaticist who understands the clinical environment and who can communicate effectively with programmers can help to prevent such problems from occurring, or can help to identify unsafe practices and remedy the situation early during system use.

Another key component of best practice in human factors is interface design. Interface design expertise is integral to assuring that the end-user experience will be satisfactory. Both software interface and user interface must be considered when designing systems. Key concepts to measure satisfaction with systems include perceived usefulness, and to a lesser extent, perceived ease of use. It is well-demonstrated that individuals (with appropriate training) will be more satisfied with a system that is difficult to use as long as the system provides the user with output that is perceived to be of value. The formally trained nurse informaticist will use guidelines such as Nielsen's heuristics[14] and IBM (Xerox Park) usability testing strategies to reveal untoward problems in early testing and thus prevent the need for workarounds after system implementation. Understanding best practice for integrating systems into workflow design are part of most formal informatics degrees and certificates. Thus, nurse informaticists trained in interface design and interface evaluation can be integral to effective system development.

In addition to software and user interface aspects of human factors design, nurse informaticists are often trained in ergonomics (e.g., physical factors in device design). These skills will be of benefit to organizational leaders who need to decide between different devices. Thus, the trained nurse informaticist should be able to oversee and guide human factors aspects of implementation.

KEY COMPONENTS OF NURSING INFORMATICS

A contention in this text is that information systems need to support the clinical judgment and workflow of all levels of end-users—be they patients, clinicians, administrators or researchers. In an ideal world, the end-user would document their health-related data at one time point only and perhaps confirm the accuracy of the data in a second step. The information system would subsequently store these data in a well-organized database making the data available for re-use at individual and/or aggregate levels, and for real-time and/or later use. This process would be designed to support both the patient and the *knowledge worker,* i.e., persons such as healthcare workers who must collect and use information to work effectively. In addition, the ideal information system must be stable, secure and perceived to be useful to patient, clinical, administrative and research stakeholders.

Towards the goal of stable, secure systems with re-usable data for managing knowledge related to nursing and patient care, several key components of nursing informatics training have been formalized. The components reflect three sciences integrated to define nursing informatics: (1) Information management and knowledge generation; (2) Information technology, including theories, structure, development, functionality, implementation and human factors assessment; and, (3) Nursing practice, including models and theories of nursing, professional nursing practice, and organizational, financial and project management. These components are included in formal nursing and other health informatics curricula. For those trained on the job, skill in these areas may have been gleaned from work experience or in-house training. The importance of these components and the way that they are relevant to nursing and organizational leadership are described in the following sections.

Information Management and Knowledge Generation

Effective information management relies on the integrity and re-usability of data. For data to have integrity (i.e., accurate, consistent and well-organized) and for it to be re-usable, standardized terminologies have been developed. These terminologies are necessary to accurately reflect "what nurses do." Many healthcare executives are aware of standardized terminologies such as the International Classification of Diseases, (ICD), Current Procedures and Treatments (CPT) and more recently, Systematized Nomenclature of Medicine Clinical Terms (SNOMED CT). ICD and CPT codes have been effective for billing purposes, but have limited use when used to characterize clinical practice. This is especially true for nursing practice in that procedures are part of a general bill rather than individual events. Towards the goal of ensuring that computerized systems accurately reflect nursing practice, several nursing terminologies have been developed. Unfortunately, these terminologies are not consistently used in clinical information systems, homegrown or vendor.

The first terminology system to be formalized in nursing was the North American Nursing Diagnosis Associations (NANDA) taxonomy, put forward by Gebbie and Lavin in 1973.[15] This taxonomy characterizes patient problems via a nursing diagnosis, and includes such elements as lack of education for patient or for family. Other standardized nursing terminologies that have since been developed are the Nursing Minimum Data set (NMDS), the clinical care classification system (CCC—formerly HHCC), Nursing Interventions Classifications (NIC) and Nursing Outcomes Classifications (NOC) to name a few.[1] Recently, the international nursing informatics community has approved a nursing reference terminology that uses standardized computer representation (object-oriented) to characterize several aspects of nursing care.[16] This is important because not only was this the first healthcare terminology to attain International Standards Organization (ISO) level of standard, but it also can provide the international community with a framework to represent nursing knowledge in clinical information systems. Standards such as these are particularly important for interoperability (i.e., the ability for information systems to *talk* to each other.) Interoperability is critical for nursing care to be communicated to all providers across a patients' care continuum.

One of the most robust standardized terminologies used in healthcare is SNOMED. In 2003, the National Library of Medicine established a five-year contract with SNOMED to provide the basic elements of the terminology for free use.[17] To date, the most important nursing terminologies have been successfully integrated into SNOMED. The efforts to standardize terminologies are consistent with the IOM reports that advocate for standardization to improve patient safety.[6]

Knowledge generation is a key component of nursing informatics. Data that are accurate, well-organized and re-usable can be closely examined for knowledge generation. Patterns of clinician or patient activities that have not previously been described can be revealed via data mining techniques that maximize the understanding of the area of interest. Data mining is important for executives who need to ensure adherence with local, state and national reporting. The nurse informaticist can help to ensure that nursing work is accurately reflected in a clinical information system and that the data will be re-usable for all levels of organizational needs.

Information Technology

The formally trained nurse informaticist understands all aspects of information technology including development and implementation, hardware, software, security, standards and protocols and telecommunication. As mentioned earlier, one of the primary roles of the nurse informaticist is as a system analyst—a translational role in which the nurse is able to translate clinician needs to information technology developers and vice versa. Nurse informaticists in such roles will have skills useful at all phases of the system development life cycle (SDLC). The SDLC includes system planning phase, system analysis, system design, system implementation and testing, and system evaluation, maintenance and support. An individual in the role of chief nurse informaticist would oversee a team that was applying the SDLC process. System planning concepts include strategic goals and priorities, vendor, product, and market analysis, resource considerations, cost-benefit analysis and establishing teams. The role of the nurse informaticists during this process includes administrative functions such as leading or participating in product evaluation and team formation for system implementation.

System analysis includes methods for needs assessment, feasibility assessment, process analysis (e.g., using process diagrams, decision trees, flow charts), functional specifications, request for proposal (RFP) development, system selection and contract issues. The role of the nurse informaticist for systems analysis might include formal needs assessment and requirements specification or might take on a more business perspective in RFP evaluation. System design includes understanding critical success factors within the scope of the SDLC. The role of the nurse informaticist during the system design phase may include database design, system quality assurance and auditing. This is different than typical hospital auditing because it refers to the quality of data from the system and is reliant on factors such as ensuring that the data are backed up, that the data can be re-used and that the data are secure.

System implementation and testing includes functions associated with initiating a new electronic system or with managing changes within an existing system. The role of the nurse informaticist towards system implementation includes user testing, policy documentation and training. System evaluation, maintenance and support include practices towards ensuring adequate user acceptance and perceived usefulness. The role of the nurse informaticist towards system evaluation, maintenance and support include operational aspects that can support upgrades and enhancements such as development of new alerts and reminders and other functions that ensure the system adequately and accurately represents the interaction between the clinician and their patients. Project management skills are critical for well-managed system implementations, and formal training in project management can facilitate a successful system implementation.

While not typically trained in computer software programming, professional nurse informaticists understand all aspects of information technology design and implementation. Knowledge of database structure and information exchange ensures that the nurse informaticist can communicate with clinicians as well as with developers. Indeed, it is the translational role of the nurse informaticist that often provides the greatest value to an organization.

Nursing Practice

Several key factors related to nursing practice impact nursing informatics. First, in most countries, trained nurses are the most populous healthcare providers. Because of this, the role of the nurse can be widely varied. Secondly, in the acute, long-term and homecare settings, nurses provide the greatest proportion of direct care to patients. This results in nurses being intermediaries between healthcare disciplines often placing the nurse in a patient advocacy role. Although healthcare is migrating towards true interdisciplinarity, the primary care giver role of the nurse remains true in most settings and must be supported by the clinical information system.

Integration of the evidence to support decision making at the point-of-care is a primary goal of organizations. Proponents of evidence practice assert that the only feasible means by which clinicians can manage the dearth of information that they are responsible to know is to have the practice recommendations fully integrated into the clinical information system.[18] Towards full integration of evidence-based practice, nurse informaticists can work with nursing practice leaders to ensure that the appropriate evidence is delivered to the appropriate individual at the appropriate time point. This might involve designing alerts or reminders for clinicians at the point-of-care or integrating national guidelines into the clinical information system.

A great deal of work has gone into defining the decision-making process of clinicians and recent work has focused on how decision-making processes affect patient safety.[19] As mentioned above, human factors play an important part in patient safety and the nurse informaticist will be able to support best practice for system design towards patient safety.

Factors related to organizational behavior, organizational change, management science and systems theory are fundamental to nursing informatics training. Many nurse informaticist programs are derived from master's level nursing administration programs, some of which provide education comparable to a Master's of Business Administration. Nurse informaticists are aware of healthcare industry trends and regulatory requirements and thus, can be integral in ensuring that the information technology supports such requirements.

NURSING INFORMATICS EDUCATION AND CERTIFICATION

Currently, formal training for nursing informatics involves obtaining a master's degree in nursing informatics or a post-master's certificate in nursing or healthcare informatics. This is consistent with the ANA definition of the informatics specialist that requires a master's degree. Most universities and many colleges with graduate level nursing programs offer master's level informatics programs, some of which can be completed online. As mentioned above, the role of the master's-prepared informatics specialist can vary widely, and is often contingent on the organization's needs. While some individuals without master's education are employed in health IT departments, the role of the nurse informaticist—particularly in leadership roles—will benefit from formal master's education.

A growing number of universities offer doctoral education in nursing informatics.

The doctoral prepared nurse informaticist possesses applied research design, analysis, and in many cases, management skills. Nurse informaticists with doctoral education are often situated in leadership roles at healthcare organizations, leadership roles in vendor organizations or in academia. Depending on the individual's specific area of research, the nurse informaticist with a doctorate might contribute to several of many organizational objectives. As mentioned earlier, an increasing number of organizations realize the potential of the doctoral prepared nurse informaticist in ensuring that nursing issues are addressed in relation to information technology. The nursing informatics community applauds this trend and is eagerly trying to ensure that supply meets the demand.

National efforts are moving towards the integration of informatics into all levels of nursing education. While technology is commonly used by students in all nursing curricula, however, not all nurses receive any introduction to nursing informatics.[20] Each level of education has increasing informatics competencies. The nurse with an Associates Degree should possess basic computer skills, the master's-prepared nurse informaticist guide a system integration and the doctoral prepared nurse informaticist possess system architecture and informatics research skills. The new registered nurse should possess at the very least basic computer skills, knowledge of some nursing terminologies such as NANDA, and perhaps NIC and NOC.

Master's-prepared nurse informaticists and baccalaureate-prepared nurses with experience or post-baccalaureate certificates are eligible to sit for certification as an Informatics Nurse. This certification is offered by the American Nurses Credentialing Center (ANCC), the certifying arm of the ANA. The ANCC certification tests for the following elements: (1) Understanding human factors; (2) Understanding system development life cycle; (3) Understanding critical elements of information technology; (4) Management of information and knowledge generation; (5) Professional practice, trends, and issues; and, (6) Models and theories of nursing, nursing management and informatics.

Many master's training programs in nursing informatics expect graduating Informatics Specialists to pursue the ANCC certification. A second certification available to nurse informaticists, is the Certified Professional in Healthcare Information and Management Systems (CPHIMS) certification exam, offered by HIMSS.

The components of the ANCC certification are similar to the elements found in the HIMSS Certified Professional in Healthcare Information and Management Systems (CPHIMS) certification exam; however, they differ in three main areas. First, the ANCC certification has more explicit expectations of human factors management (including ergonomics) and user interface design. Second, the ANCC certification tests for knowledge related to informatics theory, but the CPHIMS does not. And third, the HIMSS professional certification tests for management and leadership skills, but the ANCC certification does not. However, as mentioned previously, the master's-prepared nurse informaticist will often have business administration skills such as financial and nursing management, organizational behavior and formal leadership training.

All of these differences will be of interest to the executive because when assessing the skills of a prospective candidate, the ANCC certification does not imply management skills. However, the nurse informaticist is typically formally trained to function as a human factors expert and will be an expert in regards to nursing activities. It is important to note that neither of these certifications tests for computer programming skills; rather they test for the system analyst role, a role in which the analyst interprets end-user activities and identifies an appropriate function and appearance required for an information system. In this role, the analyst would need to understand the workflow of the clinician and would also need to know the underlying process of the computerized system.

CONCLUSION

In conclusion, nursing informatics is a robust and growing field with well-defined training programs. However, nurses and nurse informaticists have been under-utilized to date, but offer significant potential for growth in organizations. Healthcare executives who are interested in ensuring the success of clinical information system development, implementation and refinement should harness the potential of nurse informaticists to ensure that the appropriate information structures, information processes and information technology are in place to support clinical decision making in all settings.

REFERENCES

1. Saba VK, McCormick KA. *Essentials of Nursing Informatics*. 4th ed. New York, NY: McGraw-Hill Medical Pub. Division; 2006.

2. Staggers N, Thompson CB. The evolution of definitions for nursing informatics: a critical analysis and revised definition. *J Am Med Inform Assoc*. 2002;May 1;9(3):255–261.

3. Weaver CA, Delaney C, Weber P, Carr R, eds. *Nursing and Informatics for the 21st Century: An International Look at Practice, Trends and the Future*. Chicago: Health Information Management Systems Society; 2006.

4. Dykes P, Cashen M, Foster M, et al. Surveying acute care providers in the U.S. to explore the impact of HIT on the role of nurses and interdisciplinary communication in acute care settings. *JHIM*. 2006;20(2):36–44.

5. Nursing Informatics Working Group. Roles in nursing informatics. Available at: http://www.amia.org/mbrcenter/wg/ni/roles.asp. Accessed July 21, 2006.

6. Institute of Medicine. *Patient Safety: Achieving a New Standard for Care*. Washington DC: National Academies Press; 2004.

7. Institute of Medicine. *To Err is Human: Building a Safer Health System.* Washington DC: National Academies Press; 2000.

8. Institute of Medicine. *Keeping Patients Safe: Transforming the Work Environment of Nurses.* Washington, DC: National Academies Press; 2004.

9. Koppel R, Metlay JP, Cohen A, et al. Role of computerized physician order entry systems in facilitating medication errors. *JAMA.* 2005; March 9;293(10):1197–1203.

10. Garg AX, Adhikari NK, McDonald H, et al. Effects of computerized clinical decision support systems on practitioner performance and patient outcomes: a systematic review. *JAMA.* 2005;March 9;293(10):1223–1238.

11. Reynolds K, Peres A, Tatham JM. The impact on patient safety of free-text entry of nursing orders into an electronic medical record in an integrated delivery system. Paper presented at: 1: AMIA Annu Symp Proc., 2005; Washington, DC.

12. Shortliffe EH. CPOE and the facilitation of medication errors. *J Biomed Inform.* 2005;August;38(4):257–258.

13. Bates DW. Computerized physician order entry and medication errors: finding a balance. *J Biomed Inform.* Aug 2005;38(4):259–261.

14. Nielsen J. Designing Web Usability: The Practice of Simplicity. Berkeley: Peachpit Press; 1999.

15. Gebbie K, Lavin MA. Classifying nursing diagnoses. *American Journal of Nursing.* 1974;74(2):250–253.

16. International Standards Organization Tc. ISO 18104:2003: Health Informatics—Integration of a reference terminology model for nursing. 2003; December 18.

17. Mehnert R, Cravedi K. HHS launches new efforts to promote paperless health care system. Washington DC: National Institutes of Health National Library of Medicine; 2003.

18. Haynes RB. Of studies, summaries, synopsis, and systems: the "4S" evolution of services for finding current best evidence. *Evid Based Nurs.* 2005;January 1;8(1):4–6.

19. Patel VL, Currie LM. Clinical cognition and biomedical informatics: issues of patient safety. *Int J Med Inform.* Dec 2005;74(11–12):869–885.

20. Maag MM. Nursing students' attitudes toward technology: a national study. *Nurse Educ.* 2006;May–June;31(3):112–118.

CHAPTER 9

The Personal Health Record

Glenn Martin, MD

The personal health record (PHR) is an electronic, universally available, lifelong resource of health information needed by individuals to make health decisions. Individuals own and manage the information in the PHR, which comes from healthcare providers and the individual. The PHR is maintained in a secure and private environment, with the individual determining rights of access. The PHR is separate from and does not replace the legal record of any provider.[1]

This definition of a personal health record (PHR) from the American Health Information Management Association can be criticized for being prejudiced as it is limited to electronic formats. It can be dismissed as grandiose as it calls for universal access. It can even be called too optimistic as it suggests a PHR can meet all of these goals and yet still be secure and private. However, this definition is good place to begin.

Actually, it is silent on many key defining characteristics of a PHR. What will the content be and from where exactly will that information come? How current and accurate can the information be? How will the information enter the PHR? What form will the information be featured in and what will hold or transmit the PHR? In fact, all of theses issues are still open for discussion. Those discussions about the PHR should at least take place in the context of three overarching concepts:

- The players and the Terrain
- Trust
- Truth

THE PLAYERS AND THE ENVIRONMENT

Personal Health Records do not exist in a vacuum. They are held by patients, used by physicians and other healthcare providers, and operate in an increasingly electronic healthcare environment. While arguably simplistic, the way these three interact with a PHR can be characterized by the following:

Patients Are Not Medical Historians

Humans constantly demonstrate that they will not always do the right thing even if the benefits are apparent. This is especially true when they are asked to do something that will only be used infrequently and only when something bad is happening. A good example is drawing up a will or completing a healthcare proxy. In the usual situation neither is hard to do, nor are they lengthy or expensive to generate. Both documents can be of great benefit, yet many people do not complete them. The same can be said of the records organizers found in most personal financial software.

A patient's ability to understand, collect and organize medical information is usually limited. He/she cannot be expected to recognize the importance of the individual items of his/her medical history. Nor can they be expected to collect that information from a variety of providers and sources—some electronic, some paper-based—and keep it regularly maintained. Even if the PHR is easy to use, collecting the data form a variety of sources—many of which will still be on paper—can be tedious and ultimately incomplete.

There is at least one examination of layman's efforts to populate an electronic record from paper sources.[2] The authors demonstrated that accuracy of the data transfer was dependent on the type of data entry. Guided and limited fields (e.g., pull down selections) were more accurate than data that allowed for free text entry. Not surprisingly, data entries that required more knowledge and sophistication (e.g., the medical indication for a medication being prescribed) proved to be problematic. Similarly, the layman demonstrated problems in entering lab data when units (e.g., mg/ml) were needed or the normal range for the results had to be entered in order for the test to be interpretable.

Providers Have Limited Resources, Financial and Temporal

Most providers will not invest money in systems that are not proven or have a readily apparent return. Money is not the only limiting factor as providers operating in the current managed environment frequently find that their scarcest resource is time. Integration into the office workflow is a key success principle. Any successful PHR that requires a physician input has to be inexpensive and cannot take an appreciable amount of time from a provider or staff. Ideally, it would be integrated into an existing electronic medical records system, assuming the physician or hospital already has one. This does not describe the current state.

Murphy Looks over Information Systems

Information systems are complex operations with many failure points. Inaccurate information can enter the system, the software can malfunction and the hardware can crash. Murphy's Law dictates that this will happen at the worst possible time. For this discussion, however, we will limit it to those times a PHR must be created, updated or accessed. As such, a good PHR must be able to cope with systems failures; in fact, it should help overcome them. A PHR accessible only on the Internet cannot work if the network is down or cannot be reached, or if the server hosting the record is down. A PHR that has the information off-line (e.g., on a flash-drive or smart card) can work without a network. In fact, it can even help repopulate a medical record if there is truly a catastrophic failure.

TRUST

An effective PHR can only work well in an environment where trust is established, or at the very least, issues of trust are well thought out. A patient will only maintain a PHR if he/she believes that the information will be securely stored and only used for his/her benefit in circumstances with his/her approval. In the current environment, patients are bombarded by reports of massive loss of private and sensitive data. Losses have occurred in the financial and service sectors, by healthcare organizations and governmental agencies (see Table 9-1).

Losses have occurred via the Internet, corporate networks, and lost backup tapes and computers. The increasing use of flash drives has made it easier to download and transport stolen data. While it has made it easier to transport data for legitimate purposes, it also makes it more likely that those data will be lost or stolen. Robust encryption technology exists and is even available as open source freeware (e.g., Truecrypt). However, it frequently is not used or paired with utterly inadequate passwords.

A provider can only use the information on a PHR when he is convinced it actually pertains to the patient in front of him. The use of photo identification and incorporating biometric IDs will surely help achieve this confirmation. However, the complications of making identity matches from online data are well known and still an area of active concern. Furthermore, the provider must be assured that the information is reasonably complete and accurate, and that its limitations are readily apparent (e.g., date of last update, sources of information, whether sensitive information like HIV or substance abuse is maintained). While it is true that these issues exist in the standard paper environment, they are amplified by the use of electronic media.

Neither the patient nor the provider will readily accept a PHR unless access control and the uses of the information are established and enforced. Recent history has taught us a clear lesson: owners of prescribing information (large pharmacy chains and pharmacy benefit managers) have sold this information to the pharmaceutical industry. While the information has been stripped of patient identifiers, the prescribing habits of individual physicians is routinely examined and used to make marketing decisions including visits and calls by the sales force. This practice, while legal, has enraged many physicians, prompted action by multiple state and national medical societies and even prompted legislative remedies to be introduced at the state level.[3]

Patients' concerns about the use of private information that affects insurability and employability have already had an impact on HIV testing and genetic testing for susceptibility to diseases (e.g., cancer, Alzheimer's dementia). Without clear protections and adequate technological safeguards, it is likely patients will not consent to assembling a PHR—or if they do, they edit it extensively to remove pertinent and possibly life saving information. For example, there are potentially life threatening medication interactions that can occur with drugs used in the treatment of HIV infection and severe mental illness. To not include these medications or mention of the diagnoses in the record can actually increase the possibility of medical errors if the healthcare provider relies on the PHR when performing an interaction check before prescribing or dispensing.

Table 9-1: Reported Data Incidents.

(Adapted from www.IDTheftcenter.org).

2005 Data:
• 152 incidents and 57,700,000 individuals
o 11% (17) healthcare facilities/companies
o 48% (73) educational settings
2006 Data through 6/14/06:
• 93 disclosed incidents and potentially affecting more than 32,147,796 individuals
o 35% of disclosures involve educational institutions
o 23% of disclosures involve governmental or military agencies
o 19% of disclosures involve general business
o 11% of disclosures involve healthcare facilities or companies
o 12% of disclosures involve banking, credit or financial services entities
Some Health Related Losses:
UC Berkeley:
• hacked research computer
• August 2004 incident involved more than 600,000 participants in the state's In Home Supportive Services program
UCLA:
• June 2004 incident involved 145,000 blood donors via unencrypted laptop
MSMC:
• July 2005 incident involved more than 10,000 research patients with more than 6000 SSN exposed
• stolen desktop with password protected unencrypted
• Recovered and not accessed
Providence Home Services:
• January 2006 incident involved 365,000 patients via unencrypted back-up tapes
University of Pittsburgh Medical Center:
• January 2006 incident involved the demographic information of 700 patients on one of six stolen computers; medical conditions not in the file
State of Washington Health Care Authority:
• In January 2006, 6,000 health screening reminder postcards were sent to 6,000 public employees with their Social Security numbers printed on them
PricewaterhouseCoopers/University of Texas M.D. Anderson Cancer Center:
• In November of 2005, the private health information and Social Security numbers of nearly 4,000 patients were compromised after a laptop containing their insurance claims was stolen from the consultants
YMCA:
• May 2006 incident involved more than 65,000 YMCA members from Rhode Island and Seekonk, Massachusetts
• Information lost on a stolen laptop included credit-card and debit-card numbers, checking account information and Social Security numbers
• Also lost were the names and addresses of children in YMCA daycare programs and medical information about the children, such as allergies and medicine taken
Department of Veterans Affairs:
• As many as 26.5 million veterans were placed at risk of identity theft after an intruder stole an electronic data file containing their names, birth dates and Social Security numbers from the home of a Department of Veterans Affairs employee in May 2006 (The Washington Post, May 23, 2006)

TRUTH

The benefits of the widespread use of PHR's to promote patient safety and speedy, accurate and cost-effective medical care is dependent on the quality of the information provided in the record. If the information is not considered reliable, it cannot be used. If it is not considered current and appropriately comprehensive, its usefulness is seriously curtailed.

Is It Accurate and What Does That Mean?

Any physician who treats a patient with multiple medical records from multiple providers knows that the information is rarely completely consistent. There are gaps in the record and occasional contradictions. Patients may recall something one day to one provider and recall it a bit differently at a later date or in different circumstances. Significant family and early developmental history given to a psychiatrist is likely to be different than that given to a cardiologist evaluating chest pain. One entry of a side effect may very well be documented by another as an allergy. Not infrequently, a patient will report something to a physician who will subsequently conclude that it is not accurate. The amount of daily exercise or alcohol consumption being reported may not reflect reality. In the record maintained by the physician, this discrepancy may be noted and explained. How these entries are to be reconciled in a comprehensive record is not always clear, especially when it is the patient who has ownership and control of the PHR.

Corrections

Occasionally mistakes will enter a record; entries can be placed in the wrong chart, information can be misread or mistyped. Other times, interpretations of findings can change. Initial readings of radiology procedures, pathology reports and other tests can be changed in the normal course of medical care when they are reviewed by a more experienced practitioner or more information becomes available. The ability to update and correct a record, but not erase the "electronic audit trail" is needed. In addition, there should be the ability to retrieve the changes and even to functionally roll back the clock, so that it would be possible to recreate the PHR as it existed at a moment in time.

Is It Complete? Who Decides and How Do You Let Others Know?

In a perfect world, patients would feel comfortable with all necessary information being available in their PHR and all doctors would be comfortable feeding their information to it. This does not reflect reality. Some patients will only want to share some information because of privacy concerns, modesty or fear of stigmatization. A patient might decide to block his HIV status, but not know that allowing for a complete medication list— essential for maximizing patient safety by reducing medication interaction problems— actually reveals the diagnoses to a medical professional and others. Some doctors would not want to have the full diagnoses or pathology results available to all patients, as occasionally good judgment and patient preference compel less than full disclosure. How should this be recorded? Should all records be blocked from having certain information or should a notation be made that some of the record is being voluntarily withheld? Obviously, these different scenarios have different interpretations, as a clinician might conclude that a non-answer is meaningful.

Even if the record is complete, it is reasonable for a patient to withhold certain information from certain providers. Few would challenge the reasonableness of a decision not to share a history of sexually transmitted diseases with a podiatrist being consulted for a bunion. Accepting this and implementing it are two different things, however, especially if the user interface does not allow for easy access control at such a detailed level. Not giving access at all is one thing, selecting portions of a PHR to share is a much greater technical challenge.

HOW TO STORE A PHR

Paper Records

While paper records may not fall within the definition of a PHR in an electronic age, they represent a valid alternative for many individuals (see Table 9-2). Paper does have the advantage of being familiar and portable. In fact, the forms many patients are given at the beginning of an office visit to record basic health information is a rudimentary PHR. Completing a form can be done by the most unsophisticated members of the population, assuming basic literacy and access to a linguistically compatible form. It is easily edited and can be updated with minimal cost and time by anyone given access.

Table 9-2: Characteristics of Paper PHRs.

• Portable and controllable (until lost)
• Not easy to collate and summarize
• Never around when you need them
• Too much or too little
• Handwriting
• Source and timeliness of information

Paper forms do have many limitations. Updating them is not automatic and may require a dedicated and organized family archivist. They are relatively bulky and are not likely to be carried by a patient in all circumstances where a PHR would be of value. Without access to a photocopier or scanner, there is inadequate back-up of the records making loss very disruptive. If lost, the documents are easily read by the finder without need of a password or security software. Forms are generally completed with handwritten notations that may not be legible. With time, paper and ink can become difficult to read and are susceptible to environmental damage.

Paper forms are also less than ideal for integrating information from multiple sources and assembling it in an organized fashion with each update. One has only to contemplate a multi-year medication history—with repetitive scratch outs, misspelled names, and illegible dosing instructions and dates—to see the limitations. Even if a record is well maintained, there is also the risk of providing too much information. Data overload at the point-of-care can make the information almost useless as the busy clinician cannot take the time to wade through a comprehensive notebook of information.

Computer-Based Records

Clearly the equivalent of a paper history form can be placed on an individual's computer (see Table 9-3). For years, financial software has included a vital records section where one could organize the contents and locations of documents, accounts and contacts. The records remain on the individual computer but can be printed out for remote use or prepared as an electronic file for e-mail transmission.

Table 9-3: Characteristics of Computer-Based PHRs.

* Need a computer and desire to use one
* Interface has to be easy, obvious and friendly
* Still have to print it out to use it, though could e-mail it
* Hope the computer maven isn't the incapacitated patient

Unlike paper there are no issues with handwritten entries and illegibility. Well-designed, it will allow for adequate space to enter all information in correct fields and promote ready access to both a current snapshot and a historical overview of the patient's history. Backups can be done efficiently and, at least in theory, automatically. Updates could be prompted at regular intervals, either by the software or via e-mailed reminders by healthcare providers. Security can be built into the software being used or the files can be encrypted by readily available products.

The limitations of data entry remain paramount. The patient or family member has to have access to a computer and want to use it. The patient will have to take the time to assemble the necessary information and enter it. This will frequently require entering technical information in a jargon that is unfamiliar. Even if the jargon is not a problem, the provider who will eventually use the information must be wary of simple typos, transposition of numbers, and other transcription errors. A chronically ill patient with multiple specialists has the daunting task of frequent update.

As with paper, it will still require the patient to have a copy of his PHR with him when he visits the doctor or hospital. This requires planning, and in an emergency situation this may not be possible. If it is the computer user who is ill, remaining family members may not have ready access to the PHR and password, or the know-how to access and print it. It is possible to e-mail the file to a physician, but unless a secure form of transmission is readily available, there are significant security risks associated with an open transmission.

The Web

Many of the limitations of a PHR stored on a patient's personal computer can be mitigated by storing the information online using a Web-based service (see Table 9-4). If properly designed, data entry can be facilitated and storing and presenting the information in a variety of sensible formats is quite feasible. The patient does not need to remember to take his PHR with him, as it would be available from any Internet-attached device throughout the world. Linguistic challenges can be addressed by multiple versions of the forms. For example, the patient in New York completes the form in English. If he should take ill abroad, the French speaking physician in the Ivory Coast could call up the patient's PHR using the French template. The answers would be in English, but the French online version would at least have the questions and field names in French.

Table 9-4: Characteristics of Web-Based PHRs.

* Same issues of data entry
* Can it import information from other systems or the individuals' computer files?
* Who controls it and can you trust them?
* Will they stay in business?
* Need a computer and a functioning network to enter and retrieve, especially during disasters?

Storing the information remotely does raise a host of security concerns as the patient is no longer the sole holder of the record. Patients are rightly concerned about the possible loss of online records. Even if not stolen, there is precedent in the online information storage business of commercial enterprises going out of business with such rapidity that records were lost before they could be retrieved by their owners.

Security for any PHR stored online or on electronic media is a balance between competing compelling concerns. The information must be secure and unusable without permission of the patient. Yet, the information has to be readily available to healthcare workers in an emergency situation where the patient's medical condition prevents him from providing a personal identification number (PIN). Ideally, the online service provides a form of "break the glass" security where an authenticated provider can access the record without the patient's PIN, and an audit log records the emergency retrieval.

In addition, an online storage solution is only useful if the online location is accessible at all times. This requires the practitioner to have a functioning Internet hook up and for the storage site to be up and running. Even scheduled maintenance is a challenge; unlike financial sites that can safely do maintenance in the early hours of a weekend morning, a PHR may be needed 24/7. Finally, there are many situations where an accessible PHR could be life-saving, but Internet access is not guaranteed (e.g., ambulances, disaster response and blackouts).

Devices

Over the last several years, portable storage has becomes both physically smaller and quantitatively larger. Increasingly flash drives and miniature hard drives are used in the business and consumer environment. Smart cards, though not as popular in the United States as the rest of the world and with more limited data capacity, also have their place in information storage and identity authentication. PHRs can be stored on any of these media, even if that was not their original intent. For example, most MP3 players and cell phones will also allow for a data file to be stored.

The advantage that this group brings to the PHR is their easy portability and large capacity (see Table 9-5). The data entry issues outlined in the previous groups remains, as does the password control conundrum. To be most useful, the device has to be readable on a computer without special pre-installed software, and should operate on a multitude of operating systems. Portability is a two-edged sword. By carrying the device, the patient avoids the perceived risk of online storage and can be in greater control of access to the PHR. However, the patient has to remember to carry the device and avoid its loss. In addition, the updating process is another risk point in the system since the data will most likely have to be entered via a computer connection.

Form factor is important when considering an appropriate device. It has to encourage someone to carry the device, yet at the same time protect it from environmental damage. Flash drives, while small, are not tiny. Incorporating them into key rings is a popular approach. More recently, a drive and USB interface contained within a silicon bracelet has been promoted as an alternative.

Compact disks have been distributed to patients with extracts of their medical record. They do not allow for patient updates. They have the advantage of holding a great deal of information and they are inexpensive. To be useful in a portable format that a patient is likely to carry at all times, however, the smaller "business card" size CD version has to be used. Durability in a wallet remains a concern.

Table 9-5: Devices for the PHR.

Form Factors
• USB sticks, key chains, etc.
• CDs
• Smart cards
• Cell phones, I-pods, MP3 players
Considerations
• Need to carry them
• Need to update them
• Need to be able to read them
• Need to secure them from loss

Smart cards represent another form that has proven user acceptance. They are the size of a standard credit card and the incorporated integrated chip's size, location and interface are governed by accepted international standards. Data storage is limited. Typical chips hold 64k, but larger chips are now available. The chips are designed to be tamper resistant and usually incorporate some form of data encryption. The chips also contain micro-processor components that allow their use as SIM cards in phones, debit cards and identity cards. In fact, multiple uses with one card are allowed.

Combinations

It is likely that successful implementations of PHRs will combine two or more of these media. A computer is likely to be used by patients to update and maintain their cards, even if a portion of the cards are updated directly by their physician or hospital. To be useful, the information will have to be online or on the patient's person, so the stand alone computer solution has to be combined with one of the other options. For PHRs primarily stored online, a smart card or USB device may be used as the authentication to allow access, while at the same time storing information for those times when network access is not available.

For a comprehensive assemblage of available options, the following Internet site can be consulted: http:/www.myphr.com/resources/phr_search.asp (accessed June 29, 2006). Information includes links to the vendors and lost sites, with information on pricing, etc.

CONTENT AND STANDARDS

For a PHR to have the most benefits, it has to have sufficient information to be useful, organized to allow for easy access and viewing, and ideally built in such a way as to allow for interoperability with existing electronic medical records (EMRs). In the last few years, there have been several efforts underway to guide the development of PHRs in this direction.

The American Health Information Management Association and its related site, www.myPHR.org, advocates individuals to establish their own PHR using freely provided paper forms and various electronic formats. The suggested content for a PHR is found in Table 9-6. In addition to content recommendations, there are links to a variety of different products that can help assemble, organize and hold a PHR. However, standards to promote interoperability are not provided.

Table 9-6: **PHR Content (adapted from AHIMA).**

- Personal identification, including name, birth date and social security number
- People to contact in case of emergency
- Names, addresses, and phone numbers of your physician, dentist and other specialists
- Health insurance information
- Living wills and advance directives
- Organ donor authorization
- A list and dates of significant illnesses and surgeries
- Current medications and dosages
- Immunizations and their dates
- Allergies
- Important events, dates and hereditary conditions in your family history
- A recent physical examination
- Opinions of specialists
- Important tests results
- Eye and dental records
- Correspondence between you and your provider(s)
- Permission forms for release of information, operations and other medical procedures
- Any information you want to include about your health – such as your exercise regimen, any herbal medications you take and any counseling you may receive

ASTM Continuity of Care Record (standard E2369-05)

The Continuity of Care Record, CCR, is a standard specification that has been developed jointly by ASTM International, the Massachusetts Medical Society, the Health Information Management and Systems Society, the American Academy of Family Physicians, the American Academy of Pediatrics and the American Medical Association. As stated in the scope of the standard, "The Continuity of Care Record (CCR) is a core data set of the most relevant and timely facts about a patient's healthcare.[4] It is to be prepared by a practitioner at the conclusion of a healthcare encounter in order to enable the next practitioner to readily access such information. It includes a summary of the patient's health status (e.g., problems, medications, allergies) and basic information about insurance, advance directives, care documentation and care plan recommendations. It also includes identifying information and the purpose of the CCR…It is intended to foster and improve continuity of patient care, reduce medical errors, improve patients' roles in managing their health, and assure at least a minimum standard of secure health information transportability."[4]

This standard effort addresses both the content of information in the record as well as the format of the CCR. Specifically, the content is designed to be machine and human readable. The content is envisioned as being entered by the provider with the idea that the information would be used and updated by another provider when they render care at the time of a transfer or consultation. Additionally, the information would be available to the patient as a record of recent care.

The CCR core data set consists of three parts:

The Header: It contains basic information about the source and use of the information. It includes a unique CCR identifier from the provider, the date/time the record is written, the name of the patient, from and to fields, and the purpose of the record (e.g., transfer, discharge, patient record). The identifiers are neither universal patient or provider identifiers, though nothing in the standard precludes their use should they be established and accepted.

The Body: It contains patient administrative/demographic and clinical sections. Highlights of the content are found in Table 9-7. The content is comprehensive, yet generic. Clinical extensions are planned to allow for more specificity in different clinical situations. HIV and Ob/Gyn extensions are currently being developed.

Table 9-7: **Continuing Care Record Core Data Set.**

- Insurance
- Advance Directives
- Support
- Functional Status
- Problems
- Family History
- Social History
- Alerts
- Medications
- Medical Equipment
- Immunizations
- Vital Signs
- Result
- Procedures
- Encounters
- Plan of Care
- Healthcare Providers

The Footer: It contains detailed information about the "actors," that is essentially any person or organization mentioned in the record. Details about any external sources referenced in the CCR will also be included here (e.g., the location of a healthcare proxy). Free text comments that do not fit into the defined content field in the body can be entered here. Finally, there is a location for all needed digital signatures.

Interoperability

When the CCR is presented on paper, the only mandated structure is the inclusion of the core data elements. When used in an electronic format, strict adherence to a W3C XML schema and the associated Implementation Guide is required. The syntax is not specific to healthcare. There is a prohibition of the use of XML tag attributes to contain data. All data in the CCR must be tagged. Both of these decisions were made to make the CCR consistent with the general computer industry and Internet practice. All of the XML and tags within the CCR are human as well as machine-readable and the CCR stores human readable text as text strings or structured data.

By building the CCR as a collection of discrete data elements, the information can be viewed, sorted, filtered and otherwise organized without changing the content or the integrity of the data. By using the appropriate XML syntax, the CCR can be read in a Web browser, an XML aware cell phone or an XML enabled word processing document. It also allows the data elements to be reused by others as it facilitates incorporation into other medical records (even those otherwise incompatible with the source EMR) and data exchange repositories.

Harmonization

Like ASTM, Health Level Seven, Inc.(HL7 located at www.hl7.org), is another Standards Developing Organization (SDO) accredited by the American National Standards Institute (ANSI). As part of its mission to "create standards for the exchange, management and integration of electronic healthcare information," HL7 has approved Clinical Document Architecture (CDA), release 2. The CDA is a document architecture standard designed to represent medical legal healthcare encounter documents in a standardized format using XML. As such, it is a standard looking at a large variety of healthcare documents—and not just the CCR. To facilitate wide acceptance and promote industry wide functionality and interoperability, HL7 and ASTM have a Memorandum of Understanding (MOU) in place to coordinate efforts to harmonize the CDA and CCR. Out of these efforts should evolve the ability for the seamless transformation of CDA XML syntax to CCR syntax with no data loss.

Additional efforts are underway to coordinate security standards for these portable XML formats. Both ASTM and HL7 are working with a third ANSI SDO National Council for Prescription Drug Programs to harmonize the needed standards for e-Prescribing (SCRIPT).

However, even with these efforts at harmonization, the entire issue of controlled medical vocabularies remains a continuing source of frustration to achieving full interoperability. This is well laid out in the following excerpt from the Center for Healthcare Information Technology:

> To reach true data interoperability, vocabularies and semantic interoperability need to be defined and <u>tightly</u> controlled. The CDA (Version 3, under development) and the CCR are designed to support detailed semantic interoperability. There is a lack of definition, agreement and constraint, however, on existing healthcare vocabularies within the healthcare industry, which prevents CDA (Version 3, under development) and the CCR from providing constrained (interoperable) semantics. ASTM, HL7, NCPDP and X12 are all coordinating efforts with SNOMED [Systemized Nomenclature of Medicine] and other entities to define interoperable vocabularies and semantics. Note that this involves constraining and controlling the unfettered use of vocabularies and the explosion of terms within vocabularies as much as defining vocabularies. The lack of vocabulary standardization, and even more importantly, constraints, is a critical barrier to overall healthcare standard harmonization and true interoperability.[5]

USERS AND POTENTIAL USERS VIEWS

Over the last several years, online surveys have been conducted to assess the current use of PHRs and the American public's likelihood of adopting them. One of the largest studies was conducted in the spring of 2003 by the Foundation for Accountability on behalf of the Connecting for Health Initiative of the Markle Foundation.[6]

The survey solicited over 1,200 online households. Key results are as follows:

• Only 1.5 % had a PHR on their computer and an additional 0.5% had a PHR online.

- People with chronic illness were more likely to say they would use a PHR than other respondents (65% versus 58%).
- Over 60% of respondents would use one or more of the following features: e-mail communication with their doctor, tracking immunizations, check for errors in their records, transfer information to a new doctor, and getting and tracking test results.
- Over 60% of the respondents felt that a PHR could achieve one or more of the following aims: better understanding of doctors' instructions, preventing errors getting more control of their care, helping patients ask better questions, and changing how a patient takes care of themselves.
- Over 90% of respondents answered that they were very concerned about security of their PHR, though only 25% said they not use a PHR because of these concerns. Over 40% of healthy respondents would not want lab results online because of security concerns.
- Over 90% of respondents felt that their medical providers and hospitals should be able to access their PHR, but only 65% felt the same about their insurance companies. Interestingly 58% of respondents were comfortable with their doctor hosting the online PHP, but only 15% felt that way about their insurance plan and even less (12%) wanted the government as the host.

Another poll conducted in the fall of 2005 had similar results. About 60% supported the creation of an online PHR and would use it for the purposes outlined above. About 20% would not use such a service.[7]

More recently an online poll was conducted of 2,000 general consumers by Health Industry Insights, an IDC company.[8] The poll took place November/December 2005 and had a 55% response rate. The poll show how few people are actually using PHRs and some of the obstacles to widespread acceptance:

- Only 17% have used a paper or electronic PHR
- 52% have not even heard of a PHR
- Of those without a PHR over 80% are uncertain when they would start using one
- Of those with some form of PHR, 60% are on paper, 28% are on their computer and only 5% are Internet-based
- If a health plan offered a PHR with data sharing with providers, over 57% of respondents would prefer to "opt-in" to data sharing, while 26% were comfortable with an "opt-out" design.
- 62% were comfortable with having a "complete" PHR with others expressing a reluctance to include sensitive lab results or mental health and substance abuse records.

While it appears that a majority of Americans see the utility of a PHR, few have actually established one in any form. The vast preponderance of people have security concerns that would lead many to limit where they would allow the records to be stored, what they would want in those records and who they would allow to access them. Some of these decisions would limit the usefulness of the PHR, and underscore the need to address these concerns head-on if this tool for patient safety and better medical outcomes is to be widely adopted.

A CASE STUDY: SMART CARDS AT THE QUEENS HOSPITAL NETWORK

History and Design

The Queens Health Network consists of the two public hospitals and multiple affiliated clinics in the borough of Queens, New York City. The borough has a population of almost two million people and is widely considered to be the most ethnically diverse county in the United States. By the nature of their public mission, the city hospitals have an obligation to treat all comers regardless of their ability to pay. As a result, the city hospitals treat a disproportionate number of undocumented residents and transients with questionable "official" documents who historically have shown a certain fluidity of identity based on immigration, criminal and insurance pressures. In addition, there are immigrants from over one hundred countries speaking over 150 languages and dialects in Queens County—more tongues than are spoken at the United Nations. No matter how extensive the translation services are available on-site at the hospitals or readily accessible by phone, the production of a clear comprehensible medical summary at the time of care, especially emergency care, is a particular challenge in this environment.

The administration at QHN recognized that high-quality, safe patient care required a stable longitudinal identity, more so than an officially sanctioned one. From a patient care perspective, in other words, it is arguably less important to know if someone is really John Smith and more important to know his records are stored as John Smith and that he is the same John Smith from visit to visit. As such, the decision was made to use photographic ID. With that identity check in place, attention was paid to the other administrative savings that could be accrued by using this new card. In addition to embossing the patient's name and ID number, a bar code was added to the front of the card and a magnetic stripe was added to the back. The embossed information allowed for the card to be used in those paper-based activities found in some hospital areas, as well as a back-up in the event of a computer systems failure. The magnetic stripe contained the same information but was designed to allow for rapid front-desk registration while eliminating transcription errors. The bar code was included as the move to that technology to speed laboratory and pharmacy services was contemplated.

The network also realized that because of the mobility of the population and the relative close proximity of other hospitals in the borough, there was a good chance that patients received care in multiple settings. This would be especially true in the emergency room setting; an area that tended to be heavily used as the population often looked to the emergency department as the gateway for non-urgent primary care. To verify our impression that there were a substantial number of "mobile patients," we reviewed the billing records for one of our participating Medicaid managed care plans (see Table 9-8).

The review showed that over 20% of all ER visits of patients that had chosen our network as their primary healthcare provider had occurred outside of the city hospital system. Since managed care patients should be more likely to return to the home facility, the network took this number as a lower end estimate for the care-seeking mobility of the patient population.

Table 9-8: QHN 'Out of Network' ED Visits.

2002 Enrollees of a Selected Health Plan	
Vendor	ER Visits
Jamaica Hospital	348
Saint Vincent Catholic Medical Centers	317
Catholic Medical Center Physician Services, PC	244
NY Flushing Emergency Practice Plan	175
Mount Sinai Medical Center	139
NYH Medical Center of Queens	103
Wyckoff Heights Medical Center	90
Long Island Jewish Radiology	50
The Brooklyn Hospital/Caledonian	28
Brookdale Emergency Physician Associates	26
North Shore University Hospital	25
New York Presbyterian Hospital	20

In 2002, 1,847 ED visits out of 8,786 (21%) were out-of-network (non-HHC).

Within the Queens Health Network, the two hospitals had access to the complete electronic record at either facility, but this access was not available to the other emergency rooms in the borough. The city hospitals tend to treat patients that are sicker than average, primarily because of the health burden of poverty and an inability to consistently receive coordinated primary and chronic disease care. As a result, many patients are on multiple medications for multiple conditions. Given the complexity of the patients' medical care, coupled with the high percentage of those who do not use English as their primary language, the network concluded that our patients were at a higher risk of a medical miscue from adverse medication interactions, therapeutic duplications, and delayed diagnoses caused by incomplete histories and information at the point-of-care outside our network.

For all of the reasons summarized in Table 9-9, the decision was made in spring 2003 to incorporate a smart chip into the card. A standard 64k chip was selected as it was the largest readily available and felt to be large enough to record a comprehensive medical summary with room left for an EKG. The technical details of the chips and supporting hardware and software are found in Table 9-10. The key design points are that the system was smart card standard compliant and that we used off the shelf products. The credit card sized Health Connection itself is seen in Figure 9-1.

Table 9-9: What Are the Issues We Try to Confront?

- More timely information = better care
- Multi-ethnic population with more languages than the UN
- Identity confusion
  - o Common names
  - o Deliberate errors
- Multiple problems with multiple medications
- Out-of-Network ER Visits

Table 9-10: Technical Issues.

- 64k open platform Smart Card compliant with the following standards:
  - o Java Card 2.1.1
  - o Open Platform 2.0.1
  - o ISO 7816
- Application also utilizes the following:
  - o PC/SC compliant Smart Card reader
  - o Private key algorithms (3-DES)
  - o Standard Windows applications
  - o TCP/IP communications
  - o Software was written using Java and C++

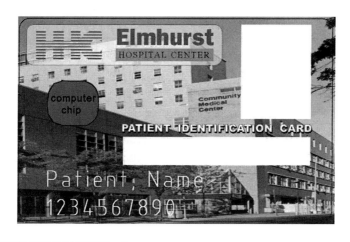

Figure 9-1: The Smart Card.

Having decided to create a card capable of storing health information, it became necessary to determine the information to be recorded and the format. The format selected was a simple text file. It required no particular viewing software, no on-site support, and it reflected the lack of clear accepted standards for such a record. Since that time, the CCR standard has evolved. It has become more accepted, reflecting a significant advance in allowing for merging of information from different sources and for more sophisticated viewing options, but still within standard browser software.

Content

Content decisions were made by polling emergency doctors within the network to determine the minimal data set that would be of use in an emergency. From those discussions, the following content was agreed to:

- Demographic information
- Emergency contacts
- Problem List and Allergies
- Active Medications
- Complete, relevant lab results

Problems were generally consistent with CPT/ICD-9 nomenclature, though free text problems were allowed. The date of the problem's activation was included, a move that was quite necessary as the network physicians do a good job adding problems, but a poor job of marking them resolved. Allergies included the type of allergen and the symptom. Active medications came from the network's EMR and included all medications prescribed at discharge, active outpatient medications or those prescribed within the last sixty days. It did not include medications from other sources. Laboratory results included standard metabolic and hematologic results, therapeutic blood levels, coagulation studies, and culture and sensitivity results. The C&S results were not written to the card if over thirty days old. For other laboratory results, the last version of any test available on the EMR was written to the card with the date they were performed.

While ED physicians were clear in their desire to have an image of an ECG on the card, this was not accomplished during the pilot. While it was possible to condense the image to an appropriate size, we were stymied by our inability to smoothly integrate the writing of the ECG information into the update workflow.

Privacy and HIPAA Considerations

A decision was made not to include financial or insurance identifiers on the card. During its initial rollout, it was felt the risk of economic data theft would adversely affect acceptance of the cards. The plan was to include the information once the cards were accepted and the security issues had been re-analyzed, post rollout. Since the information written on the card was a simple text report written from the EMR, such changes were fast and easy to accomplish. Likewise, HIV status was not included on the cards. Medications used almost exclusively in the treatment of HIV conditions were included if prescribed, as the clinicians felt the safety gains of having them included were worth the security risks.

Patient confidentiality and HIPAA concerns were addressed in the design of the program. No patient was forced to accept a Health Connections card. An informational brochure and video were developed in several languages. Before the patient sat for his picture, consent was obtained. Patients were asked to acknowledge the following statement:

> I accept the Elmhurst Health Connection Card (the "Card") and I acknowledge that it is my decision whether to disclose the information contained on the Card to another facility. I also understand that I am responsible for securing this card. In the event I become incapacitated and I am unable to communicate with my treating healthcare provider, I hereby grant consent to Elmhurst Hospital Center and participating facilities to: (1) access all of the information contained on the Card to assist in my treatment; and (2) to contact the emergency contact person contained thereon.

Non-emergent use of the card is completely controlled by the patient, as he chooses with whom to give the card to access the information. Emergency care, when the subject is unable to give consent, is covered by the statement the patient signed when accepting the card. Information on the chip was encrypted with private key algorithms (3-DES). To read the card, specific software is needed that generates the unlocking PIN from an algorithm that uses the medical record number as the source. That software was only distributed to local PCs in observed areas within the network, and eventually in two or three PCs in participating emergency rooms.

The Pilot

The goals for the pilot were to answer the following questions:

- Could a photo ID health connection card with a smart card chip be issued within the workflow of an outpatient clinic?
- Could the card be reliably updated with information from the EMR and within the workflow of the hospital?
- Would patients treated at a city hospital with a wide range of ethnic and socio-economic origins accept and use the card?
- Could other hospitals in the borough be convinced to install Health Connection card readers and software in the emergency departments?

The Health Connection smart cards were issued in the medical primary care clinic at Elmhurst Hospital. Updating was to occur at any clinic visit throughout the hospital or at the time of an inpatient discharge. For a variety of reasons, the emergency department (ED) was not a designated update location at the start of the pilot. The ED was not using the general EMR, so discharge medications would not be available at the time of update. Many lab results are still pending at time of discharge from the ED. Finally, given the nature of the ED, it was felt that a negative effect on patient flow due to updating was too a high risk to accept without adequate experience in other, less crowded areas.

Process Results

- Cards were issued beginning in August 2003. In the first two years approximately 10,000 cards were issued. Using two cameras and two card embosser/initializers, about 270 cards were issued weekly at peak periods.
- Card retention by patients has proven to be excellent. During a single two-day period, all patients registering in the clinic were reviewed. Of the 228 patients who had previously been issued cards, only two did not have their card with them at this subsequent hospital visit. In over two years, with over 14,000 cards issued, less than fifty have had to be replaced due to loss.
- Card updating has been more of a challenge. When examined, 78% of cards were updated at a clinic visit. No data is available for updates at time of discharge from inpatient service. This number reflects an assessment done outside a period of staff education or reminders about the importance of updating cards. We were pleased to see that the update process itself was easily performed by non-clinical personnel at the time of patient check out. The process takes less than a minute and requires a minimum of keystrokes. The update software checks to make sure the information being written to the card is from the appropriate medical record before allowing the write to proceed.

Patient Acceptance

As shown in Table 9-11, subjects were given an anonymous questionnaire to demonstrate their knowledge of the card and their acceptance. Only subjects with the card were polled. The results support the notion that patients were comfortable carrying a photo ID with health information stored in a chip. Their knowledge of what was actually on the card was imprecise with errors in both directions. In fact, the card held no insurance information, but it did carry basic demographic information and medical information. Subjects were in overwhelming agreement that having a card of this sort was important and agreed to use it. This is despite a significant, but clear minority of subjects who were "very concerned" about having medical information on the card. An unexpected finding was how comfortable patients were with the photo ID despite the fact that many were in the country with less than complete legal authorization. When asked follow-up questions, subjects indicated that the ID was often helpful to them when establishing their identity in non-hospital settings. At the time of the survey, most subjects did not know which hospitals could read the card. This was not surprising as deployment of the readers was still ongoing, and there was no educational attempt made by the institution to educate card carrying patients during the transaction period.

Table 9-11: **Patient Survey.**

	% English (N=32)	% Spanish (N=51)	% Total (N=83)
What information do you think is on the card?			
• Address and telephone number			
o Yes	69%	78%	75%
o No	22%	14%	17%
o Not Answered	9%	8%	8%
• Medical Information			
o Yes	72%	57%	63%
o No	9%	18%	14%
o Not Answered	19%	25%	23%
• Insurance Information			
o Yes	50%	57%	54%
o No	22%	24%	23%
o Not Answered	28%	20%	23%
Do you carry the card with you at all times?			
• Yes	75%	88%	83%
• No	16%	4%	8%
• Not Answered	9%	8%	8%
			0%
Do you have concerns about having your medical information on the card?			
• None	50%	80%	69%
• Slight	22%	12%	16%
• Very Concerned	25%	2%	11%
• Not Answered	3%	6%	5%
Would you give it to a doctor or nurse in an Emergency Room?			

	% English (N=32)	% Spanish (N=51)	% Total (N=83)
• Yes	91%	94%	93%
• No	6%	2%	4%
• Not Answered	3%	4%	4%
If you would not give it to a doctor or nurse in an Emergency Room, why not?			
• I don't want physician or nurse to see all the information about me	9%	0%	4%
• I'm not sure what is on it	16%	8%	11%
• Other reason	6%	8%	7%
• Not Answered	31%	51%	43%
Would you be willing to spend additional time at the hospital to make sure your card is updated?			
• Yes	94%	82%	87%
• No	3%	0%	1%
• Not Answered	3%	18%	12%
• 5 minutes	31%	22%	25%
• 10 minutes	13%	14%	13%
• 15 minutes	6%	20%	14%
• 20 minutes	16%	14%	14%
• 30 minutes	22%	14%	17%
• No, I would not be willing to wait extra time to update my card	3%	14%	10%
• Not Answered	0%	2%	1%
Is having a Photo ID important to you?			
• Yes	91%	100%	96%
• No	9%	0%	4%
Is having a card with your medical information on it important to you?			
• Yes	91%	92%	92%
• No	9%	4%	6%
• Not Answered	0%	4%	2%
Do you know which hospitals can read the card?			
• Yes	50%	31%	39%
• No	50%	67%	60%
• Not Answered	0%	2%	1%

Health Systems Acceptance

Issuing cards that could not be read by emergency department in other hospitals does not advance the cause of health data exchange, nor does it promote the patient safety gains of having point-of-care information access. Initially, readers were installed in the emergency departments of the nine other municipal hospitals throughout New York City. Outreach to the other hospitals in the borough of Queens was then attempted. Interestingly, the demonstration to the emergency department followed a pattern—after one minute of demonstration, the clinical utility was apparent to the clinicians and the conversation shifted to the practicalities of installing readers and discussing ways for the other institutions to issue their own cards. No institution turned down a request to install the readers. Installation involved installing the read only software on two or three PCs (usually at triage or admitting, the nursing station and a doctor's office) and connecting the smart reader, a plastic device with a USB interface costing less than $20.

Robust acceptance at a larger level has now been demonstrated by the fact that the hospitals who participated in the pilot have agreed to participate in a regional health data exchange with smart cards as an important backbone for data exchange and identity verification. In fact, two of the local hospital systems are now planning to issue their own interoperable cards as part of this project. This project has been selected for New York State matching funding as part of the HEAL NY initiative.

Because of the momentum generated by the acceptance of the card by multiple institutions in Queens, it has been possible to partner with QHN's academic affiliate, Mount Sinai School of Medicine, and our commercial partner, Siemens, to develop "the Patient Health Card" with increased functionality. Specifically, the new card system has the ability to have multiple hospitals update the card and to have the information—including an ECG—stored in a CCR compatible format. Delivery of the new card and software is expected in the third quarter of 2006. This new card will also be deployed to new facilities affiliated with Mount Sinai in New York and New Jersey.

The Future

By its very design, the pilot was not equipped to demonstrate the actual clinical and economic utility of the card. Information at the point-of-care should reduce medical errors, the need for excess tests and help avoid unnecessary admissions. All of these outcomes have the effect of reducing medical costs. Most of the benefits of data exchange at the time of the service—even if restricted to a limited data set—are outlined in Table 9-12.

Table 9-12: Patient Safety/Cost Savings.

• Avoid unnecessary testing, either by having a test result available or by better selected testing, as the information available makes the list of differential diagnoses that are much shorter and precise.
• Avoid drug-drug interactions from the inadvertent use of a drug that interacts with a substance the patient is already taking at the time of treatment.
• Avoid allergic reactions, as even food allergies can sometimes predict allergic reactions to medications (e.g., egg allergy and inoculations, seafood allergies and dyes used in radiology).
• Avoid misidentification and increase the speed of registration and treatment for all those with cards.
• Avoid unnecessary admissions from medical misadventures, as well as more complete information at the time of evaluation.

Future Functionality

As the new smart card is being developed, the ability to capitalize on the added functionality of this advanced PHR will allow for the outcomes detailed above and at the same time provide multi-application support. While still maintaining the PHR and providing point-of-care information to providers in multiple settings like nursing homes, private offices, disaster scenes and ambulances, the card may also facilitate integration with:

- Secure Electronic Prescriptions
- Disease and Case Management Programs
- Insurance Verification and Authorization
- Security/Identity component for RHIOs and NHIN

REFERENCES

1. AHIMA e-HIM Personal Health Record Work Group. The role of the personal health record in the EHR. Journal of AHIMA. 2005;July–August;76(7):64A–D. Available at: http://library.ahima.org/xpedio/groups/public/documents/ahima/bok1_027539.hcsp?dDocName=bok1_027539. Accessed on November 8, 2006.

2. Kim MI, Johnson KB. Patient entry of information: evaluation of user interfaces. *J Med Internet Res.* 2004;6:e13.

3. Zoutman DE, Ford BD, Bassili AR. A call for the regulation of prescription data mining. CMAJ 2000;163(9):1146-8; Saul S. Doctors object to gathering of drug data. New York Times. May 4, 2006.

4. ASTM E2369-05. Continuity of care record (CCR) the concept paper of the CCR. Available at: http://www.astm.org/COMMIT/E31_ConceptPaper.doc. Accessed on November 8, 2006.

5. Essential similarities and differences between the HL7 CDA/CDS and ASTM CCR. Available at: http://www.centerforhit.org/PreBuilt/chit_ccrhl7.pdf. Accessed June 29, 2006.

6. Markle Foundation. Connecting for Health: the personal health working group, final report. Available at: http://www.markle.org/downloadable_assets/final_phwg_report1.pdf. Accessed June 29, 2006.

7. Markle Foundation. Attitudes of Americans regarding personal health records and nationwide electronic health information exchange. Available at: http://www.markle.org/downloadable_assets/research_release_101105.pdf. Accessed June 29, 2006.

8. Health Industry Insights. Health industry insights consumer survey. Available at: http://www.idc.com/downloads/HIIConsumersurveyePHRs_Q&A.pdf. Accessed June 29, 2006.

CHAPTER 10

Strategy Management: Getting to the EHR

Kenneth R. Ong, MD, MPH

A USE CASE FOR STRATEGY

The hospital's executive leadership wants to improve patient safety and reduce medication errors. The chief medical officer wants computerized practitioner order entry (CPOE). The chief nursing officer wants bar code medication administration (BCMA). The vice president of quality wants clinical decision support systems (CDSS) to improve the latest pay-for-performance initiatives from the payors and the CMS. The physicians want a state-of-the-art picture archiving and communications system (PACS).

Amidst this hue and cry for information technology, the chief financial officer (CFO) reminds the leadership that capital is dear and without margin there is no mission.

Since the Balanced Budget Act of 1997, hospitals have struggled with low operating margins. Reductions in reimbursement, rising operational costs and increased bad debt expense have all hammered the bottom-line.[1] The adverse financial climate for hospitals has made investing capital scarce. At least one analyst predicts that the challenge may "resurrect strategic planning to position IT as the best solution to healthcare's persistent problems."[2]

What to do? The hospital needs a plan, a strategy that will take it on the path to the electronic medical record (EMR) (see Sidebar 10-1).[3]

Sidebar 10-1: Definition of Strategy.

"So in less formal terms, a strategy can be defined as the actions an organization is taking to close the gap between its current reality—its current markets served, offerings, processes, people, technologies, or finances—and its desired future state, documented by its long-term goals, vision, mission, or core values. Stated even more informally, strategy is what an organization or business unit is doing to get from where it is today to where it wants to be." Jim Adams[3]

STRATEGY 101

What is strategy? Quite simply, strategy can be characterized by three components:
• What you do
• What you want to become
• How you plan to get there

Strategy is about setting priorities and weighing opportunity costs. It is about choosing what to do and what not to do. Strategy operates at both corporate and unit levels. Above all, a strategy's success is ultimately judged by its implementation.[4]

Strategy is not a vision decoupled from competent analysis of reality. A convincing leader with a compelling vision is not enough. As expressed by John Humphreys:

"Today's almost mythical notion of the hero-leader demands that vision be a pre-eminent executive trait... To be sure, an organization without appropriate vision is likely to fail, but too many companies have fallen victim to the idea that managerial vision is a substitute for a complete and effective strategic examination."[5]

Commonly used constructs in strategy are mission, core values, vision statement, and goals. Simply put, a mission statement describes why a company exists or how a business unit fits into a larger organization. Core values are the guiding principles that drive a company's operations. A vision statement illustrates how the organization will fulfill its mission in the future. Goals are outcomes that are both measurable and time-bound.[6]

McNamara proposes five strategic planning models. A "basic" strategic planning model is typically for small organizations or those with minimal planning experience. It may be the first strategic plan for an organization. Developing the mission statement is the first step followed by: selecting goals; identifying approaches to achieve the goals; developing action plans; and, monitoring and updating the plan.

An issue- or goal-based model is appropriate for experienced planners and large organizations updating pre-existing plans. This model is characterized by a thorough internal and external assessment, a analysis of an organization's strengths and weaknesses and the external environment's opportunities and threats. Action plans detail resources, roles, and responsibilities for implementation. The plan may define a project multi-year budget.

The alignment model might be useful for organizations experiencing a large number of internal inefficiencies, where a plan addresses specific needs. The current commitment of resources is examined within the context of the mission. Resources are re-aligned to better serve the organization's mission.

Scenario planning may be relevant for developing strategy in the face of potential major change in direction. New regulations, changing demographics, or other external pressures can pose special challenges to an organization. Scenario planning is common to developing disaster plans for mass casualty events or avian flu epidemics. Three scenarios are crafted: a best case, worst case, and in-between scenario. A reactive strategy is fashioned for each scenario.

Finally, an "organic" (or self-organizing) model might be useful for certain corporate cultures or when senior management changes.[7] Corporate values and vision trump what might be viewed as more linear or restrictive Strength, Weakness, Opportunity, Threat (SWOT) analysis.

STRATEGY & THE ELECTRONIC MEDICAL RECORD

The complexity of health information technology (HIT) and the challenges healthcare organizations face both inside and outside their walls suggest that a more robust strategy process is needed. If strategy should be a more considered analysis than the vision of hero-leader, then planning should be that much more rigorous. Collis and Luecke describe such a strategy process, a process that expands the traditional SWOT model to incorporate implementation and performance measurement (Figure 10-1).[4]

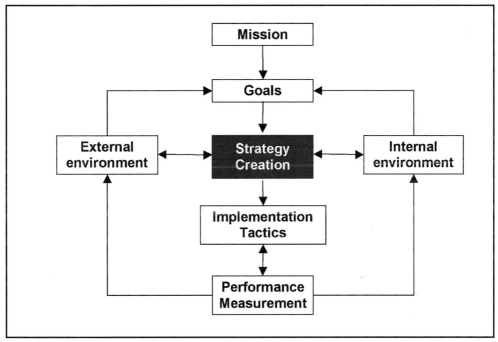

Figure 10-1: Strategy Creation.

Transforming the mission into goals is the first task. The goals should be measurable, achievable and time delimited. Without clearly defined goals, there may be no consensus on desired outcomes nor means to track the project's success or failure. For example, bar code at point of service (BCPOS)[8] for medication administration improves patient safety, but a goal of improving patient safety in and of itself would serve as an inadequate project goal. A goal of reducing medication administration errors by 20% six months after go-live could be quantified and accomplished within the defined timeline. Quantifiable goals can be measured and opportunities for improvement can be identified. They serve as a barometer for project management. In contrast, strategies that set goals that are poorly defined run the risk of failure. Overly optimistic goals that are beyond what is capable are also doomed to failure

A similar caveat applies to the size or scope of a strategy. No strategy should be so grand that it outlives the tenure of its sponsors or the attention span of its stakeholders. A project that loses its executive sponsor or its champion is a project at risk.

"[I]t's important to think five years out, plan three years out, talk two years out, and write one year out. Strategic thinking is the five-year view. It is the broad long-term direction that becomes connected to the present with the three-year plan." *Alton Brantley, MD, PhD*[9]

What makes some goals possible and others non-starters? A SWOT analysis assesses the factors both inside and outside an organization that delimit what goals are doable. The external environment poses opportunities and threats, the internal environment strengths and weaknesses (see Figure 10-2). Sample SWOT worksheets can be found on the Web.[10]

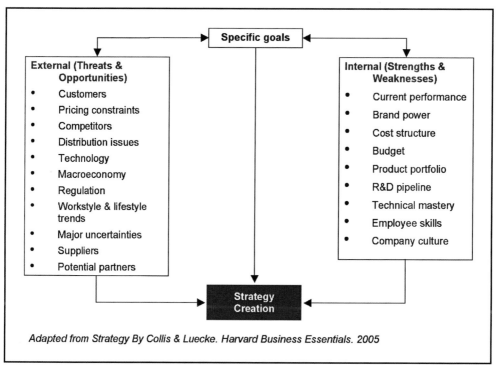

Adapted from Strategy By Collis & Luecke. Harvard Business Essentials. 2005

Figure 10-2: Internal and External Environment.

EXTERNAL OPPORTUNITIES AND THREATS

This is both the best of times and the worst of times for HIT. The opportunities and threats healthcare faces in the external environment are commonly found in the morning headlines, CNN and numerous white papers.

The opportunities are truly remarkable:

• President Bush has mentioned the importance of the electronic health record in each of his past three State of the Union addresses.[11]

• At the time of this writing, eighteen pieces of healthcare information technology legislation are before the 109th U.S. Congress.[12]

• Standardized healthcare information exchange among healthcare IT systems within the U.S. would deliver national savings of $86.8 billion annually after full implementation and would result in significant direct financial benefits for providers and other stakeholders.[13]

- Computerized practitioner order entry with clinical decision support can reduce the incidence of serious medication errors by 86%; including dose errors, frequency errors, route errors, substitution errors and allergies.[14]
- Pay for performance holds the promise of greater reimbursement for those who deliver a higher quality of care.[15]

  The external threats are formidable:
- Between 44,000 and 98,000 people die in hospitals each year as the result of medical errors. About 7,000 people per year are estimated to die from medication errors alone.[16]
- Elderly U.S. patients are prescribed improper medications in about one out of every twelve physician visits.[17]
- Overall, adults in this country receive 55% of recommended care.[18]
- Inadequate availability of patient information, such as the results of laboratory tests, is directly associated with 18% of adverse drug events.[19]
- A five-country study showed that the United States ranked poorly on care coordination, medical errors, overall rating of doctors and getting questions by providers answered. The study showed that within the U.S., 57% of patients had to tell the same story to multiple health professionals; 26% received conflicting information from different health professionals; 22% had duplicative tests ordered by different health professionals, and 25% of test results didn't reach the office in time for the patient's appointment.[20]
- While the National Health Information Network is estimated to cost $156 billion over five years, competing national concerns and their related costs vie for funding.[21] According to the Congressional Research Service in a report to Congress, war related costs could total $570 billion by 2010.[22] By including expenditures not in the CRS projection, such as lifetime healthcare and disability payments to returning veterans, replenishment of military hardware and increased recruitment costs, Bilmes and Stiglitz estimate the true costs could exceed a trillion dollars by 2010.[23] Federal aid to Louisiana for hurricane-related funding may be as much as $100 billion.[24]
- Staffing shortages in nursing, pharmacy and other health-related professions may worsen in the future.[25]
- Significant financial pressures compromise the ability for hospitals to meet these challenges. One-third of the nation's hospitals lose money overall.[26] Margins are declining. The operating margin for the average hospital was 4.04% in 2004 compared to 5.05% in 2003.[27]
- Hospitals spend a median of 2-2.49% of their operating budgets on information technology.[28] In contrast, all industries as a group spend 3.9% on IT.[29]
- Charity care has risen 30% since 1999. The growing ranks of the uninsured are associated with unreimbursed costs.[30]

INTERNAL STRENGTHS AND WEAKNESSES

Collins and Luecke suggest the three most important dimensions of an organization's strengths and weaknesses are its: (1) core competencies and processes; (2) financial condition; and, (3) management and culture. A comprehensive SWOT analysis can elucidate specific barriers to organizational change and transformation.

For example, CPOE is a complex technology that benefits from such analysis. Stablein et al developed a tool to assess hospital CPOE readiness and studied seventeen hospitals ranging in size from 75 to 906 beds. Their CPOE readiness assessment tool included such diverse components as organizational leadership, structure and culture; care standardization; order management; access to information; information technology composition; and infrastructure. While all the hospitals studied had significant gaps in one or more components, the study found that the lowest average component score was in care standardization. The highest average component score was in organizational structure and function. Organizational culture and the order management process also had low average scores. The study concluded that organizations need to develop expertise at accomplishing and sustaining change. Understanding and building CPOE readiness are an important starting point.[31]

The Medicare Quality Improvement Community (MedQIC) offers a similar tool to assess readiness for CPOE.[32] Quality improvement organizations foster its use with participating hospitals to better inform the organizational transformation necessary for successful implementation of CPOE.

The CPOE readiness assessment includes the following questions:

- Core competencies and processes: Does the IT department have one or more prior successful clinical system implementation(s)? Does or will there be a 24/7 help desk available? Do physicians know how to use a keyboard and mouse? Has the hospital been successful in changing physician behavior previously? Is there a proven multidisciplinary method for problem solving?
- Management: Do the chief executive officer, chief financial officer, chief medical officer, chief information officer, chief nursing officer and "rank and file" physicians understand the value of CPOE to patient safety and quality care? Is there a physician champion?
- Culture: Is the hospital innovative? Is the hospital a learning organization? Is the hospital tolerant of missteps in implementation?
- Financial resources: Is the hospital committed to spending up to $7.6 million for hardware and software (average costs for a 500 bed hospital) with an equal amount for installation and 20% for maintenance? Is the hospital ready to invest one or more computers for every two hospital beds?

It is axiomatic that culture eats strategy for lunch but inadequate funding is just as often as problematic, if not more so.[33] In a survey of health IT professionals in 2003, access to funding was cited as the greatest challenge to deploying patient safety technology. A high percentage of the respondents (79%) saw inadequate funding as the largest barrier to purchasing patient safety-enhancing technology.[34] Physician user resistance to technology (45%) and the maturity of the available technology (43%) were also cited as barriers to adoption. Only 14% of respondents reported that medical staff leaders offer resistance (see Figure 10-3).

Sidebar 10-2: Association Between Quality and Information Technology—
100 Most Wired Hospitals and Health Systems. [35, 36]

"The nation's 100 Most Wired hospitals and health systems have, on average, risk-adjusted mortality rates that are 7.2% lower than other hospitals. The conclusion is valid at the 99% confidence level and remains valid even after controlling the data for the size of the hospital and teaching status. However, the analysis does not establish a causal relationship between IT and outcomes."[35]

Since 1999, the American Hospital Association publication Hospitals & Health Networks has named the "100 Most Wired Hospitals and Health Systems." The one hundred are selected based on their responses to a survey and benchmarking study. The questionnaire asks hospitals to report their use of information technology in five key areas: safety and quality, customer service, business processes, workforce, public health and safety.

The survey is weighted in favor of the use of information technology for patients and customers. More than half of the points (60%) are allotted to safety and quality, customer service, public health and safety. The remaining points are given for the operational categories of business processes and work force.

Several awards are given:
- 100 Most Wired—the 100 organizations scoring highest on the survey
- Most Wireless—the 25 organizations scoring highest on the survey questions focused on wireless applications
- Most Improved—the 25 organizations not appearing on the Most Wired list whose score improved the most from 2004 to 2005
- Most Wired: Small and Rural—the 25 small and rural organizations not appearing on the Most Wired list scoring highest on the survey

Both quality and HIT investment may be dependent on a third variable—hospital finances. Encinosa and Bernard reviewed one million major surgery hospitalizations at 176 Florida hospitals from 1996 to 2000. Patients treated at the financially distressed hospitals were 13.7% more likely to have a surgery-related patient safety event than are patients treated at highly profitable hospitals (P = 0.034). Patients treated at the financially distressed hospitals also are 18.3% more likely to have a nursing-related patient safety event than patients at highly profitable hospitals (P = 0.001).[36]

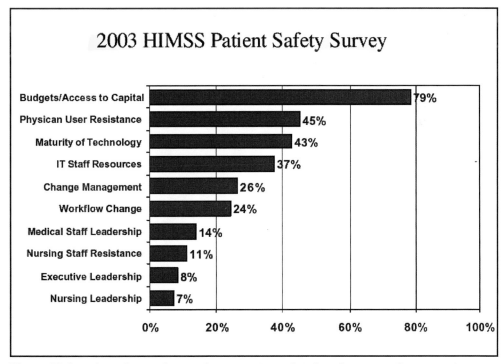

Figure 10-3: Obstacles to the Implementation of Technology to Enhance Patient Safety.

Sidebar 10-3: Greater New York Hospital Association IT Survey Demonstrates Clinical Systems as Priority and Cost as Primary Barrier.[37]

• Seventy-four individual hospitals responded to survey
• IT capital budgets not expected to increase for 2006 and 2007
• Average capital IT budget $3.9 million, median $2.8 million
• 96% ranked budget as a barrier
• 87% reported insufficient ability to support ongoing hardware and software costs as a barrier
• Reducing medical errors and promoting patient safety are top priorities for IT

EMR VS. EHR VS. CPR: A ROSE IS BUT A ROSE?

Since the electronic medical record (EMR) is often the long-term goal for an HIT strategy, it is useful to consider what an EMR is and is not. Consultant think tanks, vendors, government and other stakeholders define the EMR each in their own way. Each has aspects worth reviewing.

The terms EHR and EMR are frequently used interchangeably.[38] An even older term is the computer-based patient record, which the Institute of Medicine (IOM) defined as an essential technology for healthcare in 1991.[39] Grantors and policy makers may define EHR and EMR differently. What may appear to be subtle distinctions may decide the success or failure of a grant application.

Garets and Davis have developed an HIT adoption model comprised of eight stages:

1. All three ancillaries (laboratory, radiology and pharmacy) not installed
2. All three ancillaries are installed
3. Clinical data repository (CDR), common medical vocabulary (CMV), rudimentary clinical decision support system (CDSS) inference engine, may have Document Imaging
4. Clinical documentation (flow sheets), CDSS (error checking), PACS available outside Radiology
5. CPOE, CDSS (clinical protocols)
6. Closed loop medication administration
7. Physician documentation (structured templates), full CDSS (variance & compliance), full PACS
8. Medical record fully electronic; care delivery organization able to contribute to EHR as byproduct of EMR

An explanation of the terminology may be useful. The laboratory system manages laboratory-associated specimen testing, reporting and billing. The radiology system performs similar functions for imaging studies. The pharmacy system receives orders for and dispenses medications. In addition to being an ancillary system, pharmacy is a key component of closed loop medication administration.

The CDR is the large scale database where all patient information is stored for twenty or more years. The CDR is sometimes referred to as the heart of an EMR. It is where all laboratory and radiology results reside. It stores medication lists and clinical documentation. If the CDR is the EMR's heart, then the common medical vocabulary (CMV) is the EMR's voice. The CMV ensures that all the disparate applications agree on the same vocabulary (e.g., "Hgb" would represent 'hemoglobin' to the CDR, billing and to the laboratory.)

The rules reside in the clinical decision support system (CDSS). It is the drug-drug and drug-allergy interaction and dose-range checking in the pharmacy system. The CDSS might include a rule to enable an alert to remind a clinician if a patient more than sixty-five years old needs her Pneumovax shot or if a juvenile diabetic's hemoglobin A1c is out of control.[40,41] A CDSS is scalable. It may start with a handful of rules and later grow to dozens or hundreds of rules. Rules are a double-edged sword. If used correctly, they can improve patient safety and quality of care. If used inappropriately, they can do harm.[42] More rules are not necessarily better. Too many can result in 'alert fatigue' when the sheer volume of alerts or reminders may lead a physician to simply ignore them.

A picture archiving communications system (PACS) stores digital imaging studies. The promise of PACS for the physician is to make imaging studies available anytime from anywhere. The benefit to a hospital's operations is savings from no longer having to create and manage hard copies of imaging films. Improved accessibility to imaging studies expedites diagnosis and appropriate treatment. Like CDSS, PACS is scalable. It can start incrementally with studies that are already in a standard digital (DICOM) format, like MRI and CT scans. In later phases, studies like chest x-rays can be captured digitally, rather than on film.

Closed loop medication administration, or medication management, refers to a suite of different technologies that work in concert to reduce medication errors. The workflow starts with the physician entering an order (CPOE with CDSS); the pharmacist vetting the order in the pharmacy system; and the nurse administering the right dose of the right medication via the right route to the right patient at the right time (the five rights).[43,44] The bar code medication at point of care (BCPOC, also known as bar code medication administration, BCMA) enables the nurse to scan bar codes identifying the patient, medication and the nurse. An alert is triggered if any of the five parameters is incorrect. Radio frequency identification (RFID) is also being used in medication administration.[45] Table 10-1 represents an EMR adoption model.

Stage	Functionality	% of U.S. Hospitals
7	Medical record fully electronic; CDO able to contribute to EHR as byproduct of EMR	0.0%
6	Physician documentation (structured templates); full CDSS (variance & compliance; full PACS	0.1%
5	Closed loop medication administration	0.5%
4	CPOE, CDSS (clinical protocols)	1.9%
3	Clinical documentation (flow sheets), CDSS (error checking), PACS available outside Radiology	8.1%
2	CDR, CMV, CDSS inference engine, may have Document Imaging	49.7%
1	Ancillaries – Laboratory, Radiology, Pharmacy	20.5%
0	All three ancillaries not installed	19.3%

Table 10-1: The EMR Adoption Model (adapted from HIMSS Analytics 2006).

"Once we begin to deliver these [EMR] capabilities within the healthcare organizations, we can begin to focus on sharing patient care information [EHR] among all of the healthcare stakeholders. Currently, the hype surrounding healthcare IT has the cart before the horse. How can we discuss the potential of EHRs, much less implement them, until we have implemented effective EMRs, not only in hospitals, but in all care delivery organizations including physician practices?"[46]

The Garets and Davis model defines the EMR as the legal patient care record of the care delivery organization. In contrast, the EHR is a subset of the information in the EMR and the EHR is owned by the patient or other stakeholder (Table 10-2).

Table 10-2: The Difference Between EMR and EHR (adapted from HIMSS Analytics 2006).

Electronic Medical Records	Electronic Health Records
• The legal record of the CDO • A record of clinical services for patient encounters in a CDO • Owned by the CDO • These systems are being sold by enterprise vendors and installed by hospitals, health systems, clinics, etc. • May have patient access to some results information through a portal – but is not interactive • Does not contain other CDO encounter information	• Subset (i.e. CCR or CCD) of information from various CDOs where patient has had encounters • Owned by patient or stakeholder • Community, state, or RHIOs emerging today or nationwide in the future • Provides interactive patient access as well as the ability for the patient to append information • Connected by national health information network (NHIN)

The EHR is longitudinal, meaning that it should span the care of a patient over time across many providers. The American Society for Testing and Materials (ASTM) has developed a data model for the Continuity of Care Record (CCR) and Health Language 7's (HL7) is developing an implementation guide.[47] The data elements in the CCR would provide an overview of the patient's healthcare (see Figure 10-4).[47,48]

Though health information exchange (HIE) is possible without an EMR, HIE is certainly be more easily accomplished and cost-effective if a care delivery organization has an EMR in place. While the author attended an applicant conference in 2005 for a state-funded grant to promote HIE, one hospital representative asked the podium, "You want us to share stuff but what if we don't have the stuff to share?" He argued that without an EMR to collect and store patient information hospitals would not be able to exchange information (EHR). Any of the nearly 40% of the nation's hospitals without a clinical data repository or the other components of the EMR might have asked the same question.

A slightly different model for the EMR is offered by Gartner. Gartner is a leading provider of research and analysis about the global information technology industry. It provides data and advice to 45,000 clients worldwide representing 9,000 distinct organizations.[49]

The Gartner model defines nine core capabilities of an enterprise computer-based patient record (CPR) system. These capabilities, listed below, are also shown graphically in Figure 10-5.[50]

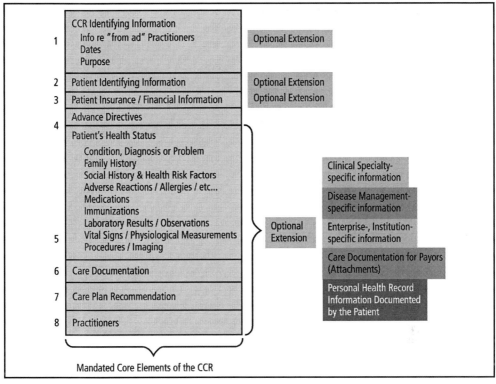

Figure 10-4: Conceptual Model of CCR Version 1, 02/08/2004.[48]

1. Clinical Data Repository

2. Support for Privacy

3. Interoperation

4. Common Medical Vocabulary / Vocabulary Server

5. Clinical Workflow

6. Clinical Decision Support

7. Document / Data Capture

8. Display / Dashboard

9. Physician Order Entry / Order Management

Figure 10-5: 9 Core Capabilities of an Enterprise CPR System.
(Adapted from Gartner's 9 Core Capabilities)

1. A clinical data repository (CDR)
2. Interoperation
3. Support for privacy
4. A controlled medical vocabulary (CMV)/vocabulary server (Voser)

5. Clinical workflow (WF)
6. Clinical decision support (CDS)
7. Clinical documentation and data capture
8. Clinical display (including clinical dashboards)
9. Order management (including practitioner order entry)

The three items the Gartner model includes that the Garets and Davis model do not are interoperation, support for privacy and clinical workflow. Interoperation is the myriad interfaces necessary for today's working information systems. Often an interface engine serves this function, serving as a hub for most if not all system interfaces. Patient demographic information from the admission, discharge and transfer (ADT) system are fed to all other hospital systems (i.e., the operating room, emergency department, blood bank, laboratory, radiology, patient accounting and pharmacy systems). The laboratory and radiology systems should feed test reports to the clinical data repository.

The support for privacy is a capability that all health information systems should enable. Various federal and state laws, like HIPAA, protect the privacy and confidentiality of patient records. An armamentarium of technologies are in play to support privacy, including authenticated and biometric logins, firewalls, virtual private networks and 128 bit encryption and audit logs of provider access to patient records, to name but a few.

An EMR should make workflow more efficient. A patient that is sent to the radiology department for an imaging study at noon should have her lunch arrive after the study, her medications held and a notice for all concerned care providers as to her location. An EMR that supports workflow should be able to coordinate all the diagnostic and therapeutic activities a patient experiences throughout her hospital stay.

Both models posed by Garets, Davis and Gartner are iterations of the CPR system the IOM defined in 1991 and refined in 1997. While the IOM described particular attributes, the subsequent models focused on technologies that would enable those attributes.

The twelve attributes that the IOM defined were:[51]

1. The CPR contains a problem list that clearly delineates the patient's clinical problems and the current status of each (e.g., is the primary illness worsening, stable or improving?).
2. The CPR encourages and supports the systematic measurement and recording of the patient's health status and functional level to promote more precise and routine assessment of the outcomes of patient care.
3. The CPR states the logical basis for all diagnoses or conclusions as a means of documenting the clinical rationale for decisions about the management of the patient's care. (This documentation should enhance use of a scientific approach in clinical practice and assist the evolution of a firmer foundation for clinical knowledge.)
4. The CPR can be linked with other clinical records of a patient—from various settings and time periods—to provide a longitudinal (i.e., lifelong) record of events that may have influenced a person's health.
5. The CPR system addresses patient data confidentiality comprehensively—in particular, it ensures that the CPR is accessible only to authorized individuals. (While

absolute confidentiality cannot be guaranteed in any system, every possible practical and cost-effective measure should be taken to secure CPRs and CPR systems from unauthorized access or abuse.)

6. The CPR is accessible for use in a timely way at any and all times by authorized individuals involved in direct patient care. Simultaneous and remote access to the CPR is possible.

7. The CPR system allows selective retrieval and formatting of information by users. It can present custom-tailored "views" of the same information.

8. The CPR system can be linked to both local and remote knowledge, literature, bibliographic or administrative databases and systems (including those containing clinical practice guidelines or clinical decision support capabilities) so that such information is readily available to assist practitioners in decision making.

9. The CPR can assist and, in some instances, guide the process of clinical problem solving by providing clinicians with decision analysis tools, clinical reminders, prognostic risk assessment and other clinical aids.

10. The CPR supports structured data collection and stores information using a defined vocabulary. It adequately supports direct data entry by practitioners.

11. The CPR can help individual practitioners and healthcare provider institutions manage and evaluate the quality and costs of care.

12. The CPR is sufficiently flexible and expandable to support not only today's basic information needs but also the evolving needs of each clinical specialty and subspecialty.

Since 1994, Andrew and Bruegel have incorporated the IOM attributes into a survey tool of fifty-four questions to query sixty-four individual EMR vendors. The vendors self-report how their EMR product fulfills the IOM attributes. The survey results are published annually.[52]

The Certification Commission for Healthcare Information Technology (CCHIT) promises to be a more objective assessment of EMR products. CCHIT is an independent, voluntary, private-sector initiative. CCHIT's mission is to accelerate the adoption of HIT by serving as an efficient, credible and sustainable product certification program. The intent is to certify for potential purchasers those products that meet criteria as EMRs.

CONCLUSION

Developing a strategy to get to the electronic health record is a key step to getting there. Strategy is crucial no matter where an organization may be on the EMR maturation ladder. Whether the plan is one, three or five years out, strategy still comes down to what you do, what you want to become, and how you plan to get there.

REFERENCES

1. Gaughan P, Pickens G. The health of our nation's hospitals, 1997–2004. *Solucient*. December 2005.

2. Bauer J. Strategic planning and information technology: back to the future all over again. *J Healthc Inf Manag*. 2005 Summer;19(3):9–11.

3. Adams J. Successfully strategic planning: creating clarity. *JHIM*. 2005;19(3):24–31.

4. Collis DJ, Luecke R. Strategy. Boston, Mass: *Harvard Business Essentials*; 2005.

5. Humphreys J. The vision thing. *MIT Sloan Management Review*. Summer 2004;45(4):96.

6. Adams J. Successful strategic planning: creating clarity. *JHIM*. 2005;19(3):24–31.

7. McNamara C. Strategic Planning. Location: The Management Assistance Program for Nonprofits. 1999.

8. Synonyms commonly used for bar code at point of service (BCPOS) are bar code medication administration (BCMA) or bar code at point of care (BCPOC).

9. Brantley A. Show strategies, plans, and strategic planning. *JHIM*. 2005;19(3):12–14.

10. New Zealand Trade and Enterprise. SWOT Analysis: A suggested outline. Available at: http://www.marketnewzealand.com/common/files/swotanalysis-worksheet2.pdf. Accessed April 1, 2006.

11. Versel N. President Bush's health-IT statement earns little ovation. *Health-IT World*. February 7, 2006. http://tmlr.net/jump/?c=18070&a=296&m=3577&p=0&t=164. Accessed November 21, 2006.

12. Health Information and Management Systems Society. Legislative crosswalk. Available at: http://www.himss.org/advocacy/news_crosswalk.asp. Accessed November 21, 2006.

13. Center for Information Technology Leadership. The Value of Healthcare Information Exchange and Interoperability. 2004.

14. Bates DW, Teich JM, Lee J, Seger D, Kuperman GJ, Ma'Luf N, Boyle D, Leape L. The impact of computerized physician order entry on medication error prevention. *J Am Med Inform Assoc*. 1999;July–August;6(4):313–21.

15. Kahn CN, Ault T, Isenstein H, Potetz L. Van Gelder S. Snapshot of hospital quality reporting and pay-for-performance under Medicare. *Health Affairs*. 2006;25;(1):148–162. Available at: http://pwchealth.com/cgi-local/hregister.cgi?link=reg/charitycare.pdf [Accessed April 1, 2006]

16. Institute of Medicine. T*o Err is Human: Building a Safer Health Care System*. Washington, DC: National Academy Press; 2000.

17. Goulding MR. Inappropriate medication prescribing for elderly ambulatory care patients. *Archives of Internal Medicine*. 2004;February 9;164(3):305–12.

18. McGlynn EA, Asch SM, Adams J, Keesey J, Hicks J, DeCristofaro A, Kerr EA. The quality of health care delivered to adults in the United States. *NEJM*. 2003;June 26;348(26):2635–2645.

19. Leape LL, Bates DW, Cullen DJ, Cooper J, Demonaco HJ, Gallivan T, et al. Systems analysis of adverse drug events. ADE Prevention Study Group. *JAMA*. 1995;274: 35–43.

20. Blendon RJ, Schoen C, DesRoches C, Osborn R, Zapert K. Common concerns amid diverse systems: healthcare experiences in five countries. *Health Aff* (Millwood). 2003;May–June;22(3):106–21.

21. Kaushal R, Blumenthal D, Poon EG, Jha AK, Franz C, Middleton B, Glaser J, Kuperman G, Christino M, Fernandopulle R, Newhouse JP, Bates DW. Cost of national health information network working group. The costs of a national health information network. *Ann Intern Med*. 2005;Aug 2;143(3):165–73.

22. Congressional Research Service. The Cost of Iraq, Afghanistan and Enhanced Base Security Since 9/11. October 7, 2005.

23. Stiglitz J, Bilmes L. The economic costs of the Iraq war. National Bureau of Economic Research Working Paper 12054. February 2006; Working paper presented at: Annual Meeting of the Allied Social Sciences Association; January 2006; Boston, MA. Available at: http://www2.gsb.columbia.edu/faculty/jstiglitz/download/2006_Cost_of_War_in_Iraq_NBER.pdf. Accessed April 7, 2006.

24. Pear R, Stolberg SG. Bush insists on approval of full aid for Louisiana. *New York Times*. March 9, 2006. http://select.nytimes.com/search/restricted/article?res=F30F12FB39550C7A8CDDAA0894DE404482 Accessed November 21, 2006.

25. American Hospital Association. The Fragile State of Hospital Finances. 2005.

26. American Hospital Association. Total, Operating and Patient Care Margins 1997 (pre-BBA) vs 2003. Annual Survey.

27. Solucient, LLC. The health of our nation's hospitals 1997–2004. December 2005. Available at: http://www.solucient.com/forms/honh.asp. Accessed April 1, 2006.

28. *Modern Healthcare.* Survey describes state of hospital IT adoption. May 19, 2005. Available at: http://www.modernhealthcare.com/chart.cms?id=376&type=surveys. (must have subscription to access.) Accessed April 6, 2006.

29. Gartner. DataQuest. Stamford, CT. August 2003.

30. PriceWaterhouse Coopers. Acts of Charity: Charity Care Strategies for Hospitals in a Changing Landscape. 2006.

31. Dona Stablein D, Welebob E, Johnson E, Metzger M, Burgess R, Classen DC. Understanding hospital readiness for computerized physician order entry. *Joint Commission on Quality and Safety Journal.* 2003;July;29(7):336–344.

32. Medqic. CPOE Readiness Assessment. Available at: http://www.medqic.org/dcs/ContentServer?cid=1122904872189&pagename=Medqic%2FMQTools%2FToolTemplate&c=MQTools. Accessed April 4, 2006.

33. Adams J. Successful strategic planning: creating clarity. *JHIM.* 2005;19(3):24–31.

34. Health Information and Management Systems Society. 2003 HIMSS Patient Safety Survey. Sponsored by McKesson Corporation. Available at: http://www.himss.org/content/files/PatientSafetyFinalReport8252003.pdf. Accessed April 4, 2006.

35. Hospitals & Health Networks. 2005 most wired survey and benchmarking study. Hospital and Health Networks. July 2005. Available at: http://www.hhnmag.com/hhnmag/jsp/articledisplay.jsp?dcrpath=HHNMAG/PubsNewsArticle/data/0507HHN_CoverStory_Landing_Page&domain=HHNMAG. Accessed April 4, 2006.

36. Encinosa WE, Bernard DM. Hospital finances and patient safety outcomes. *Inquiry.* 2005;Spring;42(1):60–72.

37. GNYHA Skyline, January 2006.

38. "Electronic health record (EHR): The current term used to refer to computerization of health record content and associated processes. Electronic medical record (EMR): A term that may be treated synonymously with computer-based patient record and/or electronic health record; often used in the US to refer to an electronic health record in a physician office setting or a computerized system of files (often scanned via a document imaging system) rather than individual data elements." Quote from material available at: http://library.ahima.org/xpedio/groups/public/documents/ahima/bok1_025042.hcsp?dDocName=bok1_025042. Accessed April 6, 2006.

39. Dick RS, Steen EB, Detmer DE, eds. *Computer-Based Patient Record: An Essential Technology for Healthcare.* Rev ed. Washington DC: Institute Of Medicine; National Academies Press; 1997. Available at: http://newton.nap.edu/catalog/5306.html. Accessed April 6, 2006.

40. Dexter PR, Perkins SM, Maharry KS, Jones K, McDonald CJ. Inpatient computer-based standing orders vs physician reminders to increase influenza and pneumococcal vaccination rates: a randomized trial. *JAMA.* 2004;November 17;292(19):2366–71.

41. Jackson CL, Bolen S, Brancati FL, Batts-Turner ML, Gary TL.A Systematic Review of Interactive Computer-assisted Technology in Diabetes Care. *J Gen Intern Med.* 2006 Feb;21(2):105–10.

42. van der Sijs H, Aarts J, Vulto A, Berg M. Overriding of drug safety alerts in computerized physician order entry. *J Am Med Inform Assoc.* 2006;March–April;13(2):138–47.

43. Bates DW, Leape LL, Cullen DJ, Laird N, Petersen LA, Teich JM, Burdick E, Hickey M, Kleefield S, Shea B, Vander Vliet M, Seger DL. Effect of computerized physician order entry and a team intervention on prevention of serious medication errors. *JAMA.* 1998;October 21;280(15):1311–6.

44. Neuenschwander M, Cohen MR, Vaida AJ, Patchett JA, Kelly J, Trohimovich B. Practical guide to bar coding for patient medication safety. *Am J Health Syst Pharm.* 2003;April 15;60(8):768–79.

45. Perrin RA, Simpson N. RFID and bar codes—critical importance in enhancing safe patient care. *J Healthc Inf Manag.* 2004;Fall;18(4):33–9.

46. Garets D, Davis M. White Paper: Electronic medical records vs. electronic health records: yes, there is a difference. HIMSS Analytics. 2006; http://www.himssanalytics.org/docs/WP_EMR_EHR.pdf. Accessed November 21, 2006.

47. Ferranti JM, Musser RC, Kawamoto K, Hammond WE. The clinical document architecture and the continuity of care record: a critical analysis. *J Am Med Inform Assoc.* 2006;Feburary 27.

48. ASTM E31.28. Continuity of care record (CCR): the concept paper of the CCR. Available at: http://www.astm.org/COMMIT/E31_ConceptPaper.doc. Accessed April 7, 2006.

49. Gartner. Stamford, CT. Available at: http://www.gartner.com/it/about_gartner.jsp. Accessed April 7, 2006.

50. Gartner. Stamford, CT. Available at: http://www.gartner.com/resources/118300/118364/the_gartner_200.pdf. Accessed April 7, 2006.

51. Institute of Medicine. The Computer-Based Patient Record: An Essential Technology for Health Care. Rev ed Washington DC: National Academies Press. 1997. Available at: http://darwin.nap.edu/books/0309055326/html/180.html. Accessed April 7, 2006.

52. Andrew W, Bruegel RB. An Exclusive Look at the EHR System Marketplace: 2005 EHR Systems Review. Compilations available at: http://health-care-it.advanceweb.com/Common/editorial/editorial.aspx?CTIID=1593. Accessed April 8, 2006.

CHAPTER 11

Software Selection

Kenneth R. Ong, MD, MPH

Why does anyone ever have to buy new software? What's wrong with the old software? Why do we need software at all? These are common questions that all of us have heard before. No doubt these are questions we may have actually asked ourselves on occasion.

Why, indeed? A project may require a new purchase of software. A hospital's strategic focus on patient safety may embark on the path to computerized practitioner order entry (CPOE) with clinical decision support system (CDSS), or closed loop medication management. The current version of a particular software product may sunset. A vendor sells a new software product and refuses to support the older version. Generations of software changed from mainframe to client server or character to Windows-driven platforms. A similar shift was seen for some products that evolved from client-server to Web-enabled. A vendor may change its underlying database from one to another (e.g., FoxPro to MS SQL Server).

The software vendor is purchased or goes out of business. Alas, their software is orphaned and left bereft of support. Even very expensive health information technology (HIT) may go the way of the eight track tape player or the Commodore 64. Merger or other enterprise-wide initiatives may drive standardization. Standardizing software across a multi-hospital system can facilitate adopting best practices and lower purchase and maintenance costs for IT. Paying multiple vendors for the same software translates into multiple contracts to manage, training associated with each software product and a Gordian knot of interfaces. Each interface can generate its own costs for maintenance and episodes of downtime.

New regulations or new accrediting standards may mandate new functionality that may only be supported by IT. The Joint Commission on Accreditation of Healthcare Organizations (JCAHO) standards for documenting pre-procedure time-outs and pain management have spurred new electronic documentation for nursing. The recent

FDA standard requiring new coding for blood product units has prompted necessary upgrades from blood bank system vendors.

BUYING SOFTWARE IS A JOURNEY

Just as best practice medication administration meets the five rights,[1] purchasing IT does as well: the right process with the right people to find the right system at the right price and for the right reasons.[2]

Sidebar 11-1: The Five Rights of Purchasing.
(adapted from Laker and Groeber).

1. The right process
2. The right people
3. The right system
4. The right price
5. The right reasons

The right reason should be the alpha and omega of every project. More in healthcare than elsewhere, IT must often serve both margin and mission. Should a clinical software system promote both patient safety and appropriate charge capture? The obvious answer is yes and yes. The right reasons should be translated into quantifiable and achievable goals. The right reason will have a quantifiable outcome. One metric that has become standard for many capital purchases is the payback period, better known as return on investment.

The right process gathers the input of all major stakeholders and ensures that an evidence-based, outcome-focused selection proceeds and that the project is aligned with the strategic plan of the organization.[3] The process often includes a software selection team comprised of both managers of the business unit or organization and the relevant executive officer(s). The software selection team may be formally charged to present its project for the approval of an executive information systems or capital expenditure approval committee. The latter committee may be responsible for approving expenses that run over the projected costs or, in that most unhappy of circumstances, terminating a project if it fails to meet its milestones, projected costs or post-go-live goals. The right selection process creates the foundations for a successful installation and maintenance.

Sidebar 11-2: The Right People for a Selection Process.

• Executive sponsor
• Project champion
• Project manager
• Representatives from other disciplines or business units relevant to the software application

The right people in the selection committee include an executive sponsor, a project champion, a project manager, and representatives from other disciplines or business units relevant to the software application. In addition to the formal process within the organization, the executive sponsor ensures through both formal and informal channels that the project has the buy-in of the organization's executive leadership. This buy-in includes not only the project budget but cooperation from other departments and business units to participate in the selection, the installation and successful continuation of the project. The larger the scope of the project, the more important that buy-in becomes.

The project manager may be from either the business unit or information systems. The project manager should be involved in both the selection and installation phases of the project. His/her role is to enumerate and assign each task, coordinate disparate and limited resources, identify potential or actual problems and deliver the project on time and within budget. Project management is a body of knowledge for which formal education and certification exists.[4] But, certification is often not the most important asset a project manager brings to the table.

Heerkens suggests the four most desired traits of a project manager are: (1) thinks like a generalist; (2) a high tolerance for ambiguity; (3) a high tolerance for uncertainty; and (4) honesty and integrity.[5] Certification marks a level of competence but experience in selecting and installing projects of similar complexity is often more reassuring.

The project champion is the person from the business unit or department who can promote and advocate others to adopt the software application, the workflow changes or the clinical transformation needed to achieve the expected project outcomes. Gladwell refers to such individuals as connectors.[6]

Rogers would categorize the ideal project champion as an early adopter: "Potential adopters look to early adopters for advice and information about an innovation. The early adopter is considered by many to be the individual to check with before adopting a new idea. This adopter category is generally sought by change agents as a local missionary for speeding the diffusion process. Because early adopters are not too far ahead of the average individual in innovativeness, they serve as a role model for many other members of a social system. Early adopters help trigger the mass when they adopt an innovation... In one sense, early adopters put their stamp of approval on a new idea by adopting it."[7]

Representatives of other relevant business units or departments should sit at the table. If their participation is important for a successful install, then they should be part of the selection process. As healthcare strives to improve quality and efficiency, collaboration and teamwork become increasingly vital. A chain is only as strong as its weakest link. Sometimes leaving just one person, one office, or one department out of the selection process can compromise a successful implementation.

The right system is the one that best enables the project's goals—be it reducing no-shows for a clinic scheduling system or reducing medication errors for a closed loop medication management system.

The conventional wisdom is that a request for proposal is the *sine qua non* for selecting the right system. In today's complex healthcare IT market, the traditional RFP is not without its problems. Laker and Groeber caution, "The classic approach is buying or building a checklist of desired features, issuing it to vendors in a request for proposal (RFP), then scoring results to see which system has the most functionality. But with today's system architectures and powerful tools, vendors can say "yes" to nearly all questions. Most vendors' RFP responses score around 90%, while actual use of system functions at client sites is maybe 50%. Plus, sales or marketing staff answer RFPs, not the programmers and analysts who really know the product."[8]

Buying software in the twenty-first century can be a little like buying a new car. When hunting for a new car today, we search the Web and newsstands for rating surveys, like Consumer Reports. We check the car manufacturer's Web site for a marketing brochure. We Google (www.google.com) online forums and blogs for opinions from consumers themselves. Whether or not they own the vehicle in question, we ask everyone we know for their opinion. We go to the car dealer to listen to that five-CD disk player with nine-speaker sound system or see first hand if the olive green looks that much cooler than the lime. During the entire journey, we share our findings with our significant other, parents and next-door neighbor. In the end, a contract is signed and we have a new car.

Online services like KLAS (www.healthcomputing.com) and MDBuyline (www.mdbuyline.com) offer consumer satisfaction rankings, product specific reports, vendor specific client commentary and more. Aunt Minnie (www.auntminnie.com) is a site devoted to imaging products and their evaluation. The number one ranking in a KLAS survey or most improved ranking are coveted. Consumer ratings are an invaluable reality check for that occasional end-user who has used the existing product forever and is convinced there is nothing better.

Critics, who are more often vendors than not, lament that customer satisfaction rating services are subject to gaming. They say that vendors with the highest rankings are only better at convincing their customers to participate in the satisfaction surveys. Yet that very same tactic is open to all vendors and fails to explain why some garner better rankings than others. The vendor's Web site should include the number of employees, annual revenues, location of the corporate headquarters, product brochures and contact information for sales. The product information from each vendor can be the starting point for developing the selection criteria rating tool for the selection team.

A vendor assessment or selection criteria rating tool has several tangible benefits. It represents a consensus within the selection team about what it expects the software to do (see "Samples: Vendor Assessment Tools" below). The "right reasons" should permeate the selection and implementation processes. Weighting the selection criteria can define what functionality has greater priority. The rating scale should be no more complicated than 1-3 or 1-5. Even numbered rating scales (e.g., 1-4 or 1-6) force evaluations that are more clearly positive or negative. Rating scales whose highest rating exceeds five or six do not necessarily add value. Categories of specifications should be rated rather than each specification itself. Selection team members find rating ten categories practical, but a hundred individual specifications impossible.

Functionality is but one section in the vendor assessment tool. Other critical sections include regulatory compliance, IT requirements and vendor characteristics. A software product that has the latest bells and whistles is at risk if its vendor's future looks dubious or if its security does not meet today's concerns for protecting health information.

Searching the Web for the latest news on vendors can uncover useful information. If one vendor purchases another with a competing product, one of the products will not fare well in the future. Learning of a company's reorganization, one should ask the vendor how that will affect their future and product support. Even a friendly acquisition may lead to a "hiccup" or temporary reduction in support services.

Demonstrations should be arranged and vendors rated with the vendor assessment tool. The tool can be used to ensure each vendor is asked to show the same specifications. The tool becomes indispensable if the products are complex in scope or if the number of demos includes three or more vendors over a span of days. A post-mortem or debriefing after each vendor's demo can help solidify areas of consensus and difference. If a product offers better support for one subset of stakeholders than another (e.g., physicians or nurses) than the team will have to decide if that trade off is worthwhile or if another product better serves all stakeholders. This advice is given full well knowing it is easier said than done.

After the scores from the vendor assessment tool are tallied, the finalists should be selected. Preliminary proposals and a list of current clients can be requested. "Due diligence" generally requires site visits and reference calls to existing clients. Both should be made without the vendor present. Be aware that it makes perfect sense for a vendor to refer the prospective customer to those current clients that are most happy with their product. Finding clients that have recently switched from one vendor to another are more useful.

The right price requires a diligent review of line items in the project plan. The project plan should be part of the contract. Training is always a key issue. The "train the trainer" option lowers travel expenses, decreases time lost to training and minimizes costs required to back-fill the staff's absence during training. A selected group of the customer's managers or super-users can be trained by the vendor on-site or at the vendor's corporate training facilities. The selected group of trainers can then train the remaining staff in the business unit or organization.

Courtesy of the Web, renting or buying software are options many vendors now offer. Back in the day of large mainframe based applications, the subscription model was common. The vendor would own and host the "heavy iron," the mainframe computers. The customer would pay a monthly or quarterly fee for access. Once again, courtesy of the World Wide Web, the application service provider (ASP) mirrors that model and offers subscription rates. The subscription model has even expanded to client-server applications. In the capital-poor environment of healthcare today, stretching the total cost of ownership over a three- to seven-year period lowers upfront capital costs. The risk of the subscription model on the part of the vendor is that the customer could decide to discontinue service before the end of the agreement. The risk for the vendor is mitigated by a mark-up in the subscription fee. In reality, the costs the customer sinks into implementation are a barrier to premature termination or changing vendors. Selecting and implementing yet another new software application is not only associated with angst, but costs and downtime.

Finally, the day arrives in a selection process when a vendor is selected. The executive sponsor and selection team present the project to the executive leadership for approval.

A successful selection process is a prelude to a successful implementation. A hasty selection can lead to missteps in implementation. The consensus required for workflow and clinical transformation is the staging platform for implementing the software and achieving the desired patient safety and business goals. Selection and planning for implementation are very much intertwined.

Sidebar 11-3: Tips for Software Selection.

Beware of software that's either nonexistent or unproven:
- Vaporware
- Visionware
- Betaware
- PPOS (PowerPoint Operating System)
- Technology on the bleeding edge (newer and riskier than the cutting edge)

If you're the type who'd hesitate to buy the first model of a new car line, you should be just as risk averse with the very latest information technology. Unless your organization classifies itself in the innovator category of the adopter distribution and has the resources to devote to developing new technology, take on "the latest and the greatest" with extreme caution.

Sidebar 11-4: Software: What's Out There.

(Adapted from Health Data Management's Software Guide).[9]

Health Data Management's Software Guide[9]

The spectrum of available health information technology and related services can be daunting to the uninitiated. Though there is always new software in development, much of what is now available is listed below:
- Application Service Provider
- Budgeting
- Claims Auditing/Analysis
- Claims Payor Management
- Claims Processors/Clearinghouse/Electronic Data Interchange (EDI)
- Claims-Related Software
- Clinical Information Systems
- Clinical Software, Specialized
- Coding & Compliance
- Computer-Based Patient Records
- Consultants
- Contract Management
- Decision Support
- Disease Management/Outcomes
- Document Management Systems
- Electronic Medical Records
- Enterprise Resource Planning (ERP)
- Financial/Billing/Patient Accounting Systems
- Hospital Acquired Infection (HAI) Monitor & Control Software System
- HIPAA Compliance
- Hospital Planning and Marketing Software
- Hospital/Healthcare Information Systems
- Interface Engines/Integration Tools
- Internet/Intranet/e-Health
- JCAHO Compliance Software System
- Laboratory
- Language Engines/Health Vocabulary
- Managed Care
- Medical Errors Prevention/Patient Safety
- Medical Staff Credentialing
- Outsourcing Services
- Picture Archive Communication System (PACS)/Radiology Systems
- Practice Management
- Scheduling
- Security
- Speech Recognition/Digital Dictation
- Telemedicine/Teleradiology Systems
- Web Portals/Web Services

SOFTWARE STRATEGIES:
BEST-OF-BREED VS. SINGLE SOURCE VS. BEST OF CLUSTER

One of the central debates in software selection is the choice between the best-of-breed and single source (see Table 11-1). The conventional wisdom argues that buying software products from a single vendor will deliver more integration. Integration means greater efficiency and cost-savings in purchasing and maintaining software. Some vendors repeat what has become the mantra of single source proponents. With a single vendor, there is but "one throat to choke" (see Figure 11-1). If there are problems with any software, the CIO has but one vendor to which to complain. The downside is there is no other vendor the customer has an existing business relationship with to act as a foil. Without competition, the customer has little negotiating cache.

Table 11-1: Best-of-Breed versus Single Source.

	Pro	Con
Best-of-Breed	Best unit or departmental functionality	• Work & cost of interfacing • Many vendors to manage
Single Source	• Integrated • "One throat to choke"	• Often poor departmental functionality • Diminished negotiating caché

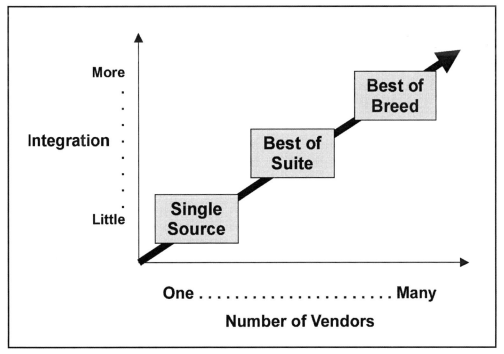

Figure 11-1: Software Selection Strategies.

Another painful reality is that the promise of integration may be illusory. One vendor may buy a compendium of different software products but fail to integrate them. Changing a menagerie of different programs into a common database with integrated logic is an expensive and time-consuming challenge.

The conventional wisdom argues that buying best-of-breed means buying the best software. Business units or departments tend to prefer selecting the best software for their particular workflow. But there are at least two trade offs. Firstly, creating and maintaining interfaces costs money. Secondly, multiple vendor relationships have to be managed. Rather than one throat to choke, there are many. When an interface has issues, one vendor may blame another leading to bewildering delays or downtime.

A third option to best-of-breed and single source is "best-of-cluster." The rationale of the "best of cluster" approach is that only a core group of software applications must be closely integrated. Applications that fall outside of the cluster need a lesser degree of integration. At the bare minimum, the cluster would include computerized practitioner order entry (CPOE), clinical decision support system (CDSS) and the pharmacy system.

The more expansive definition might include all the elements of the electronic medical record (EMR). Garets and Davis suggest the EMR environment is comprised of:[10]

- Clinical Data Repository (CDR)
- Controlled Medical Vocabulary (CMV)
- Clinical Decision Support System (CDSS)
- Clinical Documentation
- Computerized Practitioner Order Entry (CPOE)
- Pharmacy Management
- Electronic Medication Administration Record (eMAR)
- Workflow

Only a careful analysis of each care delivery organization can determine which of the three software selection strategies is right for them.

SAMPLE VENDOR ASSESSMENT TOOLS

Notes on the Vendor Assessment tools, featured in Table 11-2, Table 11-3, Table 11-4, Table 11-5, Table 11-6 and Table 11-7:

- The vendor assessment tool is but a guide for further discussion in the Selection Team. Creating the criteria for the assessment helps build consensus—not only for the selection, but for the goals for implementation. The final selection should be made in a face-to-face meeting to better solicit everyone's opinion and promote interaction.
- The rating scale is from one (very bad) through five (excellent). Though an even numbered scale forces evaluators to give negative or positive scores, it is often helpful to learn if a particular function is "good enough" or "just so-so." If vendors score similarly on some selection criteria, then other criteria may be the differentiators.
- Weighting should be determined by the Selection Team. More important criteria can be weighted with a three. The majority of criteria should be weighted one.
- Except for the sample from telehealth, all criteria were gathered from product information available to the public on vendor Web sites. Criteria should be added, removed or updated by your own selection committee.
- IT changes, innovation and changing end-user specifications drive software upgrades. Not all the product features available in the present were available in the past.
- The vendor assessment tool for telehealth was adapted from *HCA Home Telehealth & Technology News*.[11] Because telehealth was viewed as part of a greater marketing

strategy for this particular organization, Chinese, Russian and Spanish translations were required specifications.[12]

Table 11-2: Sample #1—Results Reporting & Charge Capture.

Criteria Category	Weight	Vendor A	Vendor B
Vendor characteristics			
Functionality			
Training time			
Implementation time			
Customer satisfaction			
Synchronization			
Security			
Platform			
Customizable			
Access			
Total =			

I. Vendor
   A. Ownership
   B. Established
   C. Corporate location
   D. Web site
II. Functionality
   A. Clinical results
      1. Patient list
      2. Labs with critical value alerts
      3. Micro
      4. Radiology reports
      5. Demographics
      6. Insurance information
      7. Allergies
      8. Medications
      9. Path results
      10. Consults
   B. Charge capture
      1. Customizable codes
      2. Reported ROI
      3. Reduced billing lag time
   C. Other applications:
      1. Medical reference
      2. Mobile dictation
      3. E-Prescribing
III. Training Time
IV. Implementation Time
V. Customer Satisfaction
   A. KLAS
   B. Customer references
   C. Phone calls
VI. Synchronization
   A. Wired
   B. Wireless
   C. IR
   D. Cell
VII. Security
   A. Authentication
   B. Authorization
   C. Data encryption

D. Auto logout
E. Incorrect login lockout
F. Audit trail
G. Role-based access
VIII. Platform
A. Palm
B. Pocket PC
IX. Customizable
A. Charge capture codes
B. Development kit
C. Add new patients on-fly
X. Access
A. Web
B. Handheld

Table 11-3: Sample #2—Cancer Registry.

Criteria Category	Weight	Vendor A	Vendor B	Vendor C
Functionality				
Regulation				
Training				
Vendor				
Customer satisfaction				
Hardware Specifications				
Support				
Total =				

I. Functionality
  A.   Ability to view and maintain data over time, regardless of whether the case is complete
  B.   Abstracting screens with Windows interface give you dropdown lists – listing the valid choices for the field
  C.   Accreditation & Reporting Requirements
  D.   ACOS-approved dataset and edit checks
  E.   Ad Hoc report writer for reports using data from any field, or combination of fields, from the entire database
  F.   Address labels and printable follow-up letters that can be customized using external mail merge programs
  G.   Any additional requirements of any agencies to which the hospital will be reporting (such as the state central registry or the National Cancer Database of the Commission on Cancer)
  H.   Automated daily back up procedures
  I.   Automatic abstract form printing from within the software
  J.   Comprehensive Online Help
  K.   Comprehensive, context-sensitive "Help" system built into the program for both data fields and interfield edits
  L.   Help system includes NAACCR Data Dictionary, SEER Program Manual, SEER EOD Manual, and ROADS with the surgery code appendix, all online and searchable
  M.   Data fields that can be customized for specified studies
  N.   Data Integrity Quality Control Checks
  O.   Data set requirements
  P.   Direct faxing ability to medical offices for follow up and first course of therapy information, assisting the registrars to obtain timely, accurate and complete data as required by the NYS DOH and the National Cancer Data Base with the American College of Surgeons
  Q.   Download demographic and clinical data from any department (e.g., health information management, pathology, radiation oncology)
  R.   Edit checks to ensure data accuracy and integrity
  S.   Expanded record management system with a user-friendly interface for patient record search, printing, viewing and deleting
  T.   File import and export capabilities (i.e., export of NYS DOH GENEDITS (ACoS), ASCII, and NAACCR file formats)
  U.   Follow-up letter and label merging with Microsoft Word – insert scanned letterhead to save on printing costs
  V.   Follow-up Tracking & Summary Information

W. Graphical presentations of survival data, based on multiple methods of calculating survival — all accomplished without re-keying data

X. Interface to ADT

Y. NAACCR Record Version 7, 8 and 9 transmit formats AND compliant with ROADS, NAACCR and SEER reporting requirements

Z. Physician look-up, editing and addition functions, allowing physicians to add without exiting the case

AA. Printing capabilities, including the complete patient abstract, lists of cases as specified and statistical summaries (cross tabulations) of specified cases

BB. Quality assurance notepad on every screen, for commentaries on diagnosis and follow-up

CC. Required data edits (standardized edits are advisable) and any other quality assurance considerations such as amenability to external audit

DD. Single point entry screen that provides categories for case status

EE. Mapping of Incidence Rates

FF. Statistical programs

GG. System-wide case search, to ensure each case is entered only once

HH. The latest PCE Study data evaluation items for each study done in the past five years

II. Timeline for implementation

JJ. User administration in the network environment; different user permission levels, including view-only, registrar and administrator levels

KK. User friendly data entry

LL. Whether the system will be new or a conversion

II. Regulation

  A. Compliant with New York State Cancer Registry requirements

  B. Compliance with American College of Surgeons' Commission on Cancer Approvals Standards for Cancer Programs

III. Training

  A. Initial on-site training sessions for the Cancer Registry Staff as well as interval training as needed

IV. Vendor

  A. Financial stability

  B. When company started

V. Customer satisfaction

  A. What is the registry's annual caseload?

  B. What are the advantages and disadvantages of the registry system?

  C. After the software was selected, how well did it meet the expectations of the medical and registry staff, the cancer committee, administration and IT?

  D. What are the major uses of the registry system and who uses it?

  E. What was the approximate timeline of the planning, installation, and implementation of the system?

  F. How long did it take for registry staff to learn how to use the software?

  G. How good has support been from IT and the software provider?

  H. Number of clients

  I. References

VI. Hardware Specifications

  A. Intranet vs. client server-based

  B. Hospital computer (PC) and operating system preferences

  C. Transmission/communication (modem, network) requirements

VII. Support

  A. Single and Multi User Support

  B. Cost

  C. 24/7

Table 11-4: Sample #3—Quality Measure Reporting.

Criteria Category	Weight	Vendor A	Vendor B	Vendor C	Vendor D
Quality measures supported					
Data capture and submission					
Decision support and reporting					
Training					
Customer support					
User group					
Performance improvement					
Vendor characteristics					
Totals					

I. Quality measures supported
    A. JCAHO ORYX/core measures
    B. JCAHO-CMS measures covered
        1. AMI-Acute Myocardial Infarction
        2. HF-Heart Failure
        3. PR-Pregnancy and Related Conditions
        4. PN-Pneumonia
        5. SIP-Surgical Infection Prevention
    C. CMS' National Data Repository (QNET) for 7th SOW and Market Basket Update
    D. CMS' 8th SOW Appropriate Care Measures (ACM)
    E. Hospital Quality Alliance Participant
    F. American Hospital Association's National Quality Initiative
    G. Ability to support all current and future data submission required by JCAHO, CMS and IHI
II. Data capture and submission
    A. Required source(s) of data
    B. Frequency of data submission
    C. Robust skip logic function to allow only necessary data to be entered
    D. Front-end data filters and audits to identify data entry errors at time of entry
    E. Narrow data transmission schedule to allow maximum time for chart abstraction/data entry
    F. Accessibility to real-time data to provide patient level and organization-specific reports
    G. Web-based tool populated with patient specific data (i.e., admission date/source, discharge date/status, social
        security and/or HIC numbers)
    H. Process for data updates and edits, (i.e., Does your product include real time reporting for missing data and
        performance rates?)
    I. Proven track record of reports generated and data transmitted to JCAHO and QNET in a timely manner
III. Decision support and reporting
    A. Capability to benchmark performance against a large number of hospitals and health systems
    B. By service
    C. By physician
    D. Utilization analysis
IV. Training
    A. Onsite
    B. Remote
    C. Web-based
V. Customer support
    A. Dedicated technical staff to help troubleshoot software and hardware problems
VI. User group
    A. Frequency and location of meetings
    B. Online forum: extra cost or included in base package
VII. Performance improvement
    A. Sharing "best practices"
    B. Sourcing services
    C. Consulting services
VIII. Vendor characteristics
    A. Annual revenue
    B. Number of employees
    C. Number of clients
    D. Number of years quality measure reporting product in general release

Table 11-5: Sample #4—Telehealth.

(Adapted from HCA Home Telehealth & Technology News, Volume: I Issue: 2 November 2005).

Criteria Category	Weight	Vendor A	Vendor B	Vendor C
Language • Russian • Chinese • Spanish				
Human Factors/Usability • Patient directions verbal • Patient directions in text • Ease of Use • Training Time Needed • Reporting capabilities and fees if applicable • Medication Management/Reminders • Programmability for patient education • Web-based: Yes/No • Ability and ease of transmitting data as needed • Patient Portal				
Equipment • Size/weight • Back up battery and/or operational batteries: Yes/No—# and type • Installation Time/Ease—does company offer installation/deinstallation? Fee? • Cleaning time/ease? • Equipment reliability—replacement/warranties? • Patient's/caregivers ease of use • Modem: Internal vs. External • How many peripheral devices can function at one time? # of serial ports_____ • Vendor offers equipment maintenance protocols and service intervals • Ease of connection for visit, if applicable • Reporting time: Real-time; Store and forward • Transmission carrier: POTS; Broadband; Fiber Optic; Other				
Peripherals • Medication Management • Thermometer • Stethoscope • Wireless?				
Program Design—Product Suitable for: • CHF • CAD • COPD • Wound Care • Asthma • Mental Health • HIV/AIDS • OMR/DD • Post Surgical • Long-Term Monitoring • Speech Therapy • Limited English Proficiency (LEP) or patients with low health literacy • Med Management				
Total Score				

Table 11-6: Sample #5—Emergency Department Information System.

Criteria Category	Weight	Vendor A	Vendor B	Vendor C	Vendor D	Vendor E
Registration						
Triage						
Patient Tracking						
Nurse charting						
Physician charting						
Order entry/results						
Disposition/Discharge						
Charge capture/billing						
Reporting						
Trauma registry						
Integration/Interfacing						
Printing/Fax/Scan						
Security						
Total =						

I. Registration
   A. Quick registration; discuss flow and demonstrate
   B. Number of patient identifiers; MRN#, Account #, Visit #, accept master patient index
   C. Pre-registration (e.g., ambulance, helicopter, doctor's office)
   D. Point-of-care registration: bedside, roll-a-cart, wireless
   E. ED event link – fill-in or dynamic drop down to classify ED admission event
   F. Should be able to handle a "John Doe" patient when identity is unknown with ability to merge charge when identity is learned; function limited by supervisory role
   G. Customizable: data elements, how many available
II. Triage
   A. Standard and custom flowsheets and forms
   B. Triage charting; view previous visit data and populate in current chart as appropriate (i.e., demographics, allergy history, meds)
III. Patient Tracking
   A. General Features
      1. Modification to list—custom per user, preferences; supervisor view to track staff throughput w/alerts
      2. Drill down capabilities; to chart, results
      3. Multiple patients in single bed (i.e., bed 1a and 1b)
      4. Staff level tracking (i.e., MD see patient, RN needed)
      5. Outstanding issues tracking: flag follow-up need, result discrepancies
      6. Define care areas or "units" and is there a limit of patients that can be assigned to a given care area/unit
   B. Locating a patient
      1. Passive by infrared sensors and radio frequencies
   C. Tracking encounter times
      1. Admission tracking; arrival time
      2. Time of triage
      3. Time patient is in treatment room
      4. Time patient is seen by a nurse, doctor
      5. Time medications are administered
      6. Time patient is discharged, transferred
      7. Alerts
      8. Wait times exceed user-defined values for phases of care
      9. Can wait times be defined for each care area (i.e., fast-track vs. unit six)
      10. CDC alerts
      11. Workflow
      12. Auto-queue to nurse, MD, ancillary based on documentation completion, order generation
      13. Result discrepancies (i.e., radiology)
      14. Tracking by user (i.e., worklist)

        15.Orders

        16.Tracking: orders status, result status

        17.Elapsed time of order

        18.Orders pending signatures

    D. Tracking board

        1. Views should be customizable (i.e., views for physicians, nurses and ED administration)

        2. May be specialized

        3. Visual indicators: overflow, time exceeds, pending MD, result, discharge

        4. Ability to assign patient to hall area or holding area

IV.Charting (Nursing & Physician)

    A. Supports compliance with the following standards

        1. Restraints

        2. Conscious sedation

        3. Pain assessment

        4. CMS quality measures

    B. Multiple views

        1. By function: Triage, acuity, flowsheet, assessment, meds, MAR (border patients), Dx, orders, summary, visit histories

        2. By role: Nursing, Physician, ancillary, coder, Non-ED staff (i.e., inpatient clinician)

    C. Charting elements

        1. Assessments

        2. Chief complaint

        3. History of present illness

        4. Past, Family and/or Social History

        5. Allergies (with coded allergy drop down), history

        6. Review of Systems

        7. Physical Exam; defaults for normal

        8. Nursing templates; clinical treatments, procedures, interventions, flowsheet/checklist

        9. Conscious sedation

        10.Restraint assessment

        11.Communicable diseases

        12.Domestic violence screen

        13.Condition at discharge

        14.Pain assessment and reassessment

        15.Core quality measures (pneumonia, AMI, and CHF)

        16.Age-appropriate assessment, specifically for pediatrics

        17.Syndromic surveillance

        18.Ancillary Templates: Respiratory Therapy, Case Manager, SW, chaplain, Psychiatric

        19.Documentation analyzer and guidelines: Health Care Financing Administration (HCFA) compliant, core measures, QA markers—can custom-build?

        20.Result interpretation notes

        21.Admission note

        22.Charting characteristics

    D. More than one person can work on any particular chart without the system locking

    E. Pick list/drop down menus where possible, free text, macros, radio buttons, check box, defaults

    F. Longitudinal record

    G. Templates – how many standard of each

        1. Input modalities (utility varies by function)

        2. Speech recognition

        3. PDAs

        4. Laptops

        5. Thin clients

        6. Touch screens

V. Order Entry and Results

    A. Order sets; order preferences

    B. Unread results (bolded) vs. read

    C. Alerts; Drug-drug interaction, duplicates, non-resulted

VI.Disposition / Discharge

    A. Prescriptions and medication instruction sheet

    B. Aftercare instructions and work/school notes; grade-level, multi-lingual, third party software, frequency of updates, customizable

    C. Chart completion after patient discharge

VII. Charge capture/billing

A. Automatic charge capture generated from documentation and orders

B. Code generation (e.g., CPT, E&M modifiers, calculation level of charges, HCPC, APC and custom facility supply charge codes)

C. Documentation code analysis

D. Pick-list, bar-code/supply cabinets

E. How does the charge function automate professional vs. hospital billing

VIII. Reporting

A. Census analysis: number of patients in ED by hour, shift, day, week, month, year

B. Productivity: throughput, wait time, walk-outs, result time, staff productivity, # chart completions after discharge

C. Patient Profile analysis

D. Seen in different ED areas

1. By disposition

2. By acuity

3. By diagnosis

4. By event

E. Medical Records

1. Reconciliation report; list of patients seen versus coded

F. Radiology readings

1. Accepts x-ray interpretations by emergency physician

2. Allows radiologists to flag significant discrepancies on-screen and alert on-duty ED personnel

G. Automated, HIPAA-compliant syndromic surveillance

H. Export data to third party report writer; Crystal

IX. Trauma Registry

A. Injury severity score

B. Revised trauma score

C. Weighted trauma score

D. Probability of survival score

E. Database for capture of standard trauma data

X. Integration/Interfacing

A. Bi-directional interface to the ADT (admissions, discharges and transfer) system; Quick registration from Invision to EDIM, ADT from EDIM to Invision

B. Bi-directional interfaces to support order (lab, radiology, pharmacy and cardiology, ED dispensers systems) and result communication—which systems have interfaced within each category

C. Supports multi-facility entity

D. Integrates across continuum of care

XI. Printing/Fax/Scan

A. Auto generate labels from orders (i.e., labs, patient labels)

B. Document Management – scanning external documents, consults

C. Auto fax EMR to physician office

D. Can printing be routed to printers by order type or workstation location

E. Does printing support NYS prescription law[13]

XII.   Security

A. Time-out

B. Password change

C. Multi-user workstation, sign-on and off

D. Multiple chart signatures, co-signing

E. Quick-log-in (i.e., same user at workstation, times out, input pw only)

F. Remote Access

1. Read-only (i.e., non ED personnel viewing chart)

Table 11-7: Sample #6—Surgical Management System.

Criteria Category	Weight	Vendor A	Vendor B	Vendor C
Tracking Board				
Scheduling				
Preference cards				
Perioperative documentation				
Anesthesia record interface				
Interfaces/Integration				
Clinical decision support				
Billing				
Material management/inventory				
Reports				
Implementation				
User Group				
Human factors/user-friendliness				
Financial stability of vendor				
Total				

I. Tracking Board
   A. All timestamps and events collected throughout the nursing documentation modules are available for display
   B. Easily configurable to meet the needs of each perioperative department or location ensuring HIPAA compliance and patient privacy
   C. Accurate physical tracking screens of patient/resource status, locations
   D. Big Board displays & tracking screens offer customizable views
   E. Color-coded fields alert staff to changes and warn staff of delays
   F. Stores critical checkpoints throughout surgical episode
   G. Automatically alerts staff when activities fail to meet critical checkpoint
II. Scheduling
   A. Conflict checking for equipment, staff, locations, and different ancillary department appointments
   B. Pre-defined procedure specific data entry templates that save you time when adding cases to the surgery schedule
   C. Remote communication for surgery schedule requests
   D. Automatic scheduling of related PAT activities
   E. Easy to create, flexible block time capability defined by surgeon, surgeon group and service
   F. Automatic check for credentialing of surgeons privileges by procedure
   G. Preference cards integrated with scheduling and documentation modules to improve flow of information
   H. Remote scheduling
   I. Web read-only access
   J. Multifacility enabled
   K. Integrates with ADT to provide shared demographic information
   L. Helps comply with HCFA concurrency regulations
III. Preference cards
   A. Online preference card management
   B. Exception noting
   C. Integration with a HIS billing system
   D. Integration with materials management
   E. Facility preferences automatically update as cases are moved across sites
   F. Global updates of preference cards
   G. Picklists by case, room, inventory location, day(s) with one request
   H. Cards automatically collapse for complex multi-procedure cases
   I. Easy maintenance of stock items to support preference cards
   J. Generic cards available to copy
   K. Unique pediatric features
   L. Complete multifacility functionality
IV. Perioperative documentation (pre-, intra- and post-op)

     A. JCAHO-required immediate operative note
     B. Supports Association of peri-Operative Registered Nurses' PNDS nomenclature and plan-of-care guidelines
     C. Supports JCAHO documentation (e.g., documenting "time out" for right site surgery)
     D. Post-operative documentation for nursing and QA assessments
     E. Pain-management documentation
     F. PACU and same-day surgery discharge instructions
     G. Field content is user-defined
     H. Comprehensive SMDA implant charting
     I. Demographics
     J. Allergies, medications, and surgical history
     K. Physical examination
     L. Sponge counts
     M. Review of body systems
     N. Audit trail
     O. Addendum documentation
V. Anesthesia record
     A. Controlled via touch screen, mouse, or keyboard
     B. Captures data from medical devices and displays in custom defined intervals
     C. Printed anesthesia record
VI. Interfaces/Integration
     A. Lab
     B. ADT
     C. Pharmacy
     D. Radiology
     E. Bi-Directional Materials Management Interface
VII. Clinical decision support
     A. Automatic alert via paging or e-mail to improve workflow and resource efficiency
     B. Works with pagers, PDAs, e-mail
     C. Automatic communication of E&M, ICD-9, CPT-4 and professional fee codes to billing
VIII. Billing
     A. Automation allows for flexible billing options such as time, flat fee and itemization
     B. Integrates with existing billing system automatically transferring case charges
     C. Printed billing form
     D. Change the "charge" interface without having to rely on a vendor to change it. As a result, the change becomes effective immediately
     E. Revenue maximizing decision support
     F. Combine numerous variables (payor, OR time, anesthesia time, flat rate, admission type, anesthesia type, procedure, facility, severity, room, service) to generate charges for a case
     G. Support Ambulatory Procedure Codes (APCs)
IX. Material management/inventory
     A. Item master
     B. Supply usage communication
X. Reports
     A. Inventory
     B. Equipment
     C. System includes multiple, user-defined standard reports such as: scheduling views, perioperative documents, preference cards, pick lists, and much more
     D. System includes multiple management reports such as: room utilization, surgeon utilization, block time utilization, room turnover time analysis, case cancellation analysis, case costing, and much more
     E. User-defined query tabs and icons
     F. Customized and standard reports
     G. A query builder tool
     H. Industry standard SQL language structure
     I. Full export capabilities, i.e.,, Excel and Access
     J. Intuitive user interface
     K. Schedule reports to run automatically daily, weekly, or monthly
XI. Implementation
     A. All implementation completed at customer site
     B. Implementation staff can be on site for every go-live event
     C. Ongoing operating cost
XII. User Group
     A. Active user group
     B. Regular meetings
     C. Online forum
XIII. Human factors/user-friendliness

XIV. Cost
    A. Installation time and cost
    B. Training time and cost
XV. Financial stability of vendor
    A. Year established
    B. Private versus public
    C. Number of current installations
    D. Number of full time employees
XVI. Customer satisfaction
    A. KLAS reports
    B. Reference calls ("due diligence") & site visits
        1. Lived up to expectations
        2. Vendor is improving
        3. Proactive service
        4. Contracting experience
        5. Product works as promoted
        6. Quality of:
           a) Training
           b) Implementation
        7. Support
        8. Interface services
    C. Costs/business indicators
        1. Implementation on time
        2. Implementation within budget / cost
        3. Would you buy it again
        4. Avoids nickel-and-diming
        5. Keeps all promises
        6. Would recommend to a friend / peer

REFERENCES

1. Neuenschwander M, Cohen MR, Vaida AJ, Patchett JA, Kelly J, Trohimovich B. Practical guide to bar coding for patient medication safety. *Am J Health Syst Pharm.* 2003;April 15;60(8):768–79.

2. Laker B, Groeber V. IT purchasing strategies: Make good decisions by approaching them right. *Healthcare Informatics.* 2005 Sep;22(9):48.

3. McDowell SW. Herding cats: The challenges of EMR vendor selection. *JHIM.* 2005;17(3):63–71.

4. Project Management Institute. *A Guide to the Project Management Body of Knowledge (PMBOK® Guide).* 3rd ed. New Town Square, Penn: Project Management Institute; 2006.

5. Heerkens G. *Project Management.* New York: McGraw-Hill; 2002.

6. Gladwell M. *The Tipping Point: How Little Things Can Make a Big Difference.* New York: Little Brown & Co.; 2000.

7. Rogers EM. *Diffusion of Innovations.* 4th ed. New York: Free Press; 2003.

8. Laker B, Groeber V. IT Purchasing Strategies: Make good decisions by approaching them right. *Healthcare Informatics.* 2005 Sep;22(9):48.

9. Health Data Management. 2004 software guide. Available at: http://www.healthdatamanagement.com/html/software/index.cfm. Accessed April 14, 2006.

10. Garets D, Davis M. White Paper: Electronic medical records vs. electronic health records: yes, there is a difference. *HIMSS Analytics.* 2006; http://www.himssanalytics.org/docs/WP_EMR_EHR.pdf. Accessed November 22, 2006.

11. Anonymous. Telehealth Vendor Assessment Tool from Centura Health at Home. *HCA Home Telehealth & Technology News.* 2005; November 2;I:8–9.

12. Fischman J. Bridging the language gap: Some hospitals make non-English-speaking patients feel right at home. *U.S. News and World Report.* July 9, 2006. http://www.usnews.com/usnews/health/articles/060709/17cult.htm. Accessed November 21, 2006.

13. New York State Information for a Healthy New York. Narcotic enforcement. Available at: http://www.health.state.ny.us/professionals/narcotic/. Accessed April 16, 2006.

CHAPTER 12

Project Management

Janet Bowen, MBA

> *"Strength does not come from physical capacity.*
> *It comes from an indomitable will."*
> Mahatma Gandhi (1869 – 1948)

Projects have typical cycles of scoping, planning, executing, monitoring and closure. They also have atypical and varied degrees of challenges, roadblocks and naysayers. The leadership and communication skills of the project manager are critical to the successful outcome of a project. Focus on your strengths as the leader of the project and the strengths of team resources. It is not productive to dwell on limitations, but rather recognize them and identify the appropriate resources to go beyond them. Project Managers (PMs) need to exhibit the skills of a leader by imparting vision, defining strategic goals and direction. PMs must fluently execute the skills of a manager which focuses on results, accomplishments, setting expectations and achieving success as defined by the project requirements.

Establishing a relationship with the team members and the project sponsors is essential for honest and productive communication. Projects are dynamic groups that have come together to achieve the goals and objectives defined in the charter and scope statement. People matter and the PM needs to have the skills to understand the dynamics and talents of the team and to utilize each member as effectively and as appropriate for that individual and for the role within the team. Establishing strong relationships with your team will help to better understand what motivates the team members and will help to be clear in communicating roles and expectations.

PM tools, strategy, goals and objectives—how about good old intuition? Part of project management is using good judgment—and sometimes that means changing the rules. A good time to challenge the PM rules is in the beginning of the project. Given the opportunity, challenge the team selection rule. Pick the team you want; pick a virtuoso team rather then inherit the team. Table 12-1 delineates the difference between a traditional team versus a virtuoso one.[1]

Table 12-1: Characteristics of a Traditional Team vs. a Virtuoso Team.[1]

Traditional Project Teams	Virtuoso Project Teams
Choose members based on availability	Choose members based on skills
Emphasize the needs of the team	Emphasize the needs of the individual (i.e., empowerment)
Focus on task	Focus on ideas – generates positive atmosphere enthusiasm, fun and innovation
Work individually and remotely	Work together intensively – builds team bonding, strengthens relationships
	Strives to meet expectations of highly demanding projects

TIPS FROM THE PROJECT MANAGEMENT COMMUNITY

Sometimes you learn through doing by trial and error. However, this method of learning may not afford you many repeated opportunities to serve a project as a project manager. Querying the blogs on the Web, a list of top twelve tips for project management can be crafted:[2]

1. Failure is not an option, as per Apollo 13's project leader Gene Krantz.
2. The kind of organization you are in determines the kind of leader you need to be. (I'd also add that WHERE the project is in its lifecycle and the level of project experience of your team and stakeholders also matters.)
3. A good leader has integrity (e.g., accountable), is a team player but tough when needed; and is truthful, which includes how you report project status and metrics. Don't be lazy. Push beyond your natural abilities. Get into the details. Get out of your office and talk to people.
4. Make sure that everyone in your organization can articulate what it is you're trying to accomplish. I've also heard this called "the hymn" (i.e., make sure everyone's singing the same tune from the same book.)
5. The true test of a leader is how you behave when the chips are down and things are ambiguous—including when no one is watching.
6. Your team is allowed to have morale problems; leaders are not.
7. Leaders require a sense of history. Yes, learn from the past; but understand that what you do matters in the future.
8. When faced with ethical dilemmas, apply three tests:
   a. **Newspaper** - how would you feel if it was a headline tomorrow?
   b. **Golden Rule** - how would you feel if it was done to you?
   c. **Obituary or Best Friend** - how do you want to be remembered?
9. LISTEN. One of the most essential leadership skills.
10. Create a sense of urgency. Don't under- or overestimate this tip. It might be difficult, but it will build credibility.
11. Stay on top of things; status the project often, keep things moving, and respond promptly.
12. Be persistent.

GLOBAL COMMUNITY

Never doubt that a small group of thoughtful, committed citizens can change the world.
Indeed, it is the only thing that ever has.
Margaret Mead (1901 – 1978)

As a project manager, it is important to network with your peers, join professional organizations in your industry and your profession. Membership in these groups can boost your professional image and afford you new opportunities to learn and network. As a healthcare IT professional, there are two prominent organizations that will keep you sharp and connected with trends and tools of your trade.

The Project Management Institute (PMI)
Web address: www.pmi.org

PMI is an international organization focused on project management which offers professional certification recognized worldwide. The organization has about 200,000 members represented in 125 countries. The project managers are from major industries such as aerospace, construction, healthcare and engineering. The PMI organization offers a wealth of opportunities such as online education, seminars, publications, project management volunteering, special interest groups and leadership roles.

PMI offers two professional certifications: Certified Associate in Project Management (CAPM) that requires a minimum of 1,500 hours of project management experience to be eligible to take the certification exam; and the Project Management Professional certification exam that is offered to those individuals with verifiable 7,500 hours of full life cycle PM experience. A newly offered certification offered for Program Managers is for individuals responsible for multiple projects. A PMI certification is highly-valued and enhances one's marketability in the job market.

The Healthcare Information and Management Systems Society (HIMSS)
Web address: www.himss.org

HIMSS is a national organization established in 1961 with approximately 20,000 members. Its focus is on the use of technology in healthcare and its mission is "to lead change in the healthcare information and management systems field through knowledge sharing, advocacy, collaboration, innovation and community affiliations."[3]

HIMSS has local chapters and special interest groups (SIG). Of particular interest is the Project Management SIG that focuses on healthcare project management methodology, challenges and opportunities.

Project management blogs offer an online forum of ideas and discussions. Some project managers use blogs to post project status reports since it is easily accessible by project team members and sponsors.

Some available project management Web logs are:
• http://www.pmthink.com
• http://projectized.blogspot.com
• http://www.reformingprojectmanagement.com
• http://aboutpmos.blogspot.com/

WHAT DOES A PM DO?

- Deliver projects on time and within budget
- Manage staff, customers and suppliers
- Resolve project risks, changes & issues
- Quickly complete project documentation
- Improve the quality of your deliverables

One recent job posting on the PMI Healthcare SIG site captures most of the essential skill sets that define project management:

"[M]anage sub-projects of an overall large, enterprise-wide, complex and high-profile healthcare/IT project with minimal supervision. The Project Manager is fully accountable for providing overall project management. Responsible for developing, maintaining and managing items such as project schedule, budget tracking, issue and risk management, communications planning, scope management, coordinating the efforts of the sub-project team members to meet customer requirements and overall project goals; status reporting (project team upwards to Steering Committee level). Monitors and tracks progress while ensuring quality of team deliverables. Communicates regularly to Project PMO/Steering Committee, sponsor and other stakeholders and manages the expectations of all. Keep all stakeholders informed of progress and issues. Ensures sustained buy-in at all levels to project scope and its deliverables. Apply expertise in the following project management knowledge areas:

1. *Integration Management* (e.g., project plan development, plan execution, change control management)

2. *Cost Management* (e.g., resource planning, estimating, budgeting and control)

3. *Time Management* (e.g., WBS, project schedule (MS Project), estimating, critical path identification, and tracking and control)

4. *Communication Management* (e.g., communication planning, distribution, performance reporting, closure)

5. *Scope Management* (e.g., initiation, scope planning, definition, verification, change control)

6. *Quality Management* (e.g., quality planning, assurance and control, issue identification, tracking, resolution)

7. *Risk Management* (e.g., risk planning, identification, analysis, response planning, monitoring and control)

8. *HR Management* (e.g., organization planning, team development)

9. *Procurement Management* (e.g., procurement planning, solicitation planning, solicitation/selection, contract administration and closeout)

The Project Manager will also provide mentoring as it pertains to Project Management Methodologies, processes, procedures, and tools through discussions with project team members, Information Services and other

CCHMC personnel. In addition, they will provide support in the IS Project Management Office development and process improvement initiatives.

Required Skills: Proven strong project management and leadership; excellent verbal, nonverbal, presentation, facilitation and written communication skills; strong organizational skills, mentoring/coaching and coordination skills with large complex projects. Expertise in project management methodologies with the ability to mentor in theory, as well as demonstration in the application of project management (basic project management fundamentals upwards to Sr. Project Manager levels). Proficient in scheduling (MS Project), cost, scope, contract, issue and risk identification/tracking and management. Development and management of such things as project plans, schedules, RFPs, charters, requirements definition, etc. An ability to lead and motivate people and encourage teamwork. Establish a clear vision of what determines a successful project for our internal customers. Capable of relating to diverse age and demographic backgrounds, and the ability to work well with others in a team environment. Must possess a breadth of knowledge and skills to resolve most problems independently. Demonstrate an independent work initiative, attention to detail, sound judgment, diplomacy and a professional demeanor.

Education/Work Experience: Bachelor's Degree in related discipline and/or equivalent.

Minimum of five years related experience including three years managing small to medium size and complexity projects and/or sub-projects of enterprise projects. *PM Certification and Healthcare experience a plus.*"[4]

The qualified candidates for the job description given above would have the skills sets required for every aspect of the project management lifecycle. For the project manager, the rewards are as great as the responsibilities. The dynamics of the healthcare environment and external regulatory bodies add another level of complexity to project management.

Project management can be "paper" intensive. Ideally, a project administrator would address procurement management, financial management, project setup, timesheet processing, travel arrangements, and other administrative functions that might otherwise encumber the project manager.

PROJECT MANAGEMENT OFFICE (PMO)—A CASE STUDY

Healthcare project management is changing and quickly migrating towards formalized project management. A critical change in the healthcare industry has been the creation of project management offices within the organization. The PMO functions as a governance structure that oversees all projects to ensure alignment with business strategy, appropriate project membership, adherence to project scope and expectation and monitoring of project timelines, risks and establishing a standard of quality implementation.

At the University of Illinois Medical Center (UIMC), the PMO function is within the office of the CIO. UIMC's initial step was to develop strategic IT plans. The PMO office interviewed the departments to understand current projects and priorities. "During these interviews, IS learned about departmental plans and was able to better consider how IS could support future information technology needs."[5]   The next step was to improve customer responsiveness by taking control of the customer requests by standardizing the request form, as well as the review and assignment process. The gains were realized in improved management of IT resources. The PMO office was able to define a process, implement a standard and measure the benefit from incorporating standard tools and methodology. The UMIC PMO continued to standardize tools and methodology in other areas of the project management life cycle which enabled IT to meet the growing demand of technology in healthcare.

Communication and Leadership

A quick reference guide for successful implementation of a computerized practitioner order entry system (CPOE) published by Medicare Hospital Leadership and System Improvement group cites communication as *essential*. The quick reference lists the three out of five key factors related to successful communication and leadership,[6] as shown in Table 12-2.

Table 12-2: **Factors Related to Successful Communication and Leadership.**

Build support for change • Hospital-wide support for CPOE technology is vital to its successful implementation • Hospital leaders and other "core believers" should start the process • Support of administrative leaders lends vision and supplies necessary resources • Hospital staff physicians and other personnel, including pharmacists and nurses, are individuals with detailed process knowledge, and are key to the successful adoption of the new processes • Team members from all departments involved in the practitioner ordering process must be recruited • Members who are reluctant to change and who are not technologically savvy must be included
Articulate clear, specific and realistic goals and strategies • Strategies must be developed to define and complete each step in the change process. Examples include the following steps. • Select and recruit personnel to perform the change work • Understand and define current processes • Define new processes • Develop and adopt order sets • Plan for pilot and rollout • Plan and complete staff education • Plan and complete data collection • Communicate clearly and frequently to the entire hospital staff
Identify and develop strategies for overcoming barriers to change • The number and type of barriers to change vary in each organization. Some barriers are general and commonplace, while other barriers are unique to an institution. Communication is the key to identifying most barriers to change and these barriers can be categorized into the following major areas. • Fear and inertia • "Wait and see" individuals and "core resisters" • "Workarounds"

Project Life Cycles

The typical project has a series of phases each marked by a milestone, each having particular skills sets, tools and membership participation levels. The phases are: Initiation, Planning, Executing, Controlling and Closing. Although each phase typically occurs in sequential order, phases can run in parallel or be jump-started using fast tracking methodology. The fast tracking allows controlled and planned initiation of certain activities in the next phase to start earlier thus decreasing the overall project timeline. Fast tracking methodology requires an understanding of the inherent risks in moving tasks forward and utilizing resources appropriately to achieve the intended goals.

The beginning of the project or the "Initiation" phase, occurs when the organization selects the project, identifies the roles and responsibilities of the project manager, establishes a high level scope and timeline and identifies organization or business goals. The project charter incorporates all of these parameters and is signed off by the project sponsor at the close of this phase.

The "Planning" phase is the most process intensive. It is here where a detailed project plan is constructed which requires defining of each task, activity and resource. The planning process goes through all project requirements and identifies optimal planning as well as alternate resources and plans. Establishing alternate plans will help to minimize project risks. All project stakeholders are identified. The project communication methods, budget, risk plan, quality standards and timelines are all identified in the planning phase. The planning phase is critical since the Execution, Controlling and Closing phase are executed based on the input from the planning phase. The milestone of this phase is a finalized project scope statement and a project plan. A kickoff meeting is held with the project stakeholders to communicate all key elements of the planning documents. During the course of the project there will be reiterations of the components of planning such as budget, schedule or risk identification. It is a natural occurrence in a dynamic project; however, it is the responsibility of the PM to determine reasonableness and appropriateness of the changes.

As Carolyn Wells says, "Actions lie louder than words." The "Execution" phase puts the plan into action and the team dynamics develop. This is the phase that utilizes the most resources and time; therefore, it is the most costly. The challenge here is to manage the project schedule and resources within the scope of the project.

The "Controlling" phase requires monitoring tools that effectively identify risks or quality issues emerging as the project progresses. Continuous monitoring is important to keep a pulse on the health and status of the project. A PM does not want to be blindsided by an issue that can potentially set the project back. Monitoring a project's progress is critical to achieving milestones on time and on budget. A need for change may occur during the course of a project but not without control measures which will assess the impact of the change to help determine if it is appropriate. If the project review warrants a change, then a change approval process is in order where the change is communicated to the stakeholders and the impact on the budget, scheduling, tasks or resources is clearly defined.

"Closure" is the final phase when the termination of a project is formalized. Each deliverable is reviewed and verified as completed in accordance with project requirements and the project sponsor signs a closure or acceptance document. Before all of the stakeholders disseminate and move on to either the next project or their operational roles, it is important to review the project and reflect on lessons learned. A "lessons learned" document can help identify mistakes and missed opportunities that should be prevented in subsequent projects. The lessons learned exercise can be achieved in a single meeting.

There are lessons to be learned from failed projects as well as successful ones. Both outcomes warrant a review and team discussion. The lessons can help identify and mitigate risks for next projects or help to better plan cost and resources. Learn from mistakes and go through the lessons learned exercise together as a team without finger pointing, blame or excuses. Since a lessons learned meeting can be emotionally charged, it is best to establish a project agenda, a stated objective, rules of the meeting (e.g., stay focused on tasks, not people) and then to list areas of discussion. Categorizing general project impressions, deliverables, management and timing of resources will keep the team centered and the meeting outcome more meaningful.

Project Methodology

It is important that an aim never be defined in terms of activity or methods. It must always relate directly to how life is better for everyone. . . . The aim of the system must be clear to everyone in the system. The aim must include plans for the future. The aim is a value judgment.

W. Edwards Deming (1900 – 1993)

The project methodology should be based on a standard framework such as the PMI PMBOK (Project Management Body of Knowledge) publication, a comprehensive 530-page guide of life cycle documentation standards and recommended tools for project management. ITIL (Information Technology Library) is another world-wide accepted methodology applied to the Service Delivery aspect of IT. Each PM will work within the framework established by either the PMO office or the IT Department but may modify document utilization based on either project size or most effective tools. Having a library of templates to use will decrease the PM's effort in creating the documents and will provide consistent views and content presentation to the client and the PMO office that monitors multiple projects. Maintaining a consistent methodology throughout the organization will help to facilitate clarity in all phases of the life cycle. One example is the use of a project toolkit as published by the MIT IT Department.

The MIT IT Department has published a standard project management methodology to help control and manage the number and complexity of projects. An excellent starting point is a project definition template which identifies all the necessary definition and measurement criteria. The input of data into a central repository of projects allows the PMO to monitor and manage multiple projects and helps to alert the PM if tasks are falling off track.[7] Figure 12-1 is an example of a project control book. Guidelines for project set-up and usage are defined to ensure consistency. Standard Templates and Tools are a click away.

The MIT IT PM toolkit puts all of the essentials in one location to facilitate planning. The toolkit as shown in Figure 12-2 includes a project life cycle definition and quick access to key materials, project start-up checklist, sponsor checklist, and closure.

Tools of the Trade

An apprentice carpenter may want only a hammer and saw, but a master craftsman employs many precision tools. Computer programming likewise requires sophisticated tools to cope with the complexity of real applications, and only practice with these tools will build skill in their use.

Robert L. Kruse, Data Structures and Program Design

A quick glance at the Knowledge area table in Table 12-3[8] shows the PM tools used throughout Project Management with the most intensity appearing in the Planning and Controlling phases.

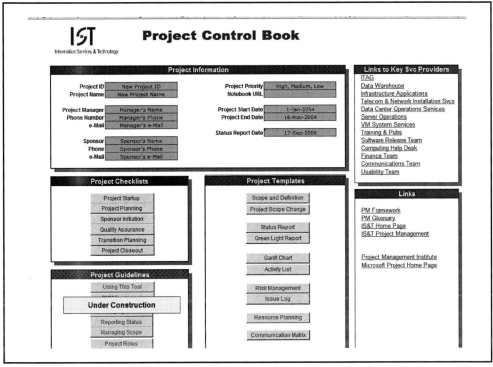

Figure 12-1: Project Control Book Example.

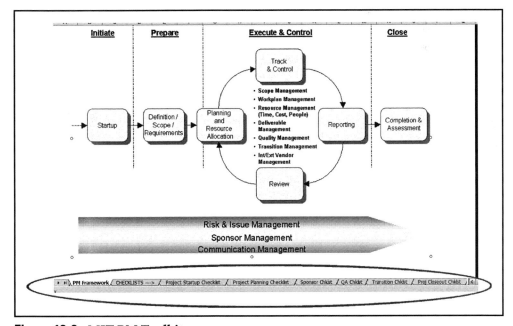

Figure 12-2: MIT PM Toolkit.

Table 12-3: The Project Knowledge Areas as defined by PMI.[8]

Knowledge Area	Initiating	Planning	Executing	Controlling	Close
Project Integration Management	Develop Project Charter Develop Preliminary Project Scope Statement	Develop Project Management Plan	Direct and Manage Project Execution	Monitor and Control Work Integrated Change Control	Close Project
Project Scope Management		Scope Planning Scope Definition Create WBS		Scope Verification Scope Control	
Project Time Management		Activity Definition Activity Sequencing Activity Resource Estimating Activity Duration Estimating Schedule Development		Schedule Control	
Project Cost Management		Cost Estimating Cost Budgeting		Cost Control	
Project HR Management		Human Resources Planning	Acquire Project Team Develop Project Team	Manage Project Team	
Project Quality Management		Quality Planning	Perform Quality Assurance	Perform Quality Control	
Project Communications Management		Communications Planning	Information Distribution	Performance Reporting Manage Stakeholders	
Project Risk Management		Risk Management Planning Risk Identification Qualitative Risk Analysis Risk Response Planning		Risk Monitoring and Control	
Project Procurement Management		Plan Purchases and Acquisitions Plan Contracting	Request Seller Responses Select Seller	Contract Administration	Contract Closure

Initiation Tools and Templates

Project selection is determined through cost benefit analysis, ROI, needs analysis, cash flow tools such as IRR and NPV, and, of course, expert judgment.

Planning Tools and Templates

The Planning phase incorporates several tools since the there are several planning areas:

• Activity planning: The WBS (work breakdown structure) is derived from the list of deliverables identified in the Initiation phase and is an effective tool that breaks down the activities in great enough detail to enable the PM to better assess cost and schedules. Either the creation of chart-like diagrams for each WBS or a numerical representation of major and minor tasks can also be used.

- Resource planning tools: HR practices, organizational structure
- Schedule planning: duration compression, resource leveling, simulation, PERT, CPM, crashing, fast tracking
- Cost Estimating tools: analogous estimating, parametric modeling, Bottoms up estimating, computerized tools
- Quality planning: Benefit/Cost analysis, benchmarking and flowcharting
- Risk planning: documentation reviews, information gathering techniques, checklists, assumption analysis, diagramming technique such as decision tree analysis
- Procurement planning: evaluation tools
- Project plan: project management software such as Microsoft project as shown in Table 12-4[9]

Table 12-4: Gantt Chart Tool in Microsoft Project.[9]

Execution and Controlling Tools and Templates

Performance reviews, variance analysis, trend analysis, earned value analysis (compares planned value with actual value), change control system and configuration management are all methods to manage and track performance.

The tools and templates listed above are part of the standard PMI toolkits recommended for each project management phase. An organization that uses standard tools and templates will find it easier to measure, monitor and manage multiple projects. Toolkits and templates also provide guidance to less experienced project managers for necessary information gathering for each phase.

CONCLUSION

Professional project management has arrived in healthcare, bringing with it standard practice methodology, guidelines, tools and organizational structure. Project management is helping the healthcare industry to achieve project successes and improve the overall management of IT projects. The healthcare market is now increasing its demand for certified project management professionals as a necessary skill set for today's environment. Healthcare delivery organizations are recognizing the importance of a project management office to oversee all projects to ensure standards and alignment with business goals and objectives. Healthcare project management is an exciting field with many challenges beyond technical. Federal regulation, academia, clinical quality, historical biases, and cultural work relationships contribute to the uniqueness of the field. Information on healthcare IT project management is widely available on the Internet, publications and through professional networks such as national and local professional organizations.

REFERENCES

1. Mektnyka K. Throw out the rules - leading an elite team on a mission requires a new approach. *Computerworld*. August 8, 2005; http://www.computerworld.com/managementtopics/management/project/story/0,10801,103697,00.html. Accessed November 21, 2006.

2. PM Think! Project Management Thought Leadership. 5 tips to becoming a great project manager. Available at: http://www.pmthink.com/2005/09/5-tips-to-becoming-great-project.htm. Accessed on September 15, 2006.

3. Healthcare Information and Management Systems Society. Available at: http://www.himss.org/ASP/aboutHimssHome.asp. Accessed on September 15, 2006.

4. Project Management Institute. Healthcare project management jobs. *Healthcare Speaks*. September 20, 2006. Available at: http://pmihealthcare.org/docs/HealthcareSpeaks. Accessed on September 22, 2006.

5. Isola M, Polikaitis A, Laureto RA. Implementation of a project management office (PMO)—experiences from year 1. *J Healthc Inf Manag*. 2006 Winter;20(1):79–87.

6. Medicare Hospital Leadership and System Improvement (HLSI). Critical Activities for Successful Implementation of CPOE Technology – Quick Reference Guide. http://www.medqic.org/dcs/BlobServer?blobcol=urldata&blobheader=multipart%2Foctet-stream&blobheadername1=Content-Disposition&blobheadervalue1=attachment%3Bfilename%3DCPOE+Quick+Reference+Guide.pdf&blobkey=id&blobtable=MungoBlobs&blobwhere=1124714932476 Accessed November 22, 2006.

7. Information Services and Technology. IS&T's project management methodology. Available at: http://web.mit.edu/ist/pmm/. Accessed on September 15, 2006. 1 Global Knowledge. An introduction to PMI's project management life cycle. White Paper; ©2006 Global Knowledge LLC. http://www.globalknowledge.com/training/olm/go.asp?find=WP_PMLifeCycle&country=United+States. Accessed November 22, 2006.

8. Global Knowledge White Paper, "An Introduction to PMI's Project Management Life Cycle"

9. *PMP Study Guide*, 2nd ed. By William Heldman, Lona Cram. ©2004 Sybex. Alameda, California.

CHAPTER 13

Quality and Health Information Technology: Key Issues for Healthcare Executives

Rachel Block

The healthcare system in the United States—and the healthcare executives who are leading it—both face mounting pressures to reduce costs or cost growth, while maintaining and expanding coverage and quality health services to all Americans. These challenges are not new, but the magnitude has grown. Today, improving healthcare quality and safety is viewed as one of the key strategies to address these entrenched problems because they have the best potential to promote greater efficiency and effectiveness of care. This may stave off harsher measures. The adoption and use of health information technology (HIT), both administrative and clinical systems, is now widely viewed as an intrinsic part of the prescription for improving the healthcare system. This chapter provides a brief historical overview of the evolving policy and operational framework for healthcare quality in the U.S.; identifies the key issues relating to quality oversight and improvement including the implications for health information technology; and describes some of the key policy and implementation challenges that lie ahead as quality measurement, reporting and improvement become increasingly tied to HIT advances.

THE CONCEPTUAL FRAMEWORK AND VISION FOR HEALTHCARE QUALITY—WHY IS HEALTH INFORMATION TECHNOLOGY SO IMPORTANT?

Today's conceptual framework for healthcare quality is comprehensive in scope, including the structure, process and outcomes of healthcare delivery.[1] When this framework was articulated more than forty years ago, there was little consensus that quality could be measured, let alone improved through systematic efforts. But, there was a small and growing body of evidence suggesting the relationships among these elements. In recent years, the definition of quality has also evolved, establishing a close relationship between *how* healthcare services are delivered and *whether* those services will achieve desired health outcomes.[2]

Having determined that it is possible to measure and evaluate quality, the healthcare field in general has nevertheless been slow to adopt the necessary steps to ensure that high quality of care is consistently delivered. The Institute of Medicine's Roundtable on Healthcare Quality concluded in 1998 that "a national focus on improving the quality of healthcare is imperative...Problems in healthcare quality are serious and extensive (and) Americans bear a great burden of harm...A major effort (is required) to rethink and reengineer how we deliver healthcare services and how we assess and try to improve the quality of care."[3]

The sense of urgency conveyed through this report was based on several well-documented concerns regarding the quality of care that is generally available to Americans today. One way to catalog these problems is through the categories of underuse, overuse and misuse of healthcare services.[3] For example, recent research has documented that adults receive about 50% of recommended preventive and primary care[4] and these gaps in care affect all segments of the population.[5] In addition, Wennberg and colleagues have written extensively about the overuse of certain medical services and procedures which can be dangerous and inefficient[6] and there is continued concern about over-prescription of antibiotics for children and adults.[7] Medication errors are a common example of misuse that results in direct patient harm.[8]

These problems are both pervasive and complex and the solutions require coordinated strategic and tactical measures. Successfully addressing these problems at an organizational and societal level requires that healthcare executives adopt a systematic and comprehensive approach, including visible and sustained leadership support; a strategic vision for healthcare that focuses on providing the safest, highest quality and most reliable care; creating organizational and professional capacity and motivation to meet and exceed that standard; adopting and publicly disclosing measures of individual and systems performance; and supporting a policy environment (including payment systems) that promotes the most effective and efficient delivery of care. HIT is an integral part of this overall approach to quality, both in terms of structural standards of care (the HIT infrastructure) as well as its contribution to process and outcomes improvement (mobilizing the information necessary to continuously measure and improve healthcare quality). Medical informatics will play a crucial supporting role to affect this transition.

A SHORT HISTORY OF QUALITY IN U.S. HEALTHCARE AND THE EMERGING ROLE OF HIT

Initial Quality Measures Focused Mainly on the Structure of Healthcare Delivery

Early efforts to formalize the methodology for quality assessment focused primarily on institutional providers, and the structure of healthcare delivery in those settings. Through the separate and sometimes coordinated efforts of the Joint Commission on

Accreditation of Healthcare Organizations (JCAHO) and the Health Care Financing Administration (HCFA, now known as the Centers for Medicare & Medicaid Services or CMS), standards were established and accrediting processes implemented for the purpose of allowing hospitals to participate in the Medicare and Medicaid programs.

At the time, there was no overall strategy or corresponding infrastructure devoted to continuously assessing or improving healthcare quality in these settings. Reports of specific problems would be investigated and, if confirmed, sanctions might apply. Neither the public or private regulation bodies, nor the providers subject to their oversight, regularly or consistently collected or publicized performance information. Medicare's one early foray into this new field—publicly reporting hospitals' mortality data—was widely criticized and quickly withdrawn, and it would be a long time before the agency reinvigorated its efforts to make quality-related information publicly available.

Soon thereafter, the concept of continuous quality improvement began to take hold in the healthcare field. During the 1990s, standards for performance measurement and continuous quality improvement were incorporated by the JCAHO and HCFA. In addition, as managed care became a popular form of organizing healthcare financing and delivery, the National Committee for Quality Assurance (NCQA) was established for the purpose of developing standards and measures for these organizations. This process followed a similar if accelerated path—first addressing structural standards and later incorporating the measurement and improvement of health plan performance. Thus, almost thirty years later, Donabedian's original formulation for assessing healthcare quality across all three dimensions of structure, process and outcomes was finally embraced by the leading standards organizations.

Performance Measurement Becomes a Major Focus in Quality

The advent of managed care helped to rapidly advance the nation's interest in quality, albeit from a negative perspective. In response to increasing calls to limit health plans' practices which were viewed as restricting access to services, President Clinton established an Advisory Commission on consumer protection and quality. In addition to proposing a consumer bill of rights, the commission found that there were limited measures of quality in general, not just for managed care. Their report called for establishing a consensus process to develop more measures of quality, as well as coordination of public and private efforts to implement those measures. These tasks were put under the auspices of two new groups—a public-private partnership to develop the measures and a federal coordinating body to drive adoption through federal health programs.[9]

The first recommendation was implemented in 1999 with the formal incorporation of the National Quality Forum (NQF). With a governance structure and membership drawn from throughout the healthcare field, NQF established a systematic and open process for evaluating and approving performance standards and measures that would address all providers and services. The NQF strategic framework board developed a comprehensive roadmap for the development, selection and use of these quality standards and measures, including information systems concepts for quality measurement that needed to be part of a national measurement and reporting system.[10]

So health information technology enters into the policy debate at this time, but more attention is focused on reconciling disparate philosophical and technical approaches to quality measurement.

The Institute of Medicine Provides a Call to Arms and a Broader Vision for Quality

Another event in 1999 had an even more profound effect in advancing quality measurement and improvement efforts, while highlighting the potential benefits of health information technology. With the publication of *To Err is Human*, the Institute of Medicine (IOM) initiated a series of widely publicized reports suggesting that problems in the safety and quality of healthcare can be largely tied to the failure of systems. Operational processes could be designed to make healthcare safer, and healthcare organizations needed to develop internal systems designed to monitor and improve safety, including the use of health information technology.[11]

Two years later, the report *Crossing the Quality Chasm* expanded on these concepts, calling for fundamental reforms in healthcare systems as captured in the brief but powerful statement, "Trying harder will not work, changing systems of care will." The report reiterates the need for standardized measures (by this time, NQF has been established), as well as payment systems changes to reward improved healthcare outcomes. HIT assumes a more prominent role in these IOM recommendations; it determined that a national health information infrastructure (NHII) was needed to support healthcare system improvement by sharing information across the healthcare system.[12]

EMR and Interoperability of Health Information Move to the Forefront

The NHII envisioned that standards-based health information exchange (HEI) provided a bridge across the quality chasm, but the field of electronic health information was still new and few data standards existed. In response, the federal Department of Health and Human Services (HHS) focused on the further development of standards to improve the quality and efficiency of data exchange across health information systems. The consolidated health informatics initiative brought together various federal health agencies to coordinate their activities and adopt common standards across federal health programs.[13] The National Committee for Vital and Health Statistics (NCVHS) provided a forum for continued discussion of data standards.[14] The IOM issued a follow-up report with recommended specifications for electronic medical records (EMR) systems.[15]

In 2004, President Bush issued an Executive Order that calls for every American to have access to electronic health records within a decade.[16] HHS created the Office of the National Coordinator for Health Information Technology in order to further advance adoption and use of electronic medical records. Shortly thereafter, HHS published its strategic framework to create the National Health Information Network (NHIN), based on the reinforcing strategies of promoting electronic medical records adoption and establishing regional health information organizations. This plan identified four broad categories of functional priorities to be addressed by health information systems interoperability, including improvements in clinical quality and population health.[17]

Quality Measurement and Reporting Are Now Central Elements of the Health Policy Agenda, But Many Issues Remain Unresolved

With the increased focus on healthcare quality, there has been a rapid expansion of quality measurement and reporting activities driven by regulatory and purchasing forces seeking greater "transparency" in healthcare. On the regulatory front, the CMS has identified priority areas, promulgated measurement specifications, and published this data in print and electronic forms. Measure sets and public reports are now available for hospitals, nursing homes, home health agencies and end stage renal disease networks.[18] In the near future, CMS will initiate voluntary data submission and eventually publish information about physician performance. On an annual basis, the federal Agency for Healthcare Research and Quality (AHRQ) publishes two national reports—one on quality measures and one on healthcare disparities—data that is drawn from a variety of sources.[19] Many private organizations collect and publish healthcare performance information as well.[20,21]

In a very short time, these efforts have achieved an important goal by providing information on a variety of quality indicators. However, the proliferation of these measurement and reporting activities also suggests a continued lack of consensus on some basic issues, including what and how to measure healthcare quality. In Crossing the Quality Chasm, IOM called for the development of a coherent set of priorities for healthcare improvement, and a corresponding set of standardized, evidence-based measures, combined with the coordination of implementation efforts (including payment systems changes) across the public and private sectors. Part of this agenda has been fulfilled: IOM developed several focus areas for healthcare improvement, and the NQF has established a process to obtain consensus on measures which to some extent are guided by those priorities.

Other parts of this agenda have proven more complex: many of the priorities identified by IOM do not yet have well-defined measures and the process of developing measures remains fragmented and uncoordinated. Similarly, there is no coordinating mechanism to ensure that measures are used consistently. The limited research completed to date suggests that public reporting has limited effect on consumer choice and more of an effect on providers, but the measures and reporting currently in use are overwhelmingly geared to consumers. Finally, there is no system in place to rationally allocate the costs of data collection, analysis and reporting. In a recent report, IOM called for renewed efforts to effect a "concerted national effort to consolidate performance measurement and reporting activities" including the creation of a National Quality Coordination Board to create such a national system.[22]

Process Improvement and Systems Redesign Have Also Become Important Parts of the Overall Quality Agenda

The concept of continuous quality improvement is not new, but its large scale application to healthcare is a recent phenomenon. Almost twenty years ago, Don Berwick proposed a new paradigm for examining healthcare quality by applying the science of industrial engineering process improvement. The pioneers of this engineering approach had demonstrated that "problems, and therefore opportunities to improve quality, had usually been built directly into the complex production processes…and even when people are at the root of the defects, the problem was generally one of poor job design, failure of leadership or unclear purpose…Real improvement in quality depends on understanding and revising the production processes on the basis of data about the processes themselves."[23] In this first article, Berwick outlines a series of steps that need to be taken at all levels of healthcare to embrace this scientific method of process improvement. Capturing, analyzing and acting on real-time information about process and outcomes are essential steps in this approach.

More recently, Berwick summarized the central law of improvement as "every system is perfectly designed to achieve the results it achieves." Improved performance is a matter of design, building the capacity of a team or organization in ways that cannot be achieved through greater effort alone. Measurement becomes a method for learning and a way to determine which systems changes are most effective and which should be discarded. By implementing the "plan-do-study-act" improvement model, testing of systems change becomes a regular activity; one which requires sustained leadership support. For healthcare managers, a key take-away point is "effective leaders challenge the status quo both by insisting that the current system cannot remain and by offering clear ideas about superior alternatives."[24]

The IOM also picked up on these themes in its report on patient safety, citing specific examples of how process improvement and information tools have enhanced airline safety practices and outcomes and their potential application to improve the safety of healthcare. They concluded that "better management of health information is a prerequisite to achieving patient safety as a standard of care…promoting systems that prevent errors from occurring in the first place and at the same time incorporating lessons learned from any errors that do occur."[25] In this regard, the IOM calls for all healthcare settings to adopt comprehensive patient safety programs that encompass: (1) case finding—identifying system failures; (2) analysis—understanding the factors that contribute to system failures; and, (3) systems redesign –making improvements in care processes to prevent errors in the future.[25]

In fact, a multitude of quality improvement strategies, methodologies and tools have been advanced in recent years, including but not limited to Six Sigma, Failure Mode and Effect Analysis, the Toyota Production System, and Root Cause Analysis, to name a few. There is some cause for concern as "competing terms, acronyms, symbols and techniques suggest a Tower of Babel—health leaders speaking different languages and using tools that do not resemble each other."[26] In this commissioned paper, the authors compare three of the leading QI approaches, and the differences and similarities become even more apparent. For example, CQI (as defined by Berwick and others) focuses on continuously improving quality with a distinct customer or patient-centered focus, while the Toyota model focuses on lean production methods that reduce costs by empowering front-line workers and eliminating waste (including errors). Finally, the goal for Six Sigma is to achieve near zero defects. While the authors conclude that each method has merits, "none will succeed in the absence of deep and sustained leadership commitment."[26] In addition, the analysis required to implement these models requires data collection and performance measurement based on a standardized taxonomy for different types of errors.

IOM takes the connection between engineering and healthcare systems even further in one of its most recent reports, pointing out that "relatively little technical talent or material resources have been devoted to improving or optimizing the operations or measuring the quality and overall productivity of the overall U.S. Healthcare System."[27] In collaboration with the National Academy of Engineering, this study calls for a formalized partnership between engineers and healthcare professionals in order to transform U.S. healthcare "from an underperforming conglomerate of independent entities...into a high-performance 'system' in which every participating unit recognizes its dependence and influence on every other unit."[27]   The report goes on to describe "opportunities and challenges for harnessing the power of systems-engineering tools, information technologies and complementary knowledge" in other science disciplines in order to achieve the IOM's quality aims.

HIT PLAYS AN IMPORTANT ROLE IN QUALITY MEASUREMENT, REPORTING AND SYSTEMS IMPROVEMENT STRATEGIES

It is clear that HIT can play an important role in meeting the challenges associated with quality measurement, reporting and improvement activities. HIT can help to reduce data collection burden and enhance the clinical content of information used for quality measurement and reporting. Current quality measurement specifications rely on a combination of claims data and clinical data based on chart review. Claims data provides a ready source of demographic and utilization data, but it has important limitations—data about services covered by other plans, or during periods when there is no insurance coverage, will not be captured in any one place. In addition, claims data does not provide some of the detailed clinical information which is important to measure and improve quality; for example, claims data would record that a lab test was conducted, but it generally will not include the values or results for the test.

Since claims data provides only some of the information needed for quality measurement and reporting, chart review is also used as a primary or supplemental data source. Chart review has several advantages—charts usually capture more clinical detail and the information is recorded regardless of whether and how the service will be paid. Because most medical records are still in paper form, there are also some drawbacks to this approach. The review of paper records to collect and report on quality measures is resource-intensive, and subject to many inconsistencies in how information is manually recorded or interpreted by the reviewer. Chart review focuses on a representative random sample of patients, providing a snapshot of the care delivered by that provider. The validity of resulting measures is highly dependent on the accuracy of the sampling methods used. This methodology produces retrospective, aggregate measures, as compared to person-level, real-time information that could immediately improve professional and personal care decisions. Finally, since separate charts are maintained in various healthcare settings, it is difficult to link data based on an episode of illness that involves more than one provider or healthcare system.

Information resources are essential to make process and systems improvement changes to improve quality. HIT can enhance and accelerate process improvements designed to reduce errors and improve outcomes in healthcare by supplying real-time, person-level data as well as supporting the use of analytic tools that can readily detect trends and performance benchmarks against specified goals. For example, health information systems are a key element in the chronic care improvement model developed by Wagner and colleagues at Group Health Cooperative of Puget Sound.[28]

Timely, standardized and accurate health information would also help providers meet new regulatory requirements relating to continuity of care and medication reconciliation. For example, access to prescription history as well as laboratory and imaging test results would help to ensure quality during admission, treatment and follow-up for common acute care conditions. The JCAHO has now established an HIT advisory panel to focus on how HIT can facilitate clinical and operational process improvement.[29] Medicare's quality improvement organizations are convening hospital workgroups focusing on HIT implementation (including bar coding, Computerized Practitioner Order Entry or CPOE, and telehealth applications), and assisting physician office practices to implement electronic medical records in conjunction with standardized quality measures.[30]

STRATEGIES TO ACCELERATE QUALITY IMPROVEMENT AND HIT ADOPTION

Since widespread adoption of quality improvement methods as well as health information technology has not been achieved, there is a growing sense of urgency to find effective strategies to spur these developments. If healthcare providers are not sufficiently motivated to adopt these measures based on improved health and safety objectives—and current payment policies may actually discourage their use—then financial incentives may be needed to stimulate and accelerate large-scale improvements in quality, safety and efficiency. HIT has been directly and indirectly incorporated among the criteria for many of these programs.

The concept of payment systems reform for quality improvement was included in the IOM's *Crossing the Quality Chasm* report, and there has been growing support for these initiatives in the public and private sectors. The Medicare Payment Assessment Commission (MedPac) which advises Congress on Medicare policy changes supports large-scale adoption of pay for performance.[31] CMS has initiated several demonstration programs—one involving hospitals, and others involving physicians and integrated care delivery organizations.[32] Leadership in the U.S. Senate reached agreement in 2005 on pay for performance legislation for Medicare,[33] but further legislative action is unlikely in the near future.

Private sector efforts to adopt pay for performance continue to expand. Bridges to Excellence was developed by several large employer groups as a means to recognize and reward physician practices for their care management practices—including the use of health information technology—as well as improved performance on selected measures.[34] The Integrated Healthcare Association in California was created to stimulate collaboration among providers and payors. In 2001, it launched its pay for performance initiative including the use of standardized measures and public reporting of performance information. HIT use was included in the initial criteria, with greater weight given to performance measures in later years.[35] The Leapfrog Group advocates for improved quality and safety in healthcare through the use of public reporting and payment incentives. Their hospital rewards program utilizes NQF standards for safe healthcare practices as well as implementation of computerized prescription order entry; several large employers and payors around the country are using this pay for performance program.[36]

At the provider level, HIT tools have proven to be effective in improving the management of chronic disease, which is a priority for public and private purchasers alike. The National Survey of Physician Organizations and the Management of Chronic Illness was developed in order to assess physicians' use of organized care management processes—including the use of health information technology and external incentives— for purposes of improving quality. Physician use of care management processes was generally low, but the study found that HIT and external incentives both increased physicians' use of these processes.[37] Another study considers the research evidence associated with various elements of the chronic care model including the use of clinical information systems interventions such as disease registries. While several components of the model have improved chronic care outcomes and reduced costs, the authors emphasize the need for payment systems changes that will strengthen the business case for providers to invest in HIT and other practice changes.[38]

Some of the new regional health information organizations are promoting the use of interoperable health information exchange in order to facilitate quality improvement and support pay for performance activities. A recent national survey identified more than one hundred of these regional organizations of which more than three-quarters of these indicated that they were implementing health information exchange in order to address "provider inefficiencies due to lack of data to support patient care."[39] Among the more advanced initiatives, almost one-third indicated they had established functions to support chronic care and disease management, and quality performance reporting has been established in more than one-quarter of these projects. An examination of the sources of funding for these projects, however, indicates limited payor or health plan involvement (just above 10%), while government grants constitute close to half of their funding.

Payors and health plans could become more engaged if these regional health information initiatives had a roadmap for how quality measures, HIT investment and incentive payments would translate into enhanced value for their healthcare expenditures. The eHealth Initiative convened national and local leaders representing provider, health plan and payor interests. They developed a set of common principles for incentives that would balance the costs and benefits of HIT investments, transition from paper to electronic sources of data for purposes of performance measurement, and reward the use of HIT that is interoperable and meets national standards as they are developed.[40]

Payment incentives could also support the use of specific HIT tools and strategies that have demonstrated effectiveness in improving healthcare quality, safety and efficiency. Could an HIT financing strategy be built on the current evidence? A recent national evidence review commissioned by the federal Agency for Health Care Research and Quality found that while there are a number of good studies and evaluations about the impact of HIT, they tend to focus on a small number of institutions and the results may not be broadly applicable across more diverse settings. In addition, the report notes that the studies provide little insight into organizational variables that may influence

HIT adoption and use. Nevertheless, the report finds that HIT has proven benefits in improved quality and safety by reducing prescription errors and increasing preventive services and adherence to clinical guidelines. While there are numerous barriers to HIT implementation cited in these studies, the authors conclude that "a major structural and ideological reorganization of clinical medicine" will be necessary if the full benefit of HIT is to be achieved.[41] Thus, payment systems changes intended to support the adoption and use of HIT need to be placed in the context of a larger strategy for healthcare systems reform.

Financing is Not the Only Barrier to HIT Adoption

Healthcare financing policies need to be updated to incorporate the investment in and use of HIT to improve quality, safety and efficiency, but financing is not the only barrier. The field of medical informatics needs to assist with implementation efforts at the individual and organizational levels, and support efforts to use HIT for purposes of quality and safety improvement. Little attention has been focused on the needs of the healthcare workforce in terms of changes in the work environment and the acquisition of new skills and competencies. Implementing quality and HIT on a larger, systemic scale requires a thorough analysis of how clinical and administrative functions are currently performed and by whom in order to develop a change strategy that integrates, rather than alienates, the healthcare workforce. Involving users in the selection and implementation of new HIT systems and applications is critical to their success. Both the smallest and largest organizations need to plan these activities carefully and adapt their strategies to their unique settings. Clinical and administrative staffs also need to be educated about privacy and security protections as well as the coding and display of electronic health information.[42] Finally, it is imperative that more professionals receive medical informatics training, as well as quality improvement techniques, in order to meet the needs of workers and organizations alike during this crucial transition to an electronic health information environment focused on systemic improvements in quality, safety and efficiency.

Major Policy Choices for HIT and Quality Remain Unresolved

There is a growing consensus that improving quality and safety is inextricably linked to the widespread adoption and use of HIT as part of a larger strategy to systematically transform the healthcare system. The trend is clear, and healthcare leaders should be focused on how, not whether, to adopt these tools and practices. But these major policy developments are still very much work in progress, and the pace and direction for future changes will be affected by whether and how these larger social and political choices are made.

- Voluntary, market-based approaches to these issues dominate today's health policy agenda. Under this paradigm, competitive forces will spur adoption and innovation with regard to quality improvement and HIT implementation. However, this will also create an uneven patchwork of solutions which may offer little consistency in public protections, uncertain return on investment, and inequitable distribution of costs and benefits. Government does not yet have clearly defined roles either promoting or enforcing greater consistency in quality and HIT efforts.

- In theory, the focus for quality improvement and HIT implementation should be on the patient or consumer. With efforts such as the Institute for Healthcare Improvement's 100k Lives Campaign, healthcare professionals and organizations are squarely facing the human consequences of healthcare systems failures. However, this focus is much less apparent in the large number of regional HIT initiatives which are forming around the country. Growing concerns about privacy and security of health information systems need to be addressed soon, or the public may thwart rather than support these efforts.
- Pay for performance can provide a link between quality improvement and financing. It is also largely untested, and there is much variation across the models that currently exist. Much work lies ahead to evaluate these models and reach consensus on the many policy and technical issues associated with these payment reforms.

REFERENCES

1. Donabedian A. Evaluating the quality of medical care. *Milbank Memorial Fund Quarterly*. 1966;44(3)66–203.

2. Lohr K, ed. *Medicare: A Strategy for Quality Assurance*. Washington DC: National Academy Press, 1990.

3. Chassin, MR, Galvin RW and the National Roundtable on Health Care Quality. The urgent need to improve health care quality. *JAMA*. September 16, 1998;280(11):1000–1005.

4. McGlynn EA, Asch SM, Adams J, et al. The quality of health care delivered to adults in the United States. *NEJM*. 2003;348:2635–2645.

5. Asch SM, Kerr EA, Keesey J, et al. Who is at greatest risk for receiving poor-quality health care? *NEJM*. 2006;354:1147–1156.

6. Wennberg, JE. Practice variations and health care reform: connecting the dots. *Health Affairs Web Exclusive*. October 7, 2004.

7. Gonzales R, Steiner JF, Sande MA. Antibiotic prescribing for adults with colds, upper respiratory tract infections and bronchitis by ambulatory care physicians. *JAMA*. 1997;278:901–904; Nyquist A-C, Gonzales R, Steiner JF, et al. Antibiotic prescribing for children with colds, upper respiratory tract infections and bronchitis: *JAMA*. 1998;279:875–877.

8. Bates DW, Cullen DJ, Laird N, et al. incidence of adverse drug events and potential adverse drug events: *JAMA*. 1995;274:29–34.

9. Advisory Commission on Health Consumer Protection and Quality in the Health Care Industry. *Quality First: Better Health Care for All Americans*. Washington DC: Government Printing Office; 1998.

10. James, B. Information systems concepts for quality measurement. *Medical Care*. 2003;41(suppl): I71–I79.

11. Institute of Medicine. *To Err is Human: Building a Safer Health Care System.*Wahington, DC: National Academy Press; 2000.

12. Institute of Medicine. *Crossing the Quality Chasm: A New Health Care System for the 21st Century*. Washington, DC: National Academy Press; 2001.

13. U.S. Department of Health and Human Services. *Consolidated Health Informatics Fact Sheet*. Available at: http://www.hhs.gov/healthit/chiinitiative.html. Accessed on April 25, 2006.

14. US Department of Health and Human Services. *National Committee on Vital and Health Statistics, Charter*. Available at http://www.ncvhs.hhs.gov/charter07.pdf. Accessed on April 25, 2006.

15. Institute of Medicine. *Key Capabilities of an Electronic Health Record System*. Washington, DC: National Academy Press; 2003.

16. Office of the President of the United States. *Incentives for the Use of Health Information Technology and Establishing the Position of National Health Information Technology Coordinator.* Presidential Executive Order. April 27, 2004. Available at: http://www.whitehouse.gov/news/releases/2004/04/20040427–4.html. Accessed on April 25, 2006.

17. US Department of Health and Human Services. *The Decade of Health Information Technology; Delivering Consumer-Centric and Information-Rich Health Care.* Available at: http://www.hhs.gov/healthit/documents/hitframework.pdf. Accessed on April 25, 2006.

18. Centers for Medicare & Medicaid Services. Examples of comparative quality performance information for home health agencies are available at: www.medicare.gov/hhcompare and hospitals are available at: http://www.hospitalcompare.hhs.gov/. Accessed on April 25, 2006.

19. Agency for Health Care Research and Quality. *2005 National Healthcare Quality Report and 2005 National Healthcare Disparities Report.* Available at: http://www.ahrq.gov/qual/. Accessed on April 26, 2006.

20. National Committee on Quality Assurance. *The State of Health Care Quality 2005.* Available at: www.ncqa.org. Accessed on April 26, 2006.

21. Health Grades. *Fourth Annual HealthGrades Hospital Quality and Clinical Excellence Study, February 2006.* Available at: www.healthgrades.com. Accessed on April 26, 2006.

22. Institute of Medicine. *Performance Measurement: Accelerating Improvement.* Washington, DC: National Academy Press; 2006.

23. Berwick D. Continuous improvement as an ideal in health care. *NEJM.* 1989;320:53–56.

24. Berwick D. A primer on leading the improvement of systems. *BMJ.* 1996;312:619–622.

25. Institute of Medicine. *Patient Safety: Achieving a New Standard of Care.* Washington, DC: National Academy Press; 2004.

26. McDonough JE, Solomon R, and Petosa L. *Quality Improvement and Proactive Hazard Analysis Models: Deciphering a New Tower of Babel.* Commissioned Paper for Institute of Medicine, Patient Safety. Washington, DC: 2004.

27. National Academy of Engineering and Institute of Medicine. *Building a Better Delivery System: A New Engineering/Health Care Partnership.* Washington, DC: National Academy Press; 2005.

28. Wagner E. Chronic disease management: what will it take to improve care for chronic illness? *Effective Clinical Practice.* 1998;1:2–4.

29. Joint Commission Establishes Healthcare Information Technology Advisory Panel . Press release, September 2005. http://www.medallies.com/downloads/JCAHOHIT.PDF.

30. Centers for Medicare & Medicaid Services. *Quality Improvement Organizations 8th Scope of Work.* Available at: http://www.cms.hhs.gov/QualityImprovementOrgs/downloads/8thSOW.pdf. Accessed on April 26, 2006.

31. Medicare Payment Advisory Commission. *Report to Congress: Medicare Payment Policy, March 2005.* available at http://www.medpac.gov/publications/congressional_reports/Mar05_TOC.pdf. Accessed on April 26, 2006.

32. Centers for Medicare & Medicaid Services. *Premier Hospital Quality Incentive Demonstration Program.* Fact sheet available at: http://www.cms.hhs.gov/HospitalQualityInits/downloads/HospitalPremierFS200602.pdf; *Medicare Health Care Quality Demonstration Program.* Fact sheet available at: http://www.cms.hhs.gov/DemoProjectsEvalRpts/downloads/MMA646_FactSheet.pdf. Accessed on April 26, 2006.

33. United States Senate. *S. 1356, the Medicare Value Purchasing Act of 2005.* Sponsored by Senator Charles Grassley (R-IA) and Max Baucus (D-MT). Available at http://thomas.loc.gov. Accessed on April 26, 2006.

34. Bridges to Excellence information available at: http://www.bridgestoexcellence.org/bte/. Accessed on April 26, 2006.

35. Integrated Healthcare Association. *Advancing Quality through Collaboration: The California Pay for Performance Program, February 2006.* Available at: http://www.iha.org/wp020606.pdf. Accessed on April 26, 2006.

36. Leapfrog Group information available at www.leapfroggroup.org. Accessed on April 26, 2006.

37. Casalino L, Gilles R, Shortell S, et al. External incentives, information technology, and organized processes to improve health care quality for patients with chronic diseases. *JAMA.* 2003;289:434–441.

38. Bodenheimer T, Wagner E, Grumbach K. Improving primary care for patients with chronic illness: the chronic care model, part 2. *JAMA.* 2002;288:1909–1914.

39. eHealth Initiative. *Emerging Trends and Issues in Health Information Exchange, 2005.* Available at: http://ccbh.ehealthinitiative.org/communities/register_download.mspx (registration is required, report is free). Accessed on April 26, 2006.

40. eHealth Initiative. *Parallel Pathways for Quality Health Care, 2005.* Available at: www.ehealthinitiative.org. Accessed on April 26, 2006.

41. Shekelle PG, Morton SC, Keeler EB. *Costs and Benefits of Health Information Technology;Evidence report/technology assessment no. 132.* Prepared by the Southern California Evidence-based Practice Center under Contract No. 290-02-0003. AHRQ Publication No.06-E006. Rockville, MD: Agency for Healthcare Research and Quality; April 2006.

42. Hersh W. Medical informatics: improving health care through information. *JAMA.* 2002;288: 1955–1958.

CHAPTER 14

Electronic Health Records: The Use of Technology to Eliminate Racial Disparities in Health Outcomes

Neil S. Calman, MD
Maxine Golub, MPH
Kwame Kitson, MD
Charmaine Ruddock, MS

Racial and ethnic disparities in health outcomes are one of the leading causes of death in this country, producing excess mortality among minority Americans in numbers that rival some of our most serious medical conditions.[1] Inequities in the quality of care received by racial and ethnic minorities have been widely documented,[1,2] leading to calls for intensified efforts to redress systematic inequalities in the healthcare system.

The Institute for Urban Family Health has had a unique opportunity to study the root causes of health disparities in the Bronx over the past four years through a community-based participatory research project known as Bronx Health REACH. During this same time, the Institute has installed the Epic system—a completely integrated electronic health record (EHR) and practice management system developed by the Epic Systems Corporation—at its family practice centers serving the Bronx community. The simultaneous initiation of these two projects has provided us with an opportunity to structure the implementation of this state-of-the-art system to address fundamental issues we identified in our work on health disparities.

In this chapter, we discuss the implementation of Epic in our network of thirteen practices: seven federally funded community health centers and six health centers that the Institute operates for our affiliated hospital system, Continuum Health. In total, this network comprises approximately 70,000 patients and produces over 180,000 primary care visits annually at four Bronx and nine Manhattan locations. We assess provider use of various features of the EHR and their views on the impact of the EHR on patient care. Findings of a recent provider survey are presented.

LESSONS FROM BRONX HEALTH REACH

Bronx Health REACH is a coalition of forty community and faith-based organizations dedicated to eliminating health disparities in the Bronx. Funded by the U.S. Centers for Disease Control, the New York State Department of Health and private funders, Bronx Health REACH has engaged in a varied portfolio of activities.[4] Early on, REACH leaders held ten focus groups to learn what community members perceived as the ways that these disparities arise from our healthcare system.[5] From these focus groups, a number of themes were identified that have informed our work over the past five years. These themes are:

- Widespread distrust and fear of the healthcare system
- Feeling undervalued and disrespected
- Difficulty communicating with doctors
- Concern about the competence of community physicians
- The importance of self-advocacy and the difficulties in practicing it
- The impact of stress and its relationship to poor health
- Obstacles to modifying lifestyles to be more health-conscious, due to the absence of health information and other factors

Mistrust

Of all these issues, the one that stood out above all others, in both the frequency that it was mentioned and in the intensity of emotion that it was presented, was the issue of mistrust that exists between patients and providers in low-income communities of color. Many describe this as "the Tuskegee Legacy," a reference to the infamous abuse of a group of African-American men over decades as medical researchers watched them deteriorate from the effects of syphilis in order to study the natural history of the disease, long after there was a known cure.[6]

Disrespect

Focus group participants frequently discussed the disrespect they felt from health providers as a major issue in their encounters with the healthcare system. People reported being treated like "ants in a line," and being told to "take a number." Examples included the failure of providers to treat them as intelligent participants in decision making about their own healthcare, and failure to share the results of labs, diagnostic tests, and specialty consultations as the providers assumed a paternalistic and authoritative role in their communications with them.

Segregation of services based on the type of health insurance one carries, or whether or not one has a "private" physician to serve as their advocate, has convinced people in our communities that they are indeed second-class citizens of the American healthcare system. The disparities that exist in private and public health insurance coverage by race serve to reinforce the community's experience that they are being treated differently because of the color of their skin.

Communication Barriers

The lack of trust articulated by focus group participants is intensified by poor communication between patients and physicians. Many participants felt that their doctors rushed through visits and made little effort to communicate. Some expressed difficulty understanding the information they received. By contrast, those who trusted their physicians expressed a sense of being listened to and having information carefully explained. The mismatch of the racial and ethnic background of the patients in communities of color and the healthcare providers who serve them also creates barriers to maximally effective, culturally sensitive communication in most cases. It also impedes linguistically competent communication in many other medical encounters.[7]

Competence

Participants in our focus groups were frequently concerned about the competence of their providers, and shared the many ways that they judged the competence of those who cared for them. Some related how they compare what their provider did for them to what their friends had experienced in similar situations, what they knew from their own reading or from mass media public health education. A few community residents reported "testing" their doctors by withholding important health information to see if the provider would ask about such problems or find them during their examination. Others spoke of leaving providers who, for example, did not refer them for an annual eye exam if they were diabetic or did not mention that they needed a mammogram even though they hadn't had one in two years.

Need for Self-Advocacy

Many of the focus group participants felt that self-advocacy is important in interactions with the healthcare system and routinely act on that belief. Others were not comfortable advocating for themselves. They expressed feeling awkward and unclear about self-advocacy, and accepted the inadequacies of the system. "You've got to have money. That's the bottom line. You got to brace yourself to that," was one man's comment.

Overall, the issues related by focus group members—almost all of who were African-American or Latino—showed that they were deeply disenfranchised in their dealings with the healthcare system. This often led to misunderstanding and/or mistrust of their provider's recommendations or the provider's rationale for a particular course of treatment. As a result, the concept of "non-adherence to provider recommendations" must be viewed in a new light.

THE EHR BRINGS ESSENTIAL CAPABILITIES TO SUPPORT PATIENT CARE

How can an electronic medical record serve to bridge this chasm of distrust and poor communication between providers and their patients? Some providers initially fear computers in the exam room as a potential added barrier to good communication and view this as a necessary evil of automating the clinical encounter. That view would lead one to shy away from EHRs, especially as a tool to improve the doctor-patient relationship. At the Institute, we decided that we would use the EHR as a major tool to bridge trust and improve communication. At every step of our planning and implementation, the focus group findings were considered and decisions regarding system configurations were made accordingly.

Restructuring Workflows to Incorporate the EHR

In the process of automating the clinical record through the installation of an EHR, all manual workflows must be reexamined and many must be reworked. This provides an opportunity to examine inefficiencies in care and places where patient communication can be improved. One example is the way that providers had to restructure their review of the patient's office record at the start of each visit.

Many providers were trained to keep the patient's chart outside their exam room so they are able to review previous encounters before going in and speaking with a patient. This gives the patients the sense that they are remembered and makes them feel less anonymous. It also serves to keep the record from being reviewed by the patient when left alone in the exam room waiting for the provider. Workflows from this paper chart model had to be dramatically restructured to avoid creating a situation where providers enter the exam room and read through computer notes without involving the patient. One solution suggested by other EHR users was to install additional terminals outside the exam rooms where providers could access their patient's charts and review them before entering the room.

Instead, we chose to redesign the encounter to put the review of prior information in the context of the current day's encounter, and to use this as an opportunity to involve the patient in his or her own care. Now providers enter the exam room unprepared by prior review of the patient's record. Their review of the record and any activity since the previous encounter is done in collaboration with the patient. Looking at the computer screen together, the provider might say, "Let's look over the note I wrote on the last visit to make sure we have followed up on all your issues." Then, "Now let's go over all the reports that have come in since your last visit ... two consult reports and your blood test results." All of our providers indicate that they encourage their patients to look at the computer screens at least some of the time, and some do this during nearly every patient visit.

Rather than being insulted by this, patients are immediately drawn into reviewing their own records with their provider at their side, where a discussion of the results and necessary follow-up are facilitated. Copies are printed for the patient to keep at home with their medical records.

Flat Panel Monitors Aid Communication

The historical view that the provider owns and controls the patient's medical record is a fiction that must be undone if we hope to involve patients in taking more responsibility for their own healthcare. We made a decision early on in our Epic planning to bring patients directly into the process of the encounter. We worked to eliminate patients' sense that their health records were not theirs, but were "owned" by the providers and practices. We specifically rejected the option of portable wireless touchpad computers, as they have screens that are visible only to the provider and are often held cradled in the provider's arm, preserving the secrecy of the paper charts they replaced.

Flat panel monitors were installed on every desk, so that all information entered into the computer would be visible to the patient as it is entered. This was a major step in eliminating the secrecy of the paper chart that patients have experienced. Patients now often read over our shoulders as we document their care, and some even correct misinformation or the misinterpretation of their statements as they see the typed words appear on the screen. Even though not all patients choose to look at the monitors, the availability they offer creates a bridge of trust and improves the provider-patient relationship.

Printers in Every Exam Room Promote Patient Education and Involvement

Another example of the critical decisions that need to be made in the set-up of hardware is the location of printers. We decided to install printers in every examination room so that information could be produced for patients as part of the encounter process. This not only improves patient flow in the health center, but also makes the vast resources of the EHR instantly available to both the patient and the provider. It also insures the confidentiality of patient information, eliminating the possibility of a document being picked up off a central printer and inadvertently handed to the wrong patient.

At the start of the encounter, while reviewing lab results and returned consult reports, the providers can print copies for their patients on the spot. The workflow used by most providers next involves a review of the nurse's notes and the vital signs taken when preparing the patient to see the provider. Vital signs, as well as all lab values, can be trended, graphed and printed for patients. The most common use of this function is the printing of progress charts of weight or blood pressure, graphing patients' improvements or lack thereof. While most of our providers still use this function infrequently, there is much variability and some providers have clearly adopted this as a standard visit activity.

It is well known that patients frequently do not take all the medications they were prescribed.[8] The EHR permits providers to review the list of current medications the patient should be taking, the quantity prescribed and when the patient should require a refill. A summary of indications and doses can be printed as well. Prescriptions are printed in the exam room, as are requests for labs and specialty consultations. Our recent survey shows that virtually all prescriptions are now written through the EHR, and that providers review printed prescriptions with their patients during most or all of their visits. All of these documents become part of a package of health information that the patient can take with them and keep as part of their personal health records.

Table 14-1 shows the results of the survey of EHR use from the healthcare provider's perspective.

Table 14-1: Survey of EHR Use by Healthcare Providers.

Providers were asked to estimate the percentage of visits that they use each of the specified features of the EHR system.

	0-10%	11-20%	21-30%	31-40%	41-50%	51-60%	61-70%	71-80%	81-90%	91-100%
Percent of visits where you encourage your patients to look at the computer screen to view information	8% (5)	5% (3)	11% (7)	8% (5)	14% (9)	3% (2)	8% (5)	19 (12)	14% (9)	11% (7)
Percent of Office Visits where you receive one or more Best Practice Alerts	17% (11)	14% (9)	19% (12)	11% (7)	12% (8)	5% (3)	6% (4)	5% (3)	6% (4)	5% (3)
Percent of Office Visits where you ignore one or more Best Practice Alerts	42% (27)	9% (6)	3% (2)	6% (4)	8% (5)	6% (4)	3% (2)	5% (3)	3% (2)	14% (9)
Percent of Best Practice Alerts you ignore overall	42% (27)	9% (6)	3% (2)	0% (0)	11% (7)	5% (3)	3% (2)	6% (4)	8% (5)	12% (8)
Percent of Prescriptions you write through the EHR	0% (0)	0% (0)	0% (0)	0% (0)	0% (0)	0% (0)	0% (0)	2% (1)	6% (4)	92% (59)
Percent of visits where you review prescriptions with your patients after they are printed	2% (1)	0% (0)	0% (0)	2% (1)	6% (4)	3% (2)	2% (1)	17% (11)	22% (14)	46% (29)
Percent of visits where you print graphs (BP, weight, labs) for your patients to take with them	44% (28)	8% (5)	8% (5)	6% (4)	8% (5)	8% (5)	8% (5)	8% (5)	2% (1)	2% (1)
Percent of visits you print educational materials from the Reference section of the EHR	12% (8)	12% (8)	12% (8)	8% (5)	12% (8)	12% (8)	12% (8)	8% (5)	5% (3)	5% (3)
Percent of Office Visits you print the After-visit summary for the patient	70% (45)	14% (9)	5% (3)	5% (3)	0% (0)	0% (0)	2% (1)	3% (2)	2% (1)	0% (0)

(From Institute for Urban Family Health – EHR User Survey – October 2005, based on an 89% response rate.)

IMPROVING TRUST AND COMMUNICATION THROUGH THE EHR

A Complete and Instantly Retrievable Clinical Record

Nothing contributes to distrust as much as having a provider who forgets critical information about their patients. Our patients have relayed examples that include providers who did not document medications they previously had given the patient (resulting in difficulty refilling the patient's prescription) and providers who forgot that they had ordered tests and had not reviewed the results since the patient's last visit. Even when prior face-to-face encounters are recorded in a paper record, the paper record rarely documents the myriad other patient encounters—requests for refills and specialty referrals, telephone calls from patients and provider's attempts to call patients regarding abnormal test results. The EHR facilitates such documentation, as it is available for recording information in almost every location in every one of our facilities and is available to providers when they are away from our network though a Virtual Private Network (VPN.) Thus, when patients return to the center, a complete record of all their activity is readily available to the provider, instilling confidence in the patient that their information is complete. Over half of our providers feel that patients view them as having improved ability to find important information in their health records and that patients view staff competency as somewhat or much better than before the installation of the EHR.

Our providers have also indicated that communication with patients, both during visits and between visits, has improved. Of the providers responding to our recent survey, 34% think that their patients feel communication in the exam room is somewhat better or much better than before the EHR. One-third of providers responded that they think patients feel communication with their provider between visits is somewhat or much better and that they get better responses to messages that they leave (see Table 14-2).

How do YOU think YOUR PATIENTS feel about your EPIC-supported practice compared to their experiences before EPIC?

Table 14-2: Patient Response to EPIC.

	Much worse now than before	Somewhat worse now than before	About the same now as before	Somewhat better now than before	Much better now than before	Don't know
Their ability to get prescriptions refilled	0% (0)	0% (0)	16% (10)	19% (12)	41% (26)	24% (15)
Their ability to get health education information	0% (0)	2% (1)	11% (7)	32% (20)	35% (22)	21% (13)
The overall competency of the staff	0% (0)	3% (2)	24% (15)	30% (19)	21% (13)	22% (14)
Your ability to find important information in their record	0% (0)	0% (0)	6% (4)	29% (18)	58% (36)	6% (4)
Your communication with them in the exam room	3% (2)	11% (7)	17% (11)	27% (17)	17% (11)	24% (15)
Their access to their own clinical information	0% (0)	0% (0)	17% (11)	33% (21)	37% (23)	13% (8)
Your communication with them between visits	0% (0)	0% (0)	13% (8)	25% (16)	43% (27)	19% (12)
Their ability to get prescriptions refills	0% (0)	0% (0)	10% (6)	27% (17)	47% (29)	16% (10)
Their ability to speak with a nurse about a health concern	2% (1)	2% (1)	35% (22)	16% (10)	14% (9)	32% (20)
Your response to messages they leave	0% (0)	3% (2)	22% (14)	24% (15)	29% (18)	22% (14)
The confidentiality of their medical record	0% (0)	3% (2)	27% (17)	13% (8)	16% (10)	41% (26)

Improved Patient Education

Most EHRs have some library of patient education material readily accessible to the provider. Epic's library is purchased from McKesson Health Solutions of Broomfield, Colorado, is largely bilingual (English/Spanish) and contains thousands of health education documents and drug information sheets. Epic facilitates the use of these educational materials for the provider by picking up key diagnoses and pharmaceutical names from the problem list, encounter diagnoses and medication lists, and suggesting educational documents that are available for immediate retrieval. In addition, hundreds of anatomical drawings are available that can be annotated by the provider on the computer and then printed for the patient. This capability completely changes the flow of information from what it had been prior to automation. It enables providers to locate information with a few keystrokes; previously, either the provider or nurse had to retrieve and copy these materials, which were used less than they are today. Despite the variable usage of printed materials by providers, we view provider feedback for expanded and improved patient educational materials as a positive sign that providers are willing to use this feature and have ideas about the type of information they would like to provide to their patients.

Patients Leave the Center with a Full Report of Their Encounter and Follow-up Recommendations

Studies of patients leaving their doctor's office indicate that they rarely have a complete understanding of what was done and what they are supposed to do next.[9] To address this, the Institute designed an "After-Visit Summary" that contains patient-friendly headings and a printout of all issues discussed in the day's encounter. The summary includes patient identifying information; a list of their measured vital signs; the chief issues as told to the nurse; the provider note; a complete problem list; a summary of active medications; any new orders written for the patient, including consultations, imaging studies and lab tests; and immunizations or medications administered in the center. While initial use of this feature is limited, providers who do use it regularly in our practice report that their patients remind them to print the After-Visit Summary if they forget to do so at the end of an encounter.

Template Letters for Follow-Up

In our experience, nothing shows our patients that we care about them as much as a call or letter from their provider. The Epic system's ability to generate pre-formatted letters is an important tool in that regard. Letterhead is scanned into the system, and letters can be generated with just a few keystrokes. Patients are routinely sent letters with their tests results and specific requests for follow-up. Templates that automatically import values from the patient's most recent laboratory results and then explain the normal value range are generated in seconds, and have been particularly helpful in improving communication with patients. Patients' contact information—home, work and mobile phone numbers—can be retrieved with a single click from anywhere in the system so a quick call can be made and documented, relaying newly received information to the patient. This type of follow-up, though time-consuming, truly makes for a patient-provider partnership that demonstrates the kind of respect and caring that patients deserve.

Quality of Care is Greatly Enhanced

EHRs and the decision-support systems that can be built into them can not only enhance the patient's sense of the providers' competence, but can actually increase that competence by running through scores of electronic checks that the human mind is incapable of doing with the same consistency and precision. One year ago, we implemented a reminder that would alert providers to recommend a pneumococcal vaccine to patients over sixty-five years of age and patients of any age with chronic pulmonary disease. This vaccine is designed to prevent pneumococcal pneumonia, a threat to the elderly and those with chronic pulmonary diseases and is recommended by the U.S. Preventive Services Task Force, indicating excellent evidence of its utility.

The results of implementing this clinical decision support can be seen in Figure 14-1. In the nine months prior to turning on this alert, our twelve facilities averaged administration of sixteen vaccines per month. A clinical decision support, or "Best Practice Alert" (BPA), was designed to remind providers at the time of a patient encounter that their patient's age or medical history warranted a vaccination and that the system could not find evidence that a pneumococcal vaccine had been ordered. In some cases, patients had been vaccinated prior to the implementation of the EHR, but to our surprise, in most cases they had not. In the first month after the BPA implementation, the number of vaccine doses given rose precipitously to 299—an eighteen-fold increase. Subsequent months saw rates that gradually declined as the population of patients for whom the vaccine is recommended quickly became immunized.

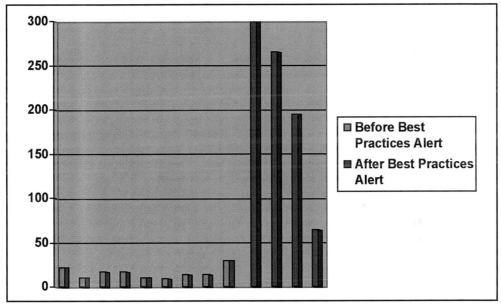

Figure 14-1: Doses of Pneumococcal Vaccine Given per Month Before and After the Introduction of Specific Best Practice Alerts.

Another BPA programmed the same month was designed to remind providers that their diabetic patients had not had an order for an ophthalmology consult in the prior twelve months or more. The results of this BPA can be found in Figure 14-2. The baseline rate for this activity was an average of 104 consultation referrals per month for the nine months prior to programming the BPA. After the BPA was implemented, the rate went to an average of 161 consults per month, a 55% increase.

How are these quality improvements related to the elimination of health disparities? The obvious answer is that improvement in the quality of our preventive care leads to improved health outcomes for our patients. But there is another effect as well.

Our REACH focus groups taught us that, in part, patients judge their providers by their adherence to what the patients understand about necessary or recommended guidelines for their care. As more is learned by people in the community about recommended standards of care, patients will increasingly measure the competence of their providers by their adherence to these standards.

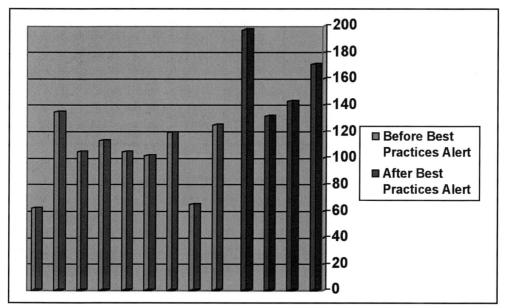

Figure 14-2: Consults to Ophthalmology for Diabetic Patients per Month
Before and After the Introduction of Specific Best Practice Alerts.

In one particularly poignant clip in a video called *Voices of Health Equality*[10] that was made by members of Bronx Health REACH, a community resident relates how she felt when a specialist she was seeing expressed surprise that she had never had an electrocardiogram even though she suffered from severe hypertension. She told the interviewer that she had been cared for by her primary care physician for years without ever having had this test offered to her. Her trust in this physician had been injured beyond repair, and she was now in search of a new source of medical care. Decision supports that remind providers of such critical errors of omission improve the quality of care and the trust the patient has in their provider.

Supporting Patient Self-Management

Physicians have no ability to change the health-related behaviors of their patients without their cooperation, and oftentimes their patients' families as well. Whether the behavior is smoking, seat belt use, overeating, lack of exercise, substance abuse or high-risk sexual behavior—without the full buy-in of the patient, there is little hope that behavior will change.

Office-based health education is a proven benefit in stimulating behavior change.[11] Yet in one study of smokers, only one-third of the patients interviewed reported ever being told to stop smoking by their regular physician.[12] In many other cases, the reimbursement system for primary care does not recognize the extraordinary time and dedication it takes to educate patients as to the dangers of their unhealthy behavior, give them the tools to change and monitor their adherence to the provider's recommendations.

In our community focus groups, patients often spoke of the brief time that providers spent with them—often commanding behavior change with a single sentence without any explanation of why or how things needed to change, let alone how to make the change itself. Patients felt rushed and uninvolved in their own care, and generally unable to fulfill their providers' request.

Our implementation of the EHR brings patients to the forefront of their own care by providing access to health education materials in English and Spanish in the exam room for review by patient and provider together in the course of each healthcare visit. Patients who understand the importance of behavioral changes are far more likely to make the necessary effort, and providers who feel that their patients are responding to their recommendations are far more likely to continue their efforts to help.

CONCLUSION

Electronic health records have great potential for improving communication between providers and their patients. There is also great potential to expand the impact of EHRs beyond the walls of the practices where they are implemented through linkages with public health agencies that provide new information to improve the health of the public.

The selection of software that is robust enough to be configured into workflows that enhance care in the manner described above is critical. Equally important are the decisions about how computers and printers are used in interactions with patients. With careful attention to these issues, EHRs can be used to effectively enhance communication.

People of color, as well as those without health insurance, get care later and often from providers who are less experienced and less likely to be board-certified.[13,14] Racial and ethnic disparities in care have been linked to delays in access to new technology, care improvements, new pharmaceuticals and state-of-the-art diagnosis and treatment.[15] In the roll out of health information technology, we must be sure that this injustice is not repeated. Government must provide funding for technology to be implemented and supported in safety-net hospitals, community health centers and public health facilities nationally, and these systems must be set up with intelligence and attention to the special needs of the populations they serve.

The Institute chose the Epic system because it allowed us to incorporate what we had learned about meeting the needs of our patients into the electronic health record system. In addition, its expandability will enable us to offer the system to other community health practices, an essential feature if complex systems are to be available to community health centers at an affordable price. Finally, its potential for integration with the public healthcare system in New York City has positioned us to participate in a number of exciting initiatives.

The Institute is committed to providing a model, not just for the integration of state-of-the-art information technology into community health practice, but for the development of multi-organizational collaborations to facilitate innovation and progress in the use of these systems in low-income communities of color. We have become the first primary care organization in New York City to collaborate with the Department of Health and Mental Hygiene to collect primary data to identify disease outbreaks and promote preventive care as part of the City's world-class Syndromic Surveillance System. This unique effort gathers data electronically from emergency departments, laboratories, pharmacies, and now, a network of primary care providers. More recently, we have partnered with the Visiting Nurse Service of New York to develop an interface with their electronic system to improve the quality of care for homebound patients.

Concern about racial disparities in health outcome in low-income communities of color has come to dominate much of the thinking about the next frontier in improving the health of these communities. In a parallel track that is not often related to concerns about health disparities, healthcare and governmental leaders have become strong advocates for advancing the use of sophisticated information technology in healthcare delivery. Using information gleaned from focus groups of community residents, and supported by literature research as well as our ongoing work on health disparities, the Institute for Urban Family Health has implemented an electronic health record in a manner that permits us to address many of the issues raised by patients about the healthcare they receive. We believe that information technology will be an increasingly valuable tool in eliminating health disparities in the community, and have, in the implementation of our electronic health record system, put that belief into practice in our community health centers in New York City.

Acknowledgements: The authors wish to thank the Tides Foundation for their support in the development of this article. We would also like to thank the members of the Bronx Health REACH Coalition for their efforts to unravel the many factors that contribute to disparities.

REFERENCES

1. Satcher D, Fryer GE, McCann J, et al. What if we were equal? A comparison of the black-white mortality gap in 1960 and 2000. *Health Affairs*. 2005;24:459–464.

2. *National Health Care Disparities Report*. Agency for Health Care Research and Quality. July 2003.

3. *Racial/Ethnic Differences in Cardiac Care: The Weight of the Evidence*. The Henry J. Kaiser Family Foundation and the American College of Cardiology Foundation. October 2002. Available at: www.kff.org.

4. Calman N. Making health equality a reality: the Bronx takes action. *Health Affairs*. 2005;24:491–498.

5. Kaplan SA, Calman, NS, Golub M, Davis JH, Ruddock, C, Billings J. Racial and ethnic health disparities; a view from the South Bronx. *JHCPU*. In press.

6. Corbie-Smith G. The continuing legacy of the Tuskegee Syphilis Study: considerations for clinical investigation. *American Journal of the Medical Sciences*. 1999;317:5–8.

7. Cooper LA, Powe NR. *Disparities in Patient Experiences, Health Care Processes, and Outcomes: The Role of Patient-Provider Racial, Ethnic, and Language Concordance*. The Commonwealth Fund. New York, NY: July 2004.

8. Safran DG, Neuman P, Schoen C. Prescription drug coverage and seniors: findings from a 2003 national survey. *Health Affairs*. Web Exclusive; April 19, 2005;W152–W166. Available at www.healthaffairs.org. Accessed June 8, 2005.

9. Lukoschek P, Fazzari M, Marantz P. Patient and physician factors predict patients' comprehension of health information. *Patient Education Counseling*. 2003;50:201–210.

10. Voices of Health Equality: A Project of Bronx Health Reach [film]. New York, NY: Bronx Health REACH in conjunction with Worldways Social Marketing; 2003.

11. See, for example, Greenlund KJ, Giles WH, Keenan NL et al. Physician advice, patient actions, and health-related quality of life in secondary prevention of stroke through diet and exercise. *Stroke*. 2002;565–570. Available at http://www.strokeaha.org. Accessed June 7, 2005; and Fries E, Edinboro P, Manion L et al. Randomized trial of a low-intensity dietary intervention in rural residents: the rural physician cancer prevention project. *American Journal of Preventive Medicine*. 2005; February;28(2):162–168.

12. Marbella AM, Riemer A, Remington P. Wisconsin physicians advising smokers to quit: results from the current population survey, 1998–1999 and behavioral risk factor surveillance system, 2000. *Wisconsin Medical Journal*. 2003;102:41–46.

13. *Access to Specialty Care: A Telephone Survey of Specialty Services in Six Hospitals*. Bronx Health REACH and The Institute for Urban Family Health. Unpublished report. New York, NY.

14. Bach PB, Hoangmai HP, Schrag D, et al. Primary care doctors who treat blacks and whites. *New England Journal of Medicine*. 2004;351:575–84.

15. See, for example, Groeneveld PW, Laufer SB, Garber AM. Technology diffusion, hospital variation, and racial disparities among elderly medicare beneficiaries: 1989–2000. *Medical Care*. 2005;43: 320–329; Sonel AF, Good CB, Mulgund J, et al. Racial variations in treatment and outcomes of black and white patients with high-risk non-ST-elevation acute coronary syndromes. *Circulation*. 2005;111: 1125–32; Feinglass J, Rucker-Whitaker C, Lindquist L, et al. Racial differences in primary and repeat lower extremity amputation: results from a multi-hospital study. *Journal of Vascular Surgery*. 2005;41:823–829; and Morris AM, Billingsley KG, Baxter NN, Baldwin L. Racial disparities in rectal cancer treatment. *Archives of Surgery*. 2004;139:151:155.

CHAPTER 15

The Road to Sustained IT Organizational Credibility

George T. Hickman, CPHIMS, FHIMSS
Kimberly A. Spire

> *"The road to hell is paved with good intentions"*
> *– Unknown.*

Albany Medical Center has undertaken a recent challenge to improve its information technology (IT) capabilities. Activities over the past two years have been substantially refocused with the intention to deliver consistent and credible outcomes. Efforts have included internal and customer-based assessments of IT processes, technologies, competencies and capabilities. Further, executive leadership worked to align a defined identity for IT for AMC.

Two years later many improvements have occurred. More so, several key implementations are now showing delivery to expectations. Yet, the IT organization remains discontented with its place on the credibility curve and continues efforts to evolve to a better place with its constituents.

Healthcare industry IT organizations are currently at varied levels of capability and competency. Factors affecting such disposition include:
• Leadership IT competency
• Clarity in expectations setting
• Competition for capital and ability to fund
• Success in past decisions
• Organizational ability to manage large scale operational changes
• Organizational competency in systems thinking (i.e., people, process, technology design and integration)

While the industry substantially hypes the state of automation when new and interesting applications are deployed, generally speaking, those successes gain recognition and are usually attributed to pioneering and well-funded organizations.

Otherwise, many IT functions seek to adequately meet expectations amidst organizational and external factors that may precede abilities to deliver and sustain improvements. The effect of this industry gap in IT performance is one whereby distance continues to grow between low and high performers, and the IT talent pool is subject to perceptions of leadership success.

In 2002, Gartner published a research paper depicting its five-level information technology (IT) credibility curve.[1] Gartner positioned that IT value to an organization is connected to its creditability and name, as well as the relationship IT has to its constituents. That relationship is a product of IT's capabilities and customer-affecting processes. The five credibility/relationship levels identified in Gartner's paper are:

1. Uncertainty
2. Skepticism
3. Acceptance
4. Trust
5. Respect

The first three levels focus on key factors within the IT function. The internal focus is necessary to assure foundational competency, capability and resourcing. The latter stages require that relational factors be active and supporting between IT and user constituents, as well as a matter of organizational culture. While all stages are inter-relational, earlier stages are more within the direct control of the IT organization and its leadership whereas the latter stages are matters of influence, relational competencies and people's desire to foster a team-based approach to IT.

When the Albany Medical Center Information Services (IS) division's newly formed management team set about marking its position on the credibility curve in early 2004, it recognized that behavioral and process changes were going to be necessary. Further, in agreeing to climb the curve, the team understood that it would need to challenge what IS brought at that time to the table when serving its constituents. IS leadership knew that a wholesale change was in the making.

BACKGROUND

The Albany Medical Center is northeastern New York's only academic health sciences center. With more than 6,500 staff members, the not-for-profit healthcare institution consists of one of New York's largest teaching hospitals, the Albany Medical Center Hospital; one of the nation's oldest medical schools, the Albany Medical College; and one of the Capital Region's most active fundraising organizations, the Albany Medical Center Foundation, Inc.

The AMC IS division is comprised of 160-plus information systems, telecommunications and clinical engineering professionals. These functions had been brought under one organizational hierarchy in recent times. While role descriptions and compensation systems had been aligned, the activities of planning, development and support varied greatly inside of IS. A change agenda would be crafted through:

- Self examination *vis-à-vis* an IS assessment
- Outside validation as provided by perceptions of constituents IS served
- Definition of an identify for IS by most-senior AMC leadership
- Strategy review, priority setting and IT plan development

Figure 15-1 portrays the overall scope for 180-day intense effort.

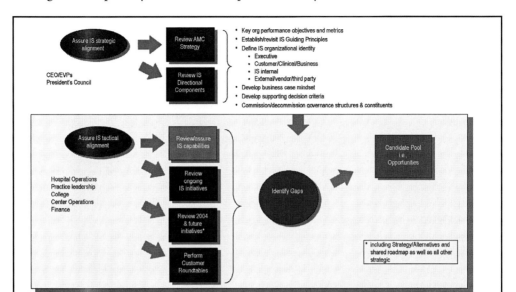

Figure 15-1: Overall Scope for AMC IS Division's 180-day Effort.

Inside-Out

The IS management team agreed to perform a 180-day assessment that would at some level examine every facet of how IS delivers products to its constituency. The toolkit utilized was developed from similar efforts based upon the experiences of a few key leaders and it followed the premise of "begin with the end in mind." Information was captured across the continuum of IS utilizing templates as may support consulting, COBIT[2] ITIL[3] and other assessment approaches. The key areas of the internal assessment included:

- Applications Management
- Infrastructure Management
- Integration Management
- IS Identity
- Key Customer Serving Processes
- Program Management
- Security

The management team agreed to perform the functional assessments on the basis of perceived competency strength. An IS executive agreed to coach each manager on her or his assessment, and the CIO served as quality review advisor during both the process and at-final drafting.

One example of assessment efforts is that which was performed for data integration. A table of all interfaces was generated that included interface name, generalized data composite, format, frequency, direction and so on. Similar, the data exchanges were schematically represented to support the review. Then, observations and recommendations were developed, as shown in Figure 15-2.

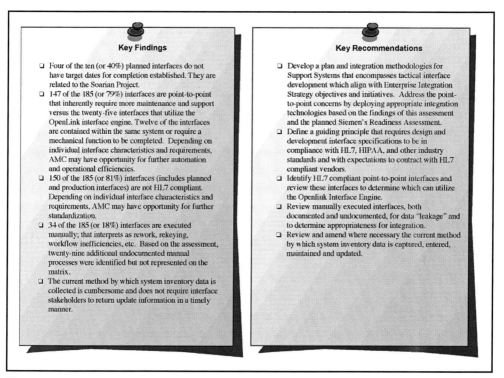

Figure 15-2: IS Assessment—Integration Management.

Upon completion of assessments for all functional areas, the aggregate recommendations were assessed for opportunities to gain efficiencies from related actions. The assessment generated around 120 significant change recommendations that were then categorized as projects and improvements within respective affinity groups or as "just do its." Examples of these change recommendations are included in Table 15-1. Thus, priorities had to be established.

We also needed to "connect" as an IS leadership team and understood that it had to happen first with personal and professional values. After the appropriate process and dialogue, we developed a list of straightforward statements of our values that we could embrace. These value statements are provided in Table 15-2.

Values are intrinsic—they cannot be forced or easily adopted. However, review of values and associated expectations are a part of our key IS recruitment process within the intended outcome that we hire with such a values commitment in mind and that we cascade the same through our organization.

Outside-In and Bottom-Up

A "customer" perception assessment was performed concurrent to the internal assessment. This assessment was comprised of two components: a survey and validation focus group dialogue. The survey was developed from a publication of the Quality Assurance Institute (QAI) regarding the top twenty attributes that define customer perceptions of information technology service organization.[4] These attributes were formed into performance statements for scoring on a 1-10 Likert scale and grouped into the following categories:

Table 15-1: **Examples of Change Recommendations.**

Key Findings	Key Recommendations	Customer Focus Group Concern
Applications Management		
• Version control and planning for all vendor package applications is an area of concern. Some vendor upgrades are automatic while other attention needs to be paid to planned upgrades for vendor applications. The following was discovered while looking at vendor applications and releases: - 49% are up to current market release - 36% are not up to current market release - 15% are not applicable or system functionality is being replaced	• AMC should stay current with vendor releases, but be proactive in installing releases based on confidence with the vendor. Decisions, roles and responsibilities should be agreed upon through Service Level Agreements (SLAs) with IS and customers.	• Proactiveness • Selection and Implementation Support
• Some AMC developed applications reside on older versions of software (e.g., Access 97) that are no longer supported.	• IS needs to develop a more rigorous proactive application update support plan for AMC-developed applications. Review should be based on current business needs and the system architecture.	• Proactiveness
• Investment in some applications focuses on departmental rather than enterprise needs. Some solutions are in place that could have enterprise capabilities (e.g., dictation).	• Business case development should review the entire workflow process prior to application technology purchases.	
• Reporting tools are in place for 74% of applications, many that have limited data extract capability and require additional support. Reporting tools are disparate across applications and include; Adhoc reporting, CoBOL, Crystal Reporting, Access, EZtrieve, Report Writer, Cold Fusion, Excel, SQL, and Focus. In some cases, even these short-list tools do not meet the enterprise needs and additional database and processes are in place for reporting.	• An enterprise wide reporting solution or suite of solutions should be implemented for reporting at AMC.	

Table 15-2: **AMC IS Values.**

We value AMC.
We honor and surpass our commitments.
We look upstream and downstream.
We are committed to one another's success.
We communicate.

- Responsiveness
- Proactiveness
- Integration, Access and Outputs
- Selection and Implementation Support
- Reliability and Performance
- Service Attitude and Communication

Further, the survey had brief sections for open responses to both tactical needs and longer-term initiatives.

The survey was delivered for completeness to a sampling of 120 medical staff and employees as identified by executive management and in consideration of how these individuals could be organized into validation groups. The survey results were summarized to support the focus group discussion that then followed. One validation technique involved understanding where Likert scores ranged broadly on particular attributes. Another factor was that of assuring expectations were managed as such dialogue strapped discussions regarding organization needs for IT.

The survey report for the customer survey and focus groups included a section of open comments as recorded during the sessions, Likert scoring by organization groups (e.g., finance, medical staff, nursing) and summaries of tactical and long-range needs. Table 15-3 includes an example of the open comments made during the focus group sessions.

Table 15-3: Current and Desired Future States—Responsiveness to Requests/ Problems.

• Call Center responsiveness is "person dependent."
• When I need to order something or need something besides call desk, I'm not sure who to call.
• Help Desk is very responsive; however, field support and "follow up takes longer."
• Because we don't have administrative access, and we believe we could handle it, we have things logged that we believe we could handle (e.g., port logging).
• Our levels of IS understanding are very different and I can feel "intimidated" by asking questions that might be too simple or by the complexity of what's asked/expected of me.
• Response time can be long—we are "dead in the water." Response may be two hours or tomorrow on a critical need.
• Don't call off hours because no one is available—"just get a recording."
• Confusion about hand offs and who calls you back based upon perceived need.
• When I call data center, they won't tell me who is on call; I have to wait for a return phone call.
• Select individuals know who to call directly to get a need.

Top-Down

The internal assessments and customer focus group reports included executive summaries. These executive summaries and the full reports were shared with the most-senior leadership including the CEO, COO, Hospital(s) Director, Dean of the Medical College and CFO with encouragement to share the same with other key leaders. Further, it was shared with select key members of the managed major IS constituencies.

Concurrently, we captured basic IS benchmarks, including IS percent of operating expense and FTE complements—both centralized and distributed. This was also compared to the application-inventory with our understanding of state in the industry. This information was used to spark an executive discussion regarding AMC's IT identity—that is, who we were and who we were seeking to be. The Gartner ABC Life-Cycle Adoption Profile was used to frame these conversations.[5] Table 15-4 provides a summary graphic of our ABC profile. In time, the executive group agreed that AMC is a B/C-type organization. But because of distributed decision making, we may have numerous A-type organization activities in play.

Table 15-4: Gartner ABC Enterprise Adoption Profiles

	TYPE A	TYPE B	TYPE C
IT Style	Cutting edge	"We go second"	Wait and see
Risk Tolerance	High	Moderate	Low
Business Use of IS	Aggressive	Balanced	Cautious
Use IS for...	Strategic advantage	Tactical edge and productivity	Utility
Change Mode	Parallel activity	Mixed	Serialized
Governance	Departmental	Hybrid	Centralized
Metrics for IS	Just in time	Value based	Efficiency
Percentage of Enterprises by Profile Type	15%	56%	29%
Percentage of Healthcare Enterprise by Profile Type	1%	15%	84%
IS Budget-to-Revenue Ratio	12%	4%	1%
IS Expense-to-Total Expense	25%	10%	2%
IS Spending Outside the IS Budget	65%	45%	50%
AMC Direct IS-to-Total Expense (fully loaded)			2.6%
AMC IS Budget-to-Revenue Ratio		4.6%	
AMC IS Expense-to-Total Expense		5.19%	
AMC IS Spending Outside the IS Budget		14% (conservative)	

(Adapted from Gartner Group, February 1997, Research Note, TV-000-225; Gartner Group, May 2000, Research Note, COM-10-8445; and, Personal Communication: Mike Davis, Gartner Group HC Practice Leader, January 2004).

To move the organization to decisions and behavior consistent with our spending capacity and risk profile, we drafted and adopted IT Guiding Principles as shown in Table 15-5. These principles were cascaded through the organization by the senior leaders to assure support.

There was also much dialogue regarding the CIO role, its authority to act and need for ongoing IT oversight. An IT oversight team was formed to address strategic direction and decisions, review and assure newly developed policies and standards, and serve as oversight for key efforts where formal oversight teams may not exist.

Through this IT executive committee, standards were developed in several areas to include desktop, server, PDA and mobile device security, as well as wireless and remote connectivity. A business case-based approach was brought to a newly formed IT planning process—one that requires understanding of strategy alignment, benefits, costs and risk profiling as elements to business unit-sponsored, and large-scale IT requests. Implementation activities that require cultural shift or significant organizational behavior change are processed through this group for alignment and tactical adjustments.

Table 15-5: AMC IT Guiding Principles.

Planning	Selection & Acquisition
1. Sponsor information technology initiatives to secure resourcing amongst AMC competing priorities. Anticipate IT demands for support of operational needs. 2. For all significant IT initiatives, identify change objectives, measures for success, risk factors and mitigators, functional and technical requirements, costs and benefits. 3. Plan for initial and ongoing licensing, support, integration, infrastructure, reporting, education, upward version migration and obsolescence replacement costs. 4. Seek to exploit Center-wide IT solutions to realize economies of scale, scope and integration as appropriate.	5. Select stable state-of-the-art technologies for most IT needs. In essence, balance the AMC IT portfolio with our ability to spend and carry risk. 6. Contract with vendors that can provide as many application solutions and integration capabilities as possible. Manage any necessary loss in functionality. 7. Buy vs. build vendor supported application solutions whenever possible. 8. Adopt a multidisciplinary, repeatable process for IT solution selection and acquisition. 9. Involve IT in requirement defining and contracting activities. Secure IS approval for information technology acquisitions (e.g., computing, biomedical, telephony). Require vendors to support AMC technology standards for infrastructure components, security, integration, interoperability, system performance and service levels.
Implementation	Ongoing Support
10. Sponsor and IS will share responsibilities for design, build, testing, training, go-lives and support consistent with a defined, AMC implementation framework. 11. Implement application package and reporting tool capabilities rather than expecting customization. 12. For all significant IT initiatives, sponsor will assess delivery of business case benefits.	13. We will all be responsible for data integrity and uses. 14. We are committed to the development of strong organizational IT competencies. 15. We support the alignment of policies, processes, performance metrics, and Customer and IS roles. 16. Balance and coordinate the demand for IT resources with operational goals and needs.

The Road to Credibility

There is a behavior health axiom that states, "A good state of mind is an inside job." The same is true for the road to credibility. Many efforts had to be internally directed to assure externally delivered outcomes.

Other elements have been put into place to support delivery including:

- **Customer/IS liaison relationship**—To address issues of communication and priority setting, a customer/IS liaison relationship was established for each business unit (see Figure 15-3). Professionals in each organization business unit were designated with this role, while a corresponding individual within IS was designated as the same. Through these critical points of contact, a venue is provided to: (1) approve or deny, and then establish priorities for requests for services; (2) review backloads for reprioritization; (3) cross-message important organizational concerns; and, (4) seek opportunities to bring business unit/IS activities into alignment.

- **eRIS**—The paper-based, duplicate fax form process of requesting system changes and new end-use assets was replaced. The electronic Request for Information Services (eRIS) system was developed by extending the help desk tool via rules-based workflow capability to deliver requests, authorization to examine, estimation respond and approval to proceed. Additionally, volume, closure and workload statistics regarding requests volumes by organizational entity can be produced. Figure 15-4 represents the flow of the electronic request from customer, IS Liaison, and information services staff vantage points.

- **Role and process clarity**—AMC needed to address ambiguity issues regarding constituent and IS roles. One way we have done that is through introduction of methods-based life-cycle approaches to IT. Both IT and customer professionals are expected or encouraged to attend dialectic courses and utilize content as made available on our intranet site.

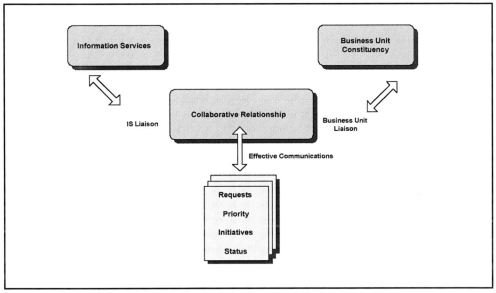

Figure 15-3: IT Governance—IS/Customer Liaison Relationship Model.

The foundation for this teaching effort comes together in three courses that we refer to as PM101, PM102 and PM103. These courses provide a life-cycle overview and reinforce the IT guiding principles, then focus on:

- General project management standards to include issues management, risk management, scope management, structure and communications
- Initial business case development, requirements definition, solution selection, negotiation and contracting
- Implementation planning, design, testing, training, go-live and ongoing support

Table 15-6 provides a snapshot of the four phases and associated stages of the life cycle.

- **Service level objectives**—Rather than overkill our measures for delivery of key IT processes and capabilities, we focused on these measures that are most service delivery affecting. These measures are regularly tracked and reviewed with the IT executive committee on a quarterly basis or as requested. The measures we track on a monthly basis are illustrated in Table 15-7.
- **Delivery of complex, enterprise systems**—All told, solid delivery of IT solutions is the most notable element of IT credibility. Developing a predictable outcome requires organization design and the requisite time to move through the full-life cycle.

In the past six weeks, AMC IS has brought live three enterprise applications:

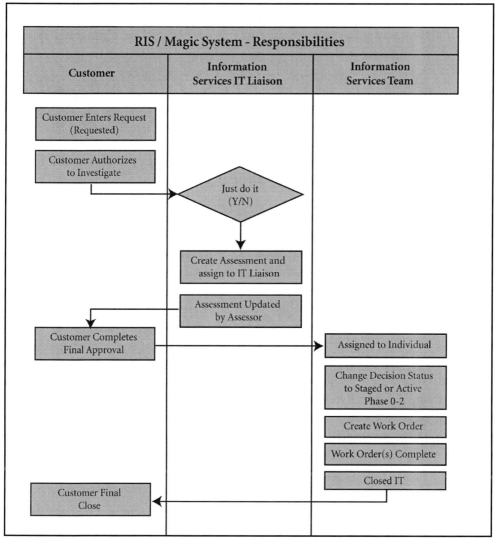

Figure 15-4: eRIS Flow.

Table 15-6: AMC IT Life Cycle—Four Phases.

Phase 0: Planning	Phase 1: Selection & Acquisition	Phase 2: Implementation	Phase 3: On Going Support
• Scope & Requirements Definition • Validation and Approval of Requirements • Recast Budget, if necessary	• Vendor Package Fit • Negotiate/ Identify Solution • Contracting/ Approval	• Project Charter, Scope Update & Planning • Design/Build/Test • Education/Training • Go Live • Post Implementation Review	• Application Maintenance (e.g., Tables, Screen Mods, Report Generation, Security Maintenance) • Technology Support • Ongoing Integration Assurance
Project and Organizational Change management spans across all phases of the IT Life Cycle.			

Table 15-7: Service Delivery Measures.

AREA	Service Level	Description	Metric	Level		
				Unacceptable	Acceptable	Exceptional
Applications and Systems *Based on Scheduled Uptime Hours of Operation	System Availability	Mainframe System & Applications Availability of critical systems	% time systems are Available	7:00 am	6:30 am	6:00 am
			Tolerance level for # events	>1	1	None
			% time Mainframe available	< 99.4%	99.4-99.7%	> 99.7%
		Client Server System & Applications Availability of critical systems	% time systems are Available	< 99.4%	99.4-99.7%	> 99.7%
			Tolerance level for # events	>1	1	None
		Network	% time network is Available	< 99.4%	99.4-99.7%	> 99.7%
			Tolerance level for # events	>1	1	None
	Scheduled Non-recurring Downtime	Quarterly effective scheduling of system downtime maintenance so customers can plan operational coverage and contingency plans.	Lead time of 14 days (Monitor significant events)	>1	1	None
			Tolerance level for # events		4 X Per Year	
Help Desk	First Level Problem Resolution – Help Desk	Calls to the Help Desk are handled quickly and efficiently.	Average speed to answer	> 35 seconds	25 – 35 seconds	< 25 seconds
			% Incoming/ Answered	< 88%	88-92%	> 92%
			% First Call Resolution	< 48%	48-53%	> 53%
Field Support	Computer Equipment Installation	Standard computer devices (PCs, printers, etc.) are installed and operational within an acceptable timeframe.	Stock		20 days	
			Stock % target date met (Monitor significant events)	< 80%	80%	>80%
			Non-Stock		40 days	
			Non-Stock % target date met (Monitor significant events)	< 80%	80%	>80%
Telephony	First Level Problem Resolution – Operators	Calls to the Operators are handled quickly and efficiently.	Avg. Speed to Answer < 6 seconds / > six seconds	< 90%	90 - 95%	> 95%
			% time PBX is available	> 10%	5 – 10%	< 5%
Clinical Engineering	Delivery of Near-full capacity/ capability	Availability of medical devices for use in clinical areas	% of devices in active service	< 95%	95-97.5%	>97.5%
			Avg. Hours of Downtime	> 95 Hrs/Day	35-94 Hrs/Day	< 35 Hrs/Day

1) **Enterprise PACS**—obsolescing five legacy stand alone PACS systems through implementation of a ubiquitously accessed enterprise system that is workflow-enabled with the radiology management system. Physician satisfaction is at a "high."

2) **Bar code-enabled, closed-loop medication administration**—implemented on an early adoption nursing unit utilizing wireless point-of-care devices and now moving through a phased deployment across the house. The early adoption unit manager stated to our CEO, "This is the best change AMC has put into place since I have worked here... I've been here for 22 years." The early benefits of stopping medication administration near-misses, improving the workflow for medication delivery and supporting medication reconciliation are evident. This system also relied upon the recent implementation of our 802.x wireless network.

3) **Web-based new generation EHR**—converted the history from a prior mainframe-based legacy system to a new generation repository and base EHR product. Additional functional modules are now staged for implementation.

   The work supporting these implementations followed our methods approaches and required interplay between significant numbers of people. While our efforts are not yet fully appreciated, life-cycle approaches and new practices are still immature. Our teams have coalesced prior to go-lives to assure success—for the sakes of the projects and AMC—most likely because of the strong individual commitments and values of our people. While a formal lessons learned assessment has not yet been conducted, it is apparent that efforts are at that sensitive juncture whereby the organization's culture and behaviors largely determine how the next-stage transition occurs. Such forward-movement hinges upon external partnerships and alliances, as well as the desire to share power in relational matters in the business of IT delivery. While role maps for life-cycle tools and other such facilitative instruments are available to support education and dialogue, these value-based changes are led from intrinsic matters of trust and desire.

   Project efforts on the immediate horizon require additional competency depth in people and process-based change and adoption of technologies need the same. Full redesign of the order-charge cycle, as well as standardization and automation of clinical documentation, present specific challenges beyond technology competencies and capabilities. Delivering the planned implementation of practitioner order entry and decision support will challenge us further. We would ponder the implications of trying to execute such large-scale organizational changes had we not progressed in fundamental and internal IT credibility. More so, we understand our heightened need for partnering and organization-wide IT competency development to deliver on such complex things. Said another way, at some level, our early efforts were really practice rounds as what happens next matters the most.

   We are hopeful that our formal lessons learned sessions will give us insights and energy to make our next implementation even better and provide us an opportunity to further grow competencies as advocates and partners with our constituents. And we are hopeful that our constituents will desire full partnership with IS—allowing us to progress to Respect on the IT credibility curve.

REFERENCES

1. Young C, Rosser B, MorelloD. *Plot Your IS Group on the IS Credibility Curve*. Stamford, CT: Gartner, Inc; 2002;1–5.

2. Control Objectives for Information and Related Technology (COBIT). COBIT is an IT governance framework and supporting toolset that allows managers to bridge the gap between control requirements, technical issues and business risks. For more information on COBIT, view: www.isaca.org/cobit.

3. Information Technology Infrastructure Library (ITIL): Originally created by the United Kingdom Government, ITIL is now used throughout the world. ITIL is the consistent and comprehensive documentation of best practice for IT Service Management. For more information on ITIL, view www.itil.co.uk.

4. Quality Assurance Institute Worldwide (QAI): The Quality Assurance Institute was founded in 1980 in the United States. QAI's founding objective was and remains to provide leadership in improving quality, productivity, and effective solutions for process management in the information services profession. For more information on QAI, view www.qaiworldwide.org.

5. Feiman J, Kirwin B, Morello D, Redman P. *Enterprise Personality Profile: Dimensions and Descriptors*. Stamford, CT: Gartner, Inc; 2004;1–5.

CHAPTER 16

Why Do Projects Fail?

Kenneth R. Ong, MD, MPH

- "Cedars-Sinai Medical Center Suspends CPOE" *Family Medicine Notes, January 23, 2003*
- "Doctors Pull Plug on Paperless System" *American Medical Association News, February 17, 2003*
- "Cedars-Sinai Doctors Cling to Pen and Paper" *The Washington Post, March 21, 2005*
- "A Big Rollout Bust" *headline from CIO.com, June 1, 2003*
- "Hospital Shuts Down CPOE System" *Health Data Management, September 29, 2005*

The suspension of Computerized Practitioner Order Entry (CPOE) at Cedars-Sinai Hospital sent digital shock waves across the nation through the e-mail threads, list services and blogs of health information technology professionals.

The $34 million, three-year CPOE project included billing and registration. CPOE was made mandatory for all physicians. Non-participating physicians risked losing staff privileges. Cedars-Sinai is a highly regarded, 952-bed hospital located in Beverly Hills, California. It is one of the top 100 "Most Wired" Hospitals.[1,2]

The list of possible reasons for the CPOE project failure is long. According to reports in the media, some physicians complained before go-live that the mandatory two hour instructor-led and online training were too long. After go-live, others reported training was too short. Of the 2,000 physicians, 85% were voluntary who may have posed a greater challenge than salaried residents. Medications misspelled in free text were not recognized. Common orders were excluded, like "clear liquids and advance diet as tolerated." There were complaints of too many questions, alerts and reminders. Reportedly rank and file physicians were not involved in design and implementation. Order entry involved too many screens with six-to-eight seconds between each screen.[3]

The CPOE initiative did have positive aspects. More than 700,000 orders for more than 7,000 patients were placed. The system performed as designed and improved quality and safety. Uptime performance and reliability met expectations. During the hiatus, the project leadership will focus on physician change management, workflow change management, system enhancement, and intensifying training and support resources.[4]

EASIER SAID THAN DONE

CPOE and clinical decision support systems (CDSS) are technologies that serve the very intricate environment of modern healthcare. Medication management is one of CPOE's primary functions. A hospital's drug formulary may contain thousands of medications with tens of thousands of possible interactions between the drugs themselves (drug-drug), patient allergies (drug-allergy), and food (drug-food). Each drug has at least two names, one chemical and one brand. Each drug has its own range of therapeutic doses for children, adults, senior and those with liver or renal impairment. A dose too small will not help; a dose too large may do more harm than good.

Sidebar 16-1: The Five Rights of Drug Administration.

• Right patient
• Right drug
• Right dose
• Right route
• Right time

Misspelling can lead to the administration of the wrong drug. The Institute of Safe Medication Practices compiles of list of agents that have been confused with one another.[5] For example, Cedax and Cidex have been confused with one another. Yet Cedax is ceftibuten, an antimicrobial given to treat infections. Cidex is a disinfectant used to cleanse endoscopes. The former is taken internally by patients. The latter is used externally on equipment.

There is still more to safe medication administration than getting the right drug.[6] The dose must be correct. A medication's therapeutic dose range may be affected by compromised liver or kidney function, body mass or age.

The route must be correct. Medications can be given via mouth, under the tongue, intravenously, subcutaneously, per rectum or intramuscularly (partial list only).

The final element of the "five rights" is time. The drug must be given at the right time to be effective or to prevent over dosage. Some drugs are better absorbed before meals; others are only tolerated after meals.

Replacing pen and paper with CPOE with a Clinical Decision Support System (CDSS) presents another set of challenges. A physician's illegible scrawl may be deftly delivered but finding the right option in a drop down list may take time to learn. A required field in an electronic medical record may force a clinician to document data he might not otherwise choose not to document in a paper-based chart.

NOT THE FIRST TIME, NOR THE LAST

The temporary setback to CPOE at Cedars-Sinai was not the first for this complex technology. Fifteen years earlier, the University of Virginia Medical Center was a pioneer when it began implementation of mandatory physician order entry in 1988.[7] In 1992, more than 550 terminals were deployed in three locations. Over 3,600 nurses, 1,200 residents, 800 medical students, and 200 attending physicians had been trained to use the new system. The program took three times longer and cost three times more than expected to install. Interestingly, the technology ("the strict, literal interpretation of rules by the computer") itself was only one of four factors that led to the system's temporary suspension. The other three factors that contributed to the "widespread organizational stress" associated with the implementation were dramatic changes in established workflow, unclear governance policies, and lack of physician understanding of the long-term strategic value of the system. Only after an executive committee with leaders from the major clinical departments was established was the initiative successfully implemented. The case study's author concludes: "[W]e may have gained a strategic and competitive advantage for the future by being forced to deal with issues of institutional change."

Failed health information system projects are not unique to the United States. The lead story on the British Broadcasting Company's evening news of October 27, 1992, was the failure of a new computer system at the London Ambulance Service.[8] The deaths of twenty to thirty people were ascribed to the failure. Areas dead to radio transmission and incorrectly pressed buttons sent incorrect ambulance locations to the system. As a consequence, too many ambulances were sent to some calls and none to others. The growing error log compromised the system further. An official inquiry found that the project was underfinanced with an inadequate timeline. The causes were several. It was unclear which of the contractors was primary and the management of the project was inadequate. The software was judged to be unfinished and unstable. The emergency backup system was untested. Training was inadequate.

On the other end of the world in 1996, a major HIT failure occurred in the New South Wales public health system in Australia.[9] An information systems steering committee commissioned a consulting firm to devise their IT strategy. The consultants recommended a "best-of-breed" approach to purchase three core systems: financial, pathology and patient administration/clinicals. Scenarios with pre-determined scripts were given to each vendor. Ultimately, a vendor was selected who had installed software in one hundred sites in the United States. Five pilot sites were selected, none of which had taken part in developing the strategy nor selecting the system. The sites pressed for more software customization than the vendor was willing to deliver. Nurses had difficulty taking time for training and not all adopted the new system. Physicians had limited time for training. Managers found the report generator inadequate. Clinicians found logging into the system cumbersome with four levels of login. Navigation was complicated with up to eleven screens and forty-three key strokes to order one test. Orders were not linked with results reporting. The character-based system appeared archaic to end-users accustomed to Windows-driven systems. The IS staff was highly dependent on vendor support. After no more than six weeks in one institution and fifteen months in another, problems continued without resolution and the $110 million project was terminated.

Aarts and Berg describe two CPOE projects in the Netherlands, where one was terminated and the other limited only to nurses and clerks.[10] A terminal emulator in a Windows environment was chosen to expand the incumbent IBM technology infrastructure. Though a mouse was adapted in the new system to replicate the light pen in the old, its movements were cumbersome. The screen was limited to a maximum of 24 X 40 characters, a fraction of the size of today's Windows or Web browser-based graphic user interfaces. One clinic nurse reported that "the characters look like Braille."

As a navigation aid in the old registration system, the patient ID number was persistently visible. The absence of such data in the new system led to delays in the ambulatory clinics. More staff was required to mitigate the computer-generated delays. The delays in the clerical workflows of the system dissuaded physicians from implementing the system's CPOE application. Inaccurate reports that underestimated patient throughput frustrated departments whose budgets were dependent on the numbers of patients treated.[11]

While the health information technology initiatives that failed in the 1990s could be ascribed to the recognized risk in building rather than buying software applications, three studies reported negative outcomes after implementing commercially developed CPOE applications. The Veterans Administration Hospital in Salt Lake City reported increased rates of adverse drug events associated with CPOE without a related clinical decision support system for drug selection, dosing and monitoring.[12] A pediatric hospital reported increased mortality after implementing CPOE that the authors attributed to issues centered on "systems integration" and "human-machine interface."[13]

The third such study, written by Koppel et al from the University of Pennsylvania, surveyed and interviewed house staff and concluded a leading CPOE system facilitated twenty-two types of medication error risks, with many reported to occur frequently.[14] The Koppel study "generated a tremendous amount of attention and discussion within the informatics community."[15] Bates cautioned that Koppel's study did not count errors or adverse events, but the perception of errors. The study failed to count errors that CPOE prevented. Thus, the study failed to demonstrate whether the medication error rate was lower or higher with CPOE. In addition, the CPOE system in use was very old (1997) and required multiple screens for many activities causing many of the problems reported. A new system has since replaced the old one.

In the same journal, Garg et al reviewed one hundred published studies on computerized clinical decision support systems (CDSS).[16] CDSS is that portion of software in HIT that provides the intelligence or the rules for an application. In most pharmacy and CPOE systems, the CDSS governs alerts for drug-drug interactions, drug-allergy interactions and dose-range checking. In an electronic medical record (EMR) in acute or ambulatory care, emergency department or other setting of care, the CDSS consists of order sets, reminders, alerts and clinical documentation. If CPOE is the hand that writes, CDSS is the brain that tells it what to write.

Garg's literature review included a broad assortment of trials. The trials were published between 1973 and 2004. While 32% of the studies provided training prior to implementation, another 42% offered training during implementation. Only 15% of the trials had a graphic user interface. The CDSS communicated its recommendations directly to the clinician via the computer in 41% of the trials and indirectly via reports placed in charts in 45%. The desired patient outcomes included cancer screening, vaccinations, and mammography. The review's authors concluded, "Many CDSS improve practitioner performance. To date, the effects on patient outcomes remain understudied and, when studied, inconsistent."

In an accompanying editorial, entitled "Waiting for Godot," the editor comments that while

> "The literature in these fields has been characterized by frequent reports of success, often accompanied by predictions of a bright new (and near) future; however, the future seems never to arrive. Behind the cheers and high hopes that dominate conference proceedings, vendor information, and large parts of the scientific literature, the reality is that systems that are in use in multiple locations, that have satisfied users, and that effectively and efficiently contribute to the quality and safety of care are few and far between."

WAITING FOR GODOT VS. THE INEVITABLE REALITY CHECK

Adherents of the Gartner theory of the Hype Cycle of Emerging Technology might argue that the surprise that accompanied the Cedars-Sinai CPOE suspension was inevitable.[17] The theory holds that there are five phases to a technology's popularity or visibility (Figure 16-1). The first phase of a Hype Cycle is the "technology trigger" or breakthrough. The media predicts that a technology may be the next big thing.

The next phase is the "Peak of Inflated Expectations" when the buzz is overpowering and expectations go far beyond reality. The third phase is the "Trough of Disillusionment" when expectations are dashed and media attention wanes. Despite the relative silence in the press, some businesses press on to better understand the actual benefits and limitations of the technology. They persist on the "Slope of Enlightenment" (see Figure 16-1).

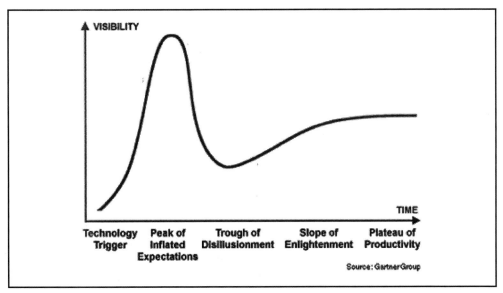

Figure 16-1: Hype Cycle of Emerging Technology.

The last and final phase is the "Plateau of Productivity." The technology has a growing history of successes. The technology has matured beyond its first generation. Its appropriate application and usefulness is better understood.

In an editorial, Wears and Berg tried to put the studies reporting contrary CPOE results in perspective: "There is a long-standing, rich, and abundant literature on the problems associated with the introduction of computer technology into complex work in other domains, as well as occasional notes in healthcare. Clearly, there is no reason to expect healthcare, that from an organizational standpoint probably the most complex enterprise in modern society, to be immune to them."[18]

Indeed, we should not be too surprised to hear of speed bumps on the path to CPOE. Research from the Standish Group in 1994 revealed that IT project failure was not unusual. Their study, the CHAOS report, revealed that 31.1% of projects were canceled before completion. Further results indicated 52.7% of projects cost 189% of their original estimates.[19]

The CHAOS report found three factors were associated with success: (1) small projects were more likely to succeed than large projects; (2) shorter time frames with early and frequent delivery of software components had a greater chance for success; and, (3) smaller project teams performed better than larger teams. The level of success was attributed to the degree of user involvement, executive management support and the participation of an experienced project manager.[20]

CPOE system installations are large, multifaceted projects. A CPOE system may cost from $8 million to $12 million.[21] Projects of similar size in Fortune 500 companies have been reported to have only an 8% success rate (see Figure 16-2).[22]

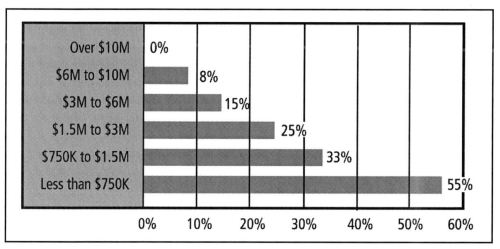

Figure 16-2: Success By Project Budget.

Another factor in the success or failure of a software installation is the quality of the software itself. KLAS, a provider of customer satisfaction reports for health information technology, conducted a recent study of vendor and provider perspectives on software quality. Sixty-one acute care providers and seven vendor executives representing twelve firms were interviewed. The providers represented 211 acute care hospitals, each with more than 200 beds. Given the aggregate number of beds, the hospitals comprised 13.5% of the industry segment.

The participating vendors were among the top twenty in customer satisfaction in 2004. They included many of the more established in health information technology, e.g, Cerner, Epic, GE, McKesson, Mediware, Misys, PeopleSoft, Per-Se, Picis, SCI Scheduling.com, Siemens and Unibased Systems Architecture.[23]

Vendors and providers ranked the characteristics of quality similarly. Stability and uptime were ranked first. Response time, ease of use, release management, maintenance cost, and certification and benchmarking followed. Though the scoring was most different for maintenance cost, providers scored each of the characteristics higher in importance than the vendors (see Figure 16-3).

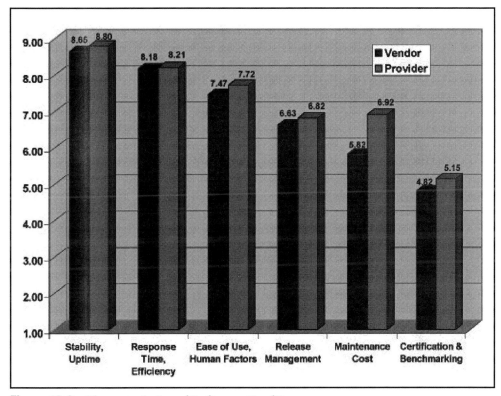

Figure 16-3: Characteristics of Software Quality.

When queried how poor software quality may impact an organization, 18%-56% of the providers acknowledged severe to intolerable negative effects on outcomes like end user disruptions, downtime of software systems, time spent recovering and fixing, testing releases and IT effort on other quality issues (see Figure 16-4).

Not all software is created equal and different vendors will have different on-time delivery rates. The more difficult the technology and the greater the clinical transformation required, the longer an application may take to install. The 2005 On-Time Delivery Report from KLAS gathered delivery times for clinical data repositories (CDR), CPOE, nurse charting, pharmacy and physician notes.[24] Physician notes projects were the most likely to be reported on-time (67%). The other project types were reported to be 45%–54 % on schedule.

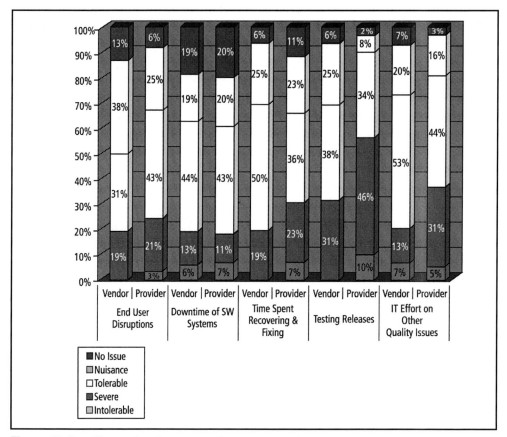

Figure 16-4: Effects of Software Quality on Provider Organizations.

Providers reported that late projects could be ascribed to vendors half the time (50%), providers 13%, and both vendors and providers 37%. CPOE projects were the most challenging, while pharmacy projects were the least. CPOE implementations were an average of twelve months late. Physician notes implementations were ten months late; nurse charting nine months late; CDR seven months late; and pharmacy five months late (see Table 16-1).

Table 16-1: On-Time Delivery of Software Projects.

Overall Averages:	Percent On-Time*	Percent Live On-Time	Percent On-Schedule	Average Months Late
CDR	45%	29%	16%	7 Months
CPOE	54%	8%	46%	12 Months
Nurse Charting	54%	20%	34%	9 Months
Pharmacy	50%	29%	21%	5 Months
Physician Notes	67%	9%	58%	10 Months

Not only clinical IT but business initiatives are challenged as well. Of the CIOs who responded, 31% reported a major delay or failure with an IT business initiative in the past eighteen months.[25] The seventy-three members (8% of total membership of 880) of the College of Health Information Management Executives took part in the survey. The most commons reasons CIOs cited for why IT business initiatives fail to produce expected value were lack of process, lack of IT alignment, and inadequate process change (51%); lack of executive ownership and accountability (49%); lack of understanding of expected business benefits (41%); communication breakdown or failure (28%); bad business objectives (24%); and, lack of outcome measurements (24%) (Figure 16-5).

	Percentage responding "most prevalent" to each underlying reason for not generating value from IT
Lack of process and IT alignment; inadequate process change	51%
Lack of executive ownership and accountability	49%
Lack of understanding of expected business benefits	41%
Communication breakdown or failure	28%
Bad business objectives	24%
Lack of outcome measurements	24%
Lack of strong or adequate project governance	23%
Failure to align business vision / goals with IT	22%
Lack of understanding of what computer users really needed	20%
Volatile situation: organization's needs changed	18%
Poor project management	17%
Costs exceeded benefits	16%
Nothing significantly improved	14%
Users did not want the IT solution	12%
Poor performance by vendor or consultant	9%
A problem of timing: the opportunity was lost	5%
Technical failure of software or hardware	0%

Figure 16-5: **When I.T. Initiatives Fail to Produce Desired Value.**
(Adapted from CHIME CIO Survey: IT Value)

Our cursory review of the literature shows that the Cedars-Sinai CPOE project suspension was neither an isolated nor an unexpected event given the prevalence of IT project failure both inside and outside healthcare. The KLAS, CHIME, and Standish Group reports established project failure as common and the surveys propose why projects fail.

KEYS TO SUCCESS

The industry press is replete with advice to those implementing HIT. One observer warns of six deadly mistakes to avoid: (1) raising expectations too high; (2) providing skimpy training; (3) doing the "big bang" implementation; (4) leaving physicians to their own devices; (5) disregarding dissidents; and, (6) giving physicians a choice.[26]

Another commentator speaks of "The Yoda Factor," admonishing those who seek CPOE to "do" rather than simply "try". The do-ers follow four basic principles: set high expectations for clinician participation and do not relent; plan for hospital-wide, phased-in implementation and stick to a unit-by-unit roll out schedule; spend massive amounts of time on workflow design, testing and training; and, have 24/7 support.[27]

Physicians who implemented CPOE successfully at University of Pennsylvania Health System, Evanston Northwestern Healthcare and Cincinnati Children's Hospital recommend ten steps for success:[28]

1. All hands on deck: Make CPOE a top organizational priority with full support from the executive leadership to unit staff.
2. Pay physician champions: Value and protect time for a physician to design, plan, and lead CPOE implementation.
3. Analyze your workflow: New, more efficient workflows should be designed to replace inefficient extant workflows.
4. Build adequate order sets: Order sets can help standardize care and speed adoption. The number of needed order sets can number in the hundreds.
5. Recognize politics: The chief medical information officer or director of medical informatics must get buy-in from the clinical department chairs.
6. Set a deadline and mean it: Delays and postponed deadlines dampen physician and organizational enthusiasm.
7. Train, train, train: Train before, during and after implementation. Train in formal sessions, online, and on the patient care units.
8. Exploit physician resistance: Go one-on-one and find out why physicians resist and use the knowledge to improve training, create more order sets, or improve usability.
9. Sell the benefits: It is about quality care and patient safety. This is not just an IT project.
10. Crack the whip: If CPOE is mandatory, enforce it.

John Glaser, the vice president and CIO of Partners HealthCare, Boston, prescribes six success factors for clinical information system implementation: (1) strong organizational vision and strategy; (2) talented and committed leadership; (3) a partnership between the clinical, administrative, and IT staffs; (4) thoughtful redesign of clinical processes; (5) excellent implementation skills, especially in project management and support; and, (6) good-to-excellent IT.[29]

Other principles provide guidance that applies to all IT projects. A round-table on IT failures at the University of Houston struck a common chord with advice given elsewhere:[30]

- Shrink the development cycle time by breaking projects into smaller bites and making sure that value is delivered at each bite
- Don't get caught in the "throwing good money after bad" trap. If value isn't being delivered, ignore the sunk costs and look only at future dollars versus benefits

- Focus attention on the opinion leaders and the change agents
- Vendors and business partners can help in diffusing technologies
- Customers may sometimes serve as a change agent
- Be sure you understand the current state completely before attempting to introduce change
- Demonstrate the value of the systems by using the worst critics as the earliest adopters
- Know to whom you are selling
- Have proper incentives for adoption
- Take advantage of beta testing opportunities
- Make sure you understand company culture and the degree that you will be affecting it
- Make your systems as reliable as is possible within the given restraints
- Develop measurement/reporting processes to monitor the success of diffusion

A number of quality improvement organizations sponsored by the Center for Medicare and Medicaid Services (CMS) offer CPOE Readiness Assessment for participating hospitals ("Identified Participant Groups"). The readiness assessment tool identifies executive and physician commitment to CPOE and analyzes the IT infrastructure readiness as well.[31]

During any software selection process, the site visits and reference calls can serve as an introduction to clients of the selected vendor who installed the product successfully. The users group can serve as a community with a depth of experience and knowledge of the product unavailable otherwise.

WHEN THINGS GO WRONG

"The best-laid plans of mice and men often go awry. "
Robert Burns

Though good planning and rigorous implementation can mitigate potential problems, problems will arise. Information technology is complicated and expensive. The nature of healthcare in the twenty-first century is in and of itself complex. Any successful IT project is the result of paying meticulous attention to workflows and people.

The tools of performance improvement can be well applied to the challenges of HIT projects. Root cause analysis, workflow diagrams, the Shewhart Cycle, Failure Modes and Effects Analysis, and cause and effect diagrams can reveal the nuances of the human–computer interface and clinical transformation.

Horsky et al applied a novel workflow analysis to study a dosing error related to computer-based ordering of potassium chloride (KCl). They reconstructed events chronologically from practitioner order entry usage logs, semi-structured interviews with involved clinicians and examined interface usability of the ordering system.[32] They found errors in the drug ordering process, confusing on-screen laboratory results review, system usability difficulties, user training problems and suboptimal display of intravenous (IV) bolus injection and medicated fluid drip orders.

In response to their findings, they determined that the screens for ordering continuous IV fluid drips and drips of limited volume needed to be clearly distinct so that the ordering of each is unambiguous; screens that list active medication orders should list IV drip orders; the laboratory results review screen needed to clearly visually indicate when the most recent results are not from the current day; an alert should be added that would inform users of existing potassium administration; another alert should be added informing users ordering potassium when there has not been a serum potassium value recorded in the past twelve hours or the most recent potassium value is greater than 4.0; and, other minor changes should be made to increase the consistency of ordering screen behavior.

Cause and effect diagrams can identify the policies, procedures, people or technology issues that need intervention.[33] Caudill-Slosberg and Weeks report a case study of inadequate coumadin therapy related to clinical documentation in an electronic medical record.[34] They employed a fishbone diagram to pinpoint opportunities for improvement (Figure 16-6).

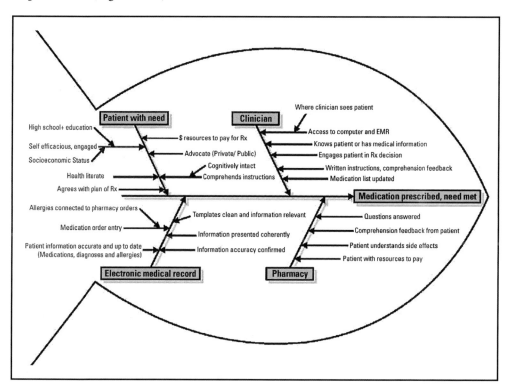

Figure 16-6: Cause-Effect Diagram of Coumadin Error.

Their analysis discovered that the ambiguity of the warfarin dosing on the medication order list resulted in inaccurate interpretation of warfarin dose and administration, the use of templates created visual barriers to identifying important information because of extraneous details, and the availability of both readable documentation and a copy-and-paste function gave false assurances that the available information was correct and facilitated its promulgation.

CONCLUSION

Knowing why projects fail can help projects succeed. No matter what the technology, getting the people, policies and workflow right are always critical. No matter how grand the plan, without scrupulous attention to execution, no innovation can succeed.

Health information technology is still maturing. Technologies like CPOE with clinical decision support systems are evolving and growing in sophistication. Ongoing research into optimizing workflow and human factors will enable smarter implementations of this essential technology in the future.[35,36,37]

REFERENCES

1. Chin T. Doctor involvement key to success of computerized order entry. *American Medical News.* March 17, 2003. http://www.ama-assn.org/amednews/2003/03/17/bisc0317.htm. Accessed November 24, 2006.

2. Versel N. Cedars-Sinai learns from its CPOE mistakes to improve workflow. *Health IT World.* September 9, 2004. http://www.bio-itworld.com/newsletters/healthit/2004/09/09/20040909_10115. Accessed November 24, 2006.

3. Connolly C. Cedars-Sinai doctors cling to pen and paper. *Washington Post.* March 21, 2005; Section A, page 1. http://www.washingtonpost.com/wp-dyn/articles/A52384-2005Mar20.html. Accessed November 24, 2006.

4. Langberg ML. Challenges to implementing CPOE. *Modern Physician.* February 1, 2003. http://www.modernphysician.com/page.cms?pageId=216. Accessed November 24, 2006.

5. Institute for Safe Medication Practices. Confused drug name list. Available at: http://www.ismp.org/Tools/confuseddrugnames.pdf. Accessed April 25, 2006.

6. Mutter M. One hospital's journey toward reducing medication errors. *Jt Comm J Qual Saf.* 2003;June;29(6):279–88.

7. Massaro TA. Introducing physician order entry at a major academic medical center: Impact on organizational culture and behavior. *Acad Med.* 1993; January;68(1):20-5.

8. Beynon-Davies P, Lloyd-Williams M. When health information systems fail. *Top Health Inf Manage.* 1999;August;20(1):66–79.

9. Souton G, Sauer C, Dampney K. Information technology in complex health services: organizational impediments to successful technology transfer and diffusion. *J Am Med Inform Assoc.* 1997;4:112–124.

10. Aarts J, Berg M. Same systems, different outcomes—comparing the implementation of computerized physician order entry in two Dutch hospitals. *Methods Inf Med.* 2006;45(1):53–61.

11. Aarts J, Doorewaard H, Berg M. Understanding implementation: the case of a computerized physician order entry system in a large Dutch university medical center. *J Am Med Inform Assoc.* 2004;May–June;11(3):207–16.

12. Nebeker JR, Hoffman JM, Weir CR, Bennett CL, Hurdle JF. High rates of adverse drug events in a highly computerized hospital. *Arch Intern Med.* 2005;165:1111–1116.

13. Watson S, Nguyen TC, Bayir H, Orr RA, Han YY, Carcillo JA, Venkataraman ST, Clark RSB. Computerized physician order entry system unexpected increased mortality after implementation of a commercially sold. *Pediatrics.* 2005;116;1506–1512.

14. Koppel R, Metlay JP, Cohen A, Abaluck B, Localio AR, Kimmel SE, Strom BL. Role of computerized physician order entry systems in facilitating medication errors. *JAMA.* 2005;Mar 9;293(10):1197–203.

15. Bates DW. Computerized physician order entry and medication errors: finding a balance. *J Biomed Inform.* 2005;Aug;38(4):259–61.

16. Garg AX, Adhikari NK, McDonald H et al. Effects of computerized clinical decision support systems on practitioner performance and patient outcomes: a systematic review. *JAMA*. 2005;293(10):1223–1238.

17. The hype cycle. Available at: http://www.gartner.com/pages/story.php.id.8795.s.8.jsp. Accessed April 22, 2006.

18. Wears RL, Berg M. Computer technology and clinical work still waiting for Godot. *JAMA*. March 9, 2005;Vol 293;No. 10:1261–1263.

19. The Standish Group International, Inc. The CHAOS report (1994). Available at: http://www.standishgroup.com/sample_research/chaos_1994_1.php. Accessed April 22, 2006.

20. Schwartz E. Six myths of IT: Myth 5—Most IT projects fail. *Infoworld*. August 13, 2004. http://www.infoworld.com/article/04/08/13/33FEmyth5_1.html. Accessed November 24, 2006.

21. First Consulting Group. Computerized physician order entry: costs, benefits and challenges. January 2003.

22. The Standish Group International, Inc. CHAOS: a recipe for success. ©1999.

23. Klas Enterprises. Software quality study: vendor and provider perspectives. January 2005.

24. Klas Enterprises. On-time delivery report 2005. August 2005.

25. College of Health Information Management Executives. 2004 CIO survey. *Modern Healthcare*. May 24, 2004. Available at: http://www.modernhealthcare.com/mediaindex.cms?type=surveys&industry=CIO%20Survey%20-%202004. Accessed April 23, 2006. Requires premium registration.

26. Baldwin G. Avoid six deadly mistakes. *Healthleaders*. January 2005;51–54. Available at: http://www.healthleadersmedia.com/magazine/view_magazine_feature.cfm?content_id=61368. Accessed April 23, 2006.

27. Gaillour FR. Why do health systems flop with CPOE? Ask Yoda: the "Yoda factor" is the difference between "trying to do CPOE" and "doing CPOE." *Physician Exec*. 2004 Mar–Apr;30(2):28–9.

28. Baldwin G. Bringing order to CPOE: 10 make or break steps. *Health Leaders*. October 2005. http://www.healthleadersmedia.com/magazine/view_magazine_feature.cfm?content_id=74158. Accessed November 24, 2006.

29. Glaser J. Success factors for clinical information system implementation. *Hospital and Health Network's Most Wired Magazine*. June 13, 2005. http://www.usafp.org/CHCSII-Files/Implementation-Files/Success%20Factors%20for%20Clinical%20Information%20System%20Implementation.pdf. Accessed November 24, 2006.

30. Information Systems Research Center, College of Business Administration, University of Houston. Project implementation, technology diffusion, adoption and acceptance: an ISRC roundtable discussion lead by Peter A. Todd and Wynne W. Chin. *ISRC Notes*. January 2001. Available at: http://www.uhisrc.com/pdf/jan01.pdf. Accessed April 23, 2006.

31. Medicare Quality Improvement Community. CPOE readiness assessment. Available at: http://www.medqic.org/dcs/BlobServer?blobcol=urldata&blobheader=multipart%2Foctet-stream&blobheadername1=Content-Disposition&blobheadervalue1=attachment%3Bfilename%3DCPOE+Readiness+Assessment.pdf&blobkey=id&blobtable=MungoBlobs&blobwhere=1127423707640. Accessed April 29, 2006.

32. Horsky J, Kuperman GJ, Patel VL. Comprehensive analysis of a medication dosing error related to CPOE. *J Am Med Inform Assoc*. 2005;12:377–382.

33. Fishbone, Ishikawa. The cause and effect diagram. Available at: http://www.isixsigma.com/library/content/t000827.asp. Accessed April 23, 2006.

34. Caudill-Slosberg M, Weeks WB. Case study: identifying potential problems at the human/technical interface in complex clinical systems. *Am J of Med Qual*. November–December 2005;200(6):353ff.

35. Feldstein A, Simon SR, Schneider J, Krail M, Laferriere D, Smith DH, Sittig DF, Soumerai SB. How to design computerized alerts to ensure safe prescribing practices. *Jt Com J on Qual and Saf.* 2004;30(11):602–613.

36. Shah NR, Seger AC, Seger DL, Fiskio JM, Kuperman GJ, Blumenfeld B, Recklet EG, Bates DW, Gandhi TK. Improving acceptance of computerized prescribing alerts in ambulatory care. *J Am Med Inform Assoc.* 2006; January–February;13(1):5–11. Epub 2005; October 12.

37. Karsh BT. Beyond usability: designing effective technology implementation systems to promote patient safety. *Qual Saf Health Care.* 2004; October;13(5):388–94.

Glossary

Adobe Acrobat: A software product from Adobe Systems that can create and edit PDFs (see PDF).

Adobe Reader: A software product from Adobe Systems that can read PDFs (see PDF).

ADT: admit-discharge-transfer, a module of an HIS that collects insurance and demographic data for a patient to enable billing.

AHIC: American Health Information Community; Michael O. Leavitt, Secretary of the Department of Health and Human Services (HHS), formed AHIC, also referred to as the Community, to help advance efforts to reach President Bush's call for most Americans to have electronic health records within ten years. The Community is a federally-chartered commission and will provide input and recommendations to HHS on how to make health records digital and interoperable, and assure that the privacy and security of those records are protected, in a smooth, market-led way. (Adapted from http://www.hhs.gov/healthit/ahic.html.)

AHIMA: American Health Information Management Association; a national organization of medical records professionals.

Alert: An alert is an application generated, automated message that may be a warning or reminder. Alerts should be actionable, enabling a recommended order or other task.

AMDIS: Association of Medical Directors of Information Systems; a national professional organization comprised of physicians with an applied informatics focus.

AMIA: American Medical Informatics Association; a national, multidisciplinary organization with an academic informatics focus.

ANSI: American National Standards Institute.

ASCII: American Standard Code for Information Interchange; an international 7-bit code for representing alphanumeric characters.

ASCII delimited: an ASCII file formatted with data field headers (column titles) separated by commas, tabs, or another alphanumeric character.

ASP: Application Service Provider; a company that provides access, via the Internet, to applications and other services that would otherwise have to reside on a local computer. ASPs offer the ability to rent applications in lieu of purchasing software.

ASTM: ASTM International is an international voluntary standards organization that develops and produces technical standards for materials, products, systems and services. It was formed in 1898 in the United States as the American Society for Testing and Materials by a group of scientists and engineers led by Charles Benjamin Dudley. They wanted to address the frequent rail breaks plaguing the fast-growing railroad industry. The group developed a standard for the steel used to fabricate rails. (Adapted from http://en.wikipedia.org/wiki/ASTM.)

Audit trail: a report that records who made what changes when to a database record; a requirement of HIPAA for protected health information (see HIPPA).

Authentication: The process of identifying an individual, usually based on a username and password. In security systems, authentication is distinct from authorization—a process of giving individuals access to system objects based on their identity. Authentication merely ensures that the individual is who he or she claims to be, but says nothing about the access rights of the individual.

Authorization: The process of granting or denying access to a network resource. Most computer security systems are based on a two-step process. The first stage is authentication, which ensures that a user is who he or she claims to be. The second stage is authorization, which allows the user access to various resources based on the user's identity.

Bar code: The machine-readable representation of the UPC. Bar codes are read by a scanner that passes over the code and registers the UPC. The width of each black line and the subsequent white space between each line coincides with the numbers of the UPC.

BCMA: bar code medication administration; bar code technology applied to medications, patients, and nursing staff. BCMA is a tool to enable the five rights to reduce medication errors (see Five Rights).

Cause and effect diagram (Ishikawa): Also called a "Fishbone Diagram," because its shape looks like a fish with the head being on the right and the tail on the left, or an "Ishikawa Diagram," after creator Kaoru Ishikawa. Tool used to make assumptions of the root-cause and/or potential or common causes, for a specific effect. Create to list all possible reasons for any given conclusion. These types of diagrams can identify the most likely reasons of a result. See the following link for more information:
http://www.sixsigmaspc.com/dictionary/causeeffectdiagram.html.

CBT: training which is delivered by computer. It can deliver lessons, provide practice and work simulations, test learners and manage training administration.

CCHIT: Certification Commission for Health Information Technology. The mission of CCHIT is to accelerate the adoption of robust, interoperable health IT throughout the U.S. healthcare system, by creating an efficient, credible, sustainable mechanism for the certification of health IT products. For physicians, as noted on the CCHIT Web site, investing in the EMR often includes uncertainty about product suitability, quality, interoperability, and data portability are very difficult to judge. A successful product certification initiative has the potential to open up the flow of health IT incentives and simultaneously reduce the risk for health IT purchasers, acting as a doubly-powerful catalyst to accelerate adoption of the EMR.

CCOW: Clinical Context Object Workgroup is a HL7 standard. It is vendor independent and allows clinical applications to share information at the point of care (http://en.wikipedia.org/wiki/CCOW).

CCR: It is a core data set to be shared between the hospital and the skilled nursing facility as the patient moves from one to the other. The information also will contain a data set of all specialties. It is hoped that the data set has the potential to reduce costs, reduce duplicate lab costs, and improve portability.

CDR: That component of a computer-based patient record (CPR) which accepts, files, and stores clinical data over time from a variety of supplemental treatment and intervention systems for such purposes as practice guidelines, outcomes management, and clinical research. May also be called a data warehouse.

CDSS: clinical decision support system; a medical knowledge system that uses items of patient data to generate a case specific advice.

CHIN: Providers and payors within a specific area who are networked to exchange medical and administrative information among them, eliminating redundant data collection and reducing paperwork. (Adapted from http://www.theebusinesssite.com/IT%20Terms/Health%20Terms.htm.) The RHIO model of health information has replaced the CHIN. One of the principal differences between the two models is the data repository. In RHIOs, the patient data resides in the repository of each of the healthcare delivery organizations. In contrast, the repository was centralized in the earlier CHIN model.

Client-server: Architecture in which an application is divided over at least two computers: the client issues requests to the server, who provides the requested data or programs.

Clinical transformation: improving clinical workflows to make them more efficient and productive. Failure to perform clinical transformation is a major reason for a software installation failure.

CMV: controlled or common medical vocabulary; scientifically validated terminology and infrastructure that enables clinicians, researchers and patients to share healthcare knowledge worldwide, across clinical specialties and sites of care (ie, SNOMED).

COW: computer on wheels (not to be confused with CCOW).

CPR: Also called electronic medical record or patient health record. Much more than a computerized medical chart, a CPR acts as a "personal health library" providing access to all resources on a patient's health history and insurance information. A CPR is a linking system rather than an independent database, it is more a process than a product. An integrated CPR will link to separate sources detailing medical history and images, laboratory results and drug allergies. Several organizations are focused on creating standards for CPRs, including common coding terminology, clinical decision support, patient confidentiality and secure data transfers.

CPT: The Current Procedural Terminology is the list maintained by the American Medical Association to provide unique billing codes for services rendered. The current version is the CPT-4. (Adapted from http://en.wikipedia.org/wiki/Current_Procedural_Terminology.)

CRT: Abbreviation of cathode-ray tube, the technology used in most televisions and computer display screens.

Database: 1. A collection of data. 2. A structured set of logically related data together with software to define the structure of the data and to obtain access to the data.

DICOM: Digital Imaging and Communications in Medicine; a communication standard to exchange text and images.

Diffusion of Innovations Theory: A broad social psychological/sociological theory that purports to describe the patterns of adoption, explain the mechanism, and assist in predicting whether and how a new invention will be successful. It is expressed in Rogers EM, *Diffusion of Innovations.* The Free Press: New York; 1962(4th ed);2003. (Adapted from http://www.amazon.com/exec/obidos/tg/detail/-/0743222091/qid=1102351028/sr=1-1/ref=sr_1_1/002-6475639-0495217?v=glance&s=books.)

ECLRS: Electronic Clinical Laboratory Reporting System; a state health department sponsored application that enables the secure transmission of reportable communicable diseases from healthcare providers to the health department. (Adapted from http://www.nyhealth.gov/professionals/reportable_diseases/eclrs/. Accessed November 22, 2006)

EMPI: An Enterprise Master Patient Index (EMPI) is a database that contains a unique identifier for every patient in the enterprise. This would include the medical centers, outpatient clinics, practice offices and rehabilitation facilities. All registration systems would look to the EMPI to obtain patient information based upon several identifiers.

Five Rights: right patient, right drug, right dose, right route and right time.

Free text entry: Natural language text without restrictions on format and word choice (in contrast to Structured Data Entry).

FTP: File Transfer Protocol: an application under TCP/IP to retrieve a file from another computer over a network.

Gigabyte: 1024 megabytes, about one billion bytes.

GIGO: Garbage in, garbage out; it means that if invalid data is entered in a computer program, the resulting output will also be invalid.

Google: Web search engine (named after a 'googol': 10100, or 1 followed by 100 zeros).

GUI: A user interface that, besides keyboard characters, may contain windows, command buttons, and icons that the user can point at to issue a command.

HEAL NY: Healthcare Efficiency and Affordability Law for New Yorkers Capital Grant Program. The "HEAL NY" Program is anticipated to be a multi-year, multi-phased program with two primary objectives:
- To identify and support development and investment in HIT initiatives on a regional level; and
- To identify and support the funding of restructuring plans undertaken in regional healthcare service delivery areas that result in improved stability, efficiency, and quality of the healthcare services in the region. (Adapted from http://www.health.state.ny.us/funding/rfa/0508190240/0508190240.pdf): Healthcare Common Procedure Coding System: based on the American Medical Association's Current Procedural Terminology (CPT). Used for reporting physician services for Medicare. Commonly pronounced Hix-Pix. (Adapted from http://en.wikipedia.org/wiki/HCPCS.)

Heuristic logic: problem-solving method closely resembling human reasoning, in which a decision is reached after following paths of yes or no decisions using heuristics, that is informal rules of thumb.

HIMSS: Healthcare Information and Management Systems Society; the largest national professional organization devoted to healthcare information technology.

HIPAA: the Health Insurance Portability and Accountability Act of 1996 protects health insurance coverage for workers and their families when they change or lose their jobs. Establishes national standards for electronic healthcare transactions and national identifiers for providers, health plans and employers. It also addresses the security and privacy of health data.

HITSP: Healthcare Information Technology Standards Panel; The HITSP functions as an open partnership of the public and private sectors and reaches across the entire healthcare community. (Adapted from http://www.ansi.org/standards_activities/standards_boards_panels/hisb/hitsp.aspx?menuid=3.)

HL7: Health Level 7; a healthcare specific communication standard for data exchange between computer applications.

Home-grown: Software that has been developed by the client. While home-grown applications may well fit the needs of the client, they must be maintained by the client and may not be competitive with vendor products that must respond to the demands of the market place (see "Shrink-wrapped" or "Off the shelf" software).

HTML: Mark-up Language: the language that describes WWW-documents and included links.

HTTP: Hypertext Transfer Protocol; the protocol for moving hypertext files across the Internet.

Human factors: The field of effort and body of knowledge devoted to the adaptation and design of equipment for efficient and advantageous use by people considering physiological, psychological and training factors (see Usability).

Integration: The process that allows separate functions to use a common technology and database, pass data and information without requiring translation, reformatting or duplicate entry; enables cross-functional views and management.

Interface: A common boundary between two different software applications, two pieces of equipment or between a piece of equipment and a human being.

Internet: A worldwide network of computer networks. It provides exchange of information by e-mail, bulletin boards, file access and transfer, etc.

Interoperability: Ability to manage data and functions from different platforms.

Intranet: A private network inside a company or organization that uses the same kinds of software that you would find on the public Internet, but only for internal use.

IOM: Institute of Medicine; an organization within the National Academy of Sciences that acts as an advisor in health and medicine and conducts policy studies relevant to health issues. The IOM coined the term "computer-based patient record" and emphasizes its importance for future healthcare management and delivery.

IP address: 32-bit number that uniquely identifies a computer connected to the Internet.

IR: infrared; The most common home automation use of IR is in hand-held remote controls for TVs, images and CD Players. Infrared light is invisible to the human eye and cannot penetrate walls.

IRR: Internal rate of return. The internal rate of return (IRR) is defined as the interest rate that gives a net present value (NPV) of zero. The NPV is calculated from an annualized cash flow by discounting all future amounts to the present (Adapted from http://en.wikipedia.org/wiki/Internal_rate_of_return.)

Java: A computer programming language invented by Sun Microsystems. Using Java, Web developers create small programs called "applets" that allow Web pages to include animations, calculators, scrolling text, sound effects and games.

Kilobyte: 2(superscript 10) or 1024 bytes.

Knowledge base: a collection of stored facts, heuristics, and models that can be used for problem solving.

LAN: local area network; a group of computers and other devices in a relatively limited area (such as a single building) that are connected by a communications link, which enables any device to interact with any other device on the network.

LCD: Liquid Crystal Display. The type of display found on digital watches and laptop computers. Their major advantage is low power consumption, leading to long battery life for portable devices.

Legacy system: a computer system that remains in use after an organization installs new systems.

LOINC: Logical Observation Identifiers, Names, and Codes. A database protocol aimed at standardizing laboratory and clinical codes for use in clinical care, outcomes management, and research. Developed by the Regenstrief Institute for Healthcare, LOINC is touted as a middleman solution to potential translation problems between labs that use HL7 reporting and recipient systems that may not be able to translate such data. (Adapted from http://www.payorid.com/glossary.asp.)

Lossless compression: a mathematical technique for reducing the number of bits needed to store data that allows recreation of the original data.

Lossy compression: a mathematical technique for reducing the number of bits needed to store data that results in loss of information.

Malware: Malware (a portmanteau of "malicious software") is any software program developed for the purpose of causing harm to a computer system, similar to a virus or Trojan horse (Adapted from http://en.wikipedia.org/wiki/Malware.)

MBWA: Managers walk around the company, getting a "feel" for people and operations; stopping to talk and to listen. Sometimes known as Management by

Walking Around and Listening (MBWAL). This management style is based on the HP Way developed by entrepreneur Dave Packard, co-founder of Hewlett-Packard.

Medical Informatics New York: a professional organization of chief medical information officers and directors of medical informatics in the greater New York metropolitan area. (Adapted from http://www.medinfony.org.)

Megabyte: 2(superscript 10) or 1,048,576 bytes.

Moore's Law: The observation made in 1965 by Gordon Moore, co-founder of Intel, that the number of transistors per square inch on integrated circuits had doubled every year since the integrated circuit was invented. Moore predicted that this trend would continue for the foreseeable future. In subsequent years, the pace slowed down a bit, but data density has doubled approximately every 18 months, and this is the current definition of Moore's Law, which Moore himself has blessed. Most experts, including Moore himself, expect Moore's Law to hold for at least another two decades.

MPI: the module of a healthcare information system used to uniquely identify a patient within the system.

National Health Information Network (NHIN): The infrastructure that interconnects regional health information organizations (RHIOs). (Adapted from http://www.os.dhhs.gov/healthit/goals.html.)

NLM: National Library of Medicine, the sponsor of Medline and a significant source of Federal funding for healthcare IT.

NPV: Net present value. The difference between the discounted present value of benefits and the discounted present value of costs. (Adapted from http://www.nps.navy.mil/drmi/definition.htm.)

Occam's razor: Originally propounded by the English philosopher, William of Occam (1300-1349), as: *Entia non sunt multiplicanda praeter necessitatem*. Translated, it means: *Entities should not be multiplied more than necessary*. In other words, the simplest explanation is the one that is most likely to be correct, or KISS (keep it simple, stupid!). Adapted from http://en.wikipedia.org/wiki/Occam's_razor.)

Off-the-shelf software: See "shrink-wrapped."

Oracle: Based in Redwood, California, Oracle Corporation is the largest software company whose primary business is database products. Historically, Oracle has targeted high-end workstations and minicomputers as the server platforms to run its database systems. Its relational database was the first to support the SQL language, which has since become the industry standard.

PACS: Picture archiving and communication system: a system for digital acquisition, storage and retrieval of images.

PBCC: Problem between chair and computer (slang); a self-deprecating or insulting reference that suggests a problem is due to end-user ignorance.

PDA: Personal Digital Assistant; a small hand-held computer that in the most basic form, allows you to store names and addresses, prepare to-do lists, schedule appointments, keep track of projects, track expenditures, take notes and do calculations. Depending on the model, you also may be able to send or receive e-mail; do word processing; play MP3 music files; get news, entertainment and stock quotes from the Internet; play video games; and have an integrated digital camera or GPS receiver. In healthcare, patient results reporting and charge capture applications may be integrated into a PDA.

PDF: Short for Portable Document Format, a file format developed by Adobe Systems. PDF captures formatting information from a variety of desktop publishing applications, making it possible to send formatted documents and have them appear on the recipient's monitor or printer as they were intended. To view a file in PDF format, you need Adobe Reader, a free application distributed by Adobe Systems.

Petabyte: 2 to the 50th power (1,125,899,906,842,624) bytes. A petabyte is equal to 1,024 terabytes.

PHIN MS: Public Health Information Network Messaging System; used to transmit public health data in a secure fashion. (Adapted from http://www.cdc.gov/phin/messaging/systems/2003_04_23_An%20Overview%20of %20the%20PHINMS.pdf.)

PHR: The personal health record is a medical record owned and kept by the patient accessible via the Internet and / or in the form of a device, like a flash drive or smart card.

PIN: A personal identification number (PIN) is a numeric value that is used in certain systems to gain access, and authenticate. PINs are a type of password. (Adapted from http://en.wikipedia.org/wiki/Personal_identification_number. Accessed November 22, 2006)

Pixel: Contraction of "picture element": the smallest part of a digital picture.

Point-of-care system: a system that allows for the entry and retrieval of patient-specific data at the bedside.

PPOS: PowerPoint Operating System (slang); a pejorative reference to advertised software that may not exist in reality (see Vaporware).

QIO – Quality Improvement Organization: QIOs are independent, community-based organizations working to improve healthcare quality in every state and territory in the U.S. QIOs have three-year, performance-based contracts with the

Medicare program and work in every setting of care, including pharmacies and health plans. (Adapted from http://www.cms.hhs.gov/QualityImprovementOrgs/.)

Query: To request information from a database.

RAM: Random-access memory: the most common computer memory which can be used by programs to perform necessary tasks while the computer is on.

RCA: root cause analysis; determining what actually caused a failure, as opposed to what appears to have been the cause. A strategy used to identify the most basic or causal factor(s) that contribute to variations in performance. Most often used to identify causal factors that underlie a sentinel event or major unusual incident.

Read-only access: Ability to read a file or record in a database without the ability to modify it.

Read-write access: Ability to read and change a file or record in a database.

Reminder: An alert that informs an end-user to perform a given task. Reminders are commonly used for preventive medicine alerts (ie, annual flu vaccinations for those at risk).

Remote access: Access to a software application outside an organization. Remote access to patient results reporting via the Internet is a core technology that can improve patient safety and expedite patient care.

Required field: a form field that must be filled in order to submit the form.

Results reporting: often includes laboratory tests, radiology reports and dictations.

RFID: radio frequency identification; refers to the technology that uses devices attached to objects that transmit data to an RFID receiver. These devices can be attached to patients, medications, hospital gurneys, ECG machines, portable x-ray machines, and other devices or people. RFID has advantages over bar codes such as the ability to hold more data, the ability to change the stored data as processing occurs, does not require line-of-sight to transfer data and is very effective in harsh environments where bar code labels won't work.

RHIO: regional health information organization; an often public-private enterprise that seeks to share patient information between different healthcare providers.

ROM: Read-Only Memory: This is a computer's unchangeable memory. It's used to store programs that start the computer and run diagnostic functions.

SDO: Standards developing organization, like ANSI.

Shrink-wrapped: a software product that can be readily installed with little or no customization. Customization incurs additional development costs and may complicate future software version upgrades. (Also "turn-key" or "off-the-shelf").

SNOMED: Systematized Nomenclature of Human and Veterinary Medicine. A standardized vocabulary system for medical databases. Current modules contain more than 144,000 terms and are available in at least twelve languages.

SOAP: A SOAP note is written by healthcare providers after examining a patient. The length and focus of each component of a SOAP note varies depending on the specialty; for instance, a surgical SOAP note is likely to be much briefer than a medical SOAP note, and will focus on issues that relate to post-surgical status (eg, it will often be noted whether the patient has passed gas, because if they have, it is considered by many physicians to be safer to allow them to eat.) (Adapted from http://en.wikipedia.org/wiki/Subjective_Objective_Assessment_Plan.)

SQL: Structured Query Language; SQL is a standard interactive and programming language for getting information from and updating a database.

SQL Server: Microsoft's commercial database product that competes with Oracle (see Oracle).

SSO: Single Sign On refers to a single identity that is shared across multiple systems. (Adapted from http://webapp.lab.ac.uab.edu/wiki/mlist/index.php/MlistGlossary.)

Structured data entry: Context-sensitive data entry in which the clinician completes part of a form presented on a screen by selecting from the screen a term that is related to the patient's problem or to the answer to a foregoing question (ie, drop-down menu, radio buttons, check boxes).

Syndromic surveillance: investigational approach where health department staff, assisted by automated data acquisition and generation of statistical alerts, monitor disease indicators in real-time or near real-time to detect outbreaks of disease earlier than would otherwise be possible with traditional public health methods. (Adapted from http://www.cdc.gov/mmwr/preview/mmwrhtml/su5301a3.htm.)

Telemedicine: The delivery of healthcare at a distance, increasingly via the Internet.

Teleradiology: Provision of remote radiology image interpretation.

Terabyte: One trillion bytes, one million megabytes, or one thousand gigabytes.

Turn key system: a computer system that is purchased from a vendor and that can be installed and operated with minimal modification.

Unique identifier: a string of characters that uniquely identifies an individual or database record.

URL (unique resource locator): address of an information resource on the Web.

Usability: Usability is a generic term that refers to design features that enable something to be user-friendly.

USB: Universal Serial Bus: a protocol for transferring data to and from digital devices. Many digital cameras and memory card readers connect to the USB port on a computer.

Validation: verification of correctness; also refers to programming that enables required fields.

Vaporware: A slang term for software which has been announced and perhaps even demonstrated, but has not been delivered to commercial customers.

Venn diagram: A graphical representation of all objects of a class (a set) by closed figures showing relationships between subsets.

VeriSign: VeriSign is the dominant certification authority on the Internet at the present time.

Voice recognition: The technology by which sounds, words or phrases spoken by humans are converted into electrical signals, and these signals are transformed into coding patterns that can be identified by a computer.

VPN: A Virtual Private Network, or VPN, is a private communications network usually used within a company, or by several different companies or organizations, communicating over a public network. VPN message traffic is carried on public networking infrastructure (eg, the Internet) using standard (often insecure) protocols. (Adapted from http://en.wikipedia.org/wiki/Virtual_private_network.)

WAN: wide area network; a network that connects computers distributed over long distances.

WiFi: The popular name for 802.11x wireless networking. This standard replaces the cables in an Ethernet network.

Worm: A self-replicating program that reproduces itself over a network.

WYSIWYG: Characteristic of a program or application which displays formatted material on the screen so that it looks the same as it will appear when printed out.

XML: Extensible Markup Language; a flexible way to create standard information formats and share both the format and the data on the World Wide Web.

Index

A

*Page numbers with *f* indicate figures; page numbers with *t* indicate tables; page numbers with *n* indicate notes.